Resource CD-ROM

for

Hands Heal

Communication, Documentation, and Insurance Billing for Manual Therapists

THIRD EDITION

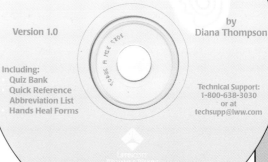

Resource CD-ROM for

Hands Heal

Communication, Documentation, and Insurance Billing for Manual Therapists, Third Edition

Version 1.0

by
Diana Thompson

Including:
- Quiz Bank
- Quick Reference
- Abbreviation List
- Hands Heal Forms

Technical Support:
1-800-638-3030
or at
techsupp@lww.com

Copyright © 2006
Lippincott Williams & Wilkins,
A Wolters Kluwer Co.
All rights reserved.

As a bonus for you, Lippincott Williams & Wilkins has included an interactive CD-ROM with tools to enhance your learning and your practice!

This resource is the perfect tool to help you prepare for exams, to reinforce what you have learned, and to make your paperwork easier.

The CD-ROM includes:

- A quiz tool with approximately 225 multiple-choice questions so you can test your knowledge and study for tests. Choose study mode or test mode, and even e-mail your results to your instructor. A comprehensive exam is offered and rationales are given so you can understand the reasoning behind the correct answer.

- The blank forms from the book that you can print out and use and practice.

- Quick-reference list including symbols and abbreviations commonly used in documentation.

For technical support, contact 1-800-638-3030 or techsupp@lww.com.

LIPPINCOTT WILLIAMS & WILKINS

HANDS HEAL

Communication, Documentation, and Insurance Billing for Manual Therapists

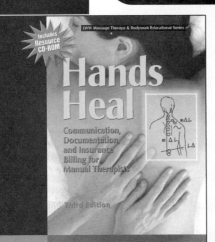
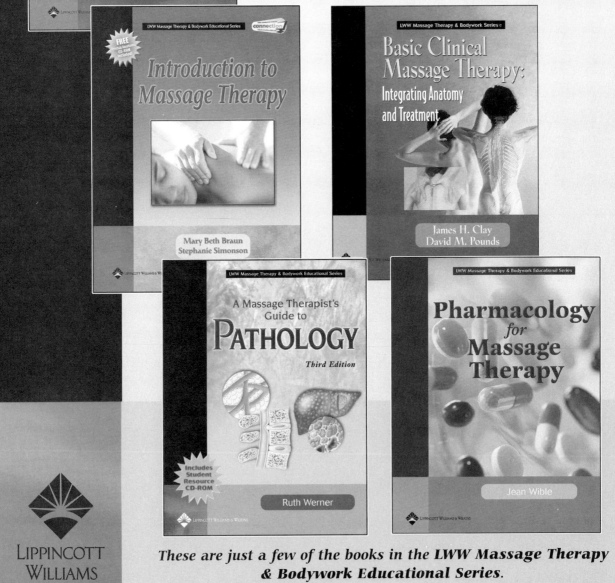

Hands Heal

Communication, Documentation, and Insurance Billing for Manual Therapists

THIRD EDITION

Diana L. Thompson

Licensed Massage Practitioner
Seattle, Washington

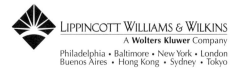

LIPPINCOTT WILLIAMS & WILKINS
A **Wolters Kluwer** Company

Philadelphia • Baltimore • New York • London
Buenos Aires • Hong Kong • Sydney • Tokyo

Executive Editor: Peter J. Darcy
Managing Editor: Anne Seitz, Hearthside Publishing Services
Editorial Coordinator: Katherine Staples
Marketing Manager: Christen Murphy
Associate Production Manager: Kevin P. Johnson
Compositor: Schawk, Inc.
Printer: Courier

Second Edition, 2002

Library of Congress Cataloging-in-Publication Data

Thompson, Diana L.
    Hands heal : communication, documentation, and insurance
  billing for manual therapists / Diana L. Thompson. — 3rd ed.
      p. cm.
    ISBN 0-7817-5757-6 (alk. paper)
    1. Massage therapy—Practice.   1. Title
    [DNLM: 1. Massage—organization & administration. 2. Massage
    —economics. 3. Practice Management—organization & administration.
    4. Interpersonal Relations. 5. Medical Records—standards.
    WB 537 T469h 2006]
    RM722.T48 2006
    615.8'22'068—dc22

                                        2005010880

To purchase additional copies of this book, call our customer service department at **(800) 638-3030** or fax orders to **(301) 223-2400.** International customers should call **(301) 223-2300.**

Visit Lippincott Williams & Wilkins on the Internet: http://www.LWW.com. Lippincott Williams & Wilkins customer service representatives are available monday–Friday from 8:30 AM to 6:00 PM, EST.

05 06 07 08 09
1 2 3 4 5 6 7 8 9 10

I dedicate this edition to my beautiful wife, Jackie, who patiently loved me during this personal growth experience called writing. You *espejo* my soul.

Foreword

The licensed massage practitioner has so much to offer the individual consumer and the health care community. More and more massage practitioners are realizing the importance of their work and creating greater awareness and momentum about the benefits of massage therapy. Despite the gains that are being made with individual consumers, non-massage health care practitioners and insurers remain reluctant to embrace massage therapy as an integral part of modern health care. This reluctance stems from a list of issues, including lack of practice guidelines and standards of care, perceptions of professionalism, effective chart note documentation, and responsiveness to the communication needs of other health care professionals.

Seen in this light, Diana Thompson's book is a very timely and much-needed bridge to overcome these real and perceived obstacles surrounding practice guidelines, professionalism, treatment protocol, and documentation. Diana Thompson brings forth unending experiences in understanding patient needs, figuring out what is important to the referring doctor, and satisfying insurance companies in the paperwork process. She brings practical information to life by blending years of experience, stories, and humor that undoubtedly will make this book required reading for all massage students, as well as for those practitioners wanting to work more closely with medical doctors, osteopaths, chiropractors, and physical therapists. It will also help practitioners have an easier time when dealing with insurance companies.

The value of this book is multidimensional for massage practitioners and the massage profession. Practitioners will find practical, simple, and easy-to-use information and forms that comprehensively capture relevant information. Paperwork will become more efficient and effective. The profession benefits immensely because the book raises the bar on expectations within and outside the massage profession concerning communication, documentation, and professionalism.

Hands Heal facilitates the mission of each licensed massage practitioner and massage therapy association that seeks greater access for the consumer to obtain massage treatment and care and relief for illness, injury, and disease, as well as for those wishing to obtain maximum health. Diana Thompson has made a very valuable contribution. It is now up to each licensed massage practitioner, massage therapy organization, and massage school to join her in advancing a most worthy cause.

Richard H. Adler
Attorney-at-Law, Editor

Preface

Background of Hands Heal *and Manual Therapy*

Hands Heal was conceived in the early 1990s. At that time, complementary and alternative medicine was receiving a lot of press and catching the attention of mainstream health care systems. Massage therapists, bodyworkers, movement therapists, and energy workers were receiving patient referrals from physicians, many for the first time. Increasingly, manual therapy services were being covered by insurance plans.

Not everyone in allopathic medicine greeted the complementary providers with open arms. Skepticism was widespread. Many questioned the validity of manual therapies. Insurance carriers demanded statistics and scientific studies proving that treatment was curative and not palliative. Few were found. Independent medical examinations were implemented early in personal injury cases, and health insurance utilization review boards audited practitioners, in attempts to deny or to limit the use of manual therapies.

In this atmosphere of litigation and peer reviews, charting focused on proving the legitimacy of the practitioners and their modalities. I wrote the first edition of *Hands Heal* to prepare massage therapists for the charting requirements of those skeptical times. My information was based on years of experience in the early stages of the integration of massage therapy into health care. My teachers were chiropractors, attorneys, and insurance adjusters. I have been videotaped for depositions, been given testimony in court, have submitted narratives to lawyers, and have seen my charts reviewed by utilization management panels. On the upside, when my claims were denied, the decisions were reversed after I submitted convincing progress reports. I filed liens in county courthouses and requested letters of guarantee from attorneys, and, as a result, I received payment in full when others were being asked to cut their bills in half. I wanted to share what I had learned.

Much has changed in a short time. Manual therapies are now considered a viable treatment option for many people and are a covered benefit in an increasing number of insurance plans across the United States. As a result of this widespread integration of manual therapies into private health care benefit packages, charting requirements have also changed. The focus of documentation is shifting from legitimizing the practitioners and validating manual modalities to proving that the treatments improve patient outcomes and cost less than traditional treatments. The shift demands progress-oriented functional outcomes reporting, a style of charting recently adopted by physical therapists and other health care providers. Progress is apparent when the patient's quality of life improves. Quality of life is measured through functional outcomes—the patient's increased ability to participate in activities of daily life.

xii

HANDS HEAL:
COMMUNICATION,
DOCUMENTATION,
AND INSURANCE BILLING
FOR MANUAL THERAPISTS

Current research supports the emphasis on functional outcomes. A randomized trial studying the effects of various alternative therapies in treating persistent low back pain was conducted at the Center for Health Studies in Washington State. Dan Cherkin, PhD, Senior Scientific Investigator, concluded that therapeutic massage is an effective treatment for persistent low back pain because massage significantly improved the patient's ability to function (for example, ability to walk up stairs and put on socks). There was not a statistically significant reduction in symptoms, though there was a correlation between massage and the reduction of medication (Cherkin D, Eisenberg D, Street J, et al. Randomized trial comparing traditional Chinese medical acupuncture, therapeutic massage, and self-care education for chronic low back pain. Arch Intern Med 2001;161). When we, as manual therapists, persist in trying to demonstrate patient progress through a reduction in symptoms, we are less able to provide our patients with encouraging results or to prove the curative nature of our modalities. When we demonstrate patient progress through improved function, however, we will validate manual modalities successfully.

This shift in charting is exciting. Practitioners and patients alike enjoy the focus on improving function. Setting functional goals and charting functional outcomes engages patients in their healing, inviting them to participate in all levels of healing. Functional outcomes reporting fits into a SOAP format with few adjustments, and the second edition of *Hands Heal* made the transition to functional outcomes reporting easy.

Regarding terminology, it is not my intent to offend anyone with my choice of words. Therefore, I wish to explain my terminology. My goal is to be inclusive and representative of the diversity within complementary health care professions. However, the words I choose may not be the terms you use in your practice. Please insert words appropriate to your profession and beliefs where you find it necessary to do so. For example, I refer to manual therapists as *practitioners* or *health care providers*; you may call yourselves *educators* or *therapists*. I use the term *patients*; you may prefer *clients* or *students*. I say *referring health care provider* instead of *primary care provider*, so as not to imply that physicians are the only acceptable primary care.

Changes in the Second and Third Editions

In addition to the inclusion of functional outcomes, several significant changes appear in the second and third editions of *Hands Heal*. First, I replaced *massage therapy* with *manual therapy* in the subtitle. My intent was to include all hands-on healing arts. The term *manual therapy* embraces all forms of soft tissue, spinal, and bioenergetic manipulation, as well as postural re-education. Soft tissue manipulation is the primary technique of massage therapy and physical therapy and is part of the extensive array of bodywork specialties. Chiropractors and osteopaths practice spinal manipulation. Bioenergetic manipulation specialists focus on the energetic fields of the body, including Reiki, therapeutic touch, and Polarity. Postural re-education specialists use Feldenkrais, Aston-Patterning, and the Alexander Technique, to name a few.

The second change to the subtitle is the inclusion of communication and insurance billing with documentation. These topics are natural and necessary additions. Communication and the therapeutic relationship are integral to documentation; we have nothing to write if we are not engaged with our patients. Patients are involved in every level of healing, from providing information to choosing and implementing their care. Their involvement hinges on our relationship with them; if we are honest, respectful, and encouraging, they may trust us and open themselves to change. My intent throughout the second edition was to emphasize building productive relationships with those ultimately responsible for healing—the patient—and shift the focus away from our need to prove that we are legitimate health care providers. Skillful communication enables us to accomplish and document patient outcomes, the only proof we need.

Insurance billing was included at the persistent urging of my colleagues. At first, the task was overwhelming. Once I committed to the project, however, it became clear what was needed. Many texts on insurance billing specialize in the regulations of a particular state and provide information that is quickly outdated. This book provides tools that are universally applicable to the verification and reimbursement needs of personal injury, workers' compensation, and private health insurance billing across the United States. It does not provide information detailing the modalities that insurance plans cover, nor does it instruct you on the CPT codes to use. State regulations vary and plans differ in their inclusion of manual therapies. Instead, *Hands Heal* teaches how to communicate with the individual carriers, verify each patient's benefits, complete the billing forms accurately, record payments, and resolve or appeal unpaid claims. This information is not time-sensitive, because you learn the skills necessary to adapt to changing codes and procedures.

In the third edition, I have included additional coding information and coverage of HIPAA regulations. Although most manual therapists do not have to be HIPAA-compliant—because they do not store or transmit patient health care information electronically—all practitioners should understand and follow its Privacy Rules. It is important for all of us to protect every patients' confidential health information. In addition, HIPAA requires standardized coding; specifically, CPT codes that identify types of health care services and ICD-9 codes that categorize the patient's health condition. You will find a list of physical medicine and rehabilitation CPT codes that manual therapists commonly provide on the Insurance Verification form, as well as a discussion of CCI code bundling, which determines code pairs that cannot be billed on the same date of treatment. For those patients who come to you for treatment but are self-referred (meaning there is no referring HCP to provide you with a formal diagnosis), I have listed ICD-9 codes (in Appendix E) that refer to common musculoskeletal symptoms. You can select codes from this list that best represent the symptoms you are treating. Use them to complete the HCFA 1500 billing form for reimbursement.

In addition, there are changes to the SOAP format. In the second and third editions, the SOAP format is no longer modified for massage therapists. Traditionally, the Assessment section of the SOAP chart is the place for recording the practitioner's diagnosis of the patient's condition. Massage therapists do not have diagnostic scope. Therefore, I previously advocated using the Assessment section to record the changes in the patient data that resulted from the massage. With the inclusion of functional outcomes reporting, the Assessment section is allocated to recording functional goals. As a result, massage therapists no longer need to modify the SOAP format to make use of all categories. Continue to omit the diagnosis from the Assessment section unless your scope of practice permits it. Record the results of your treatment in the Objective section of the SOAP chart, which is consistent with other health care professions. Use the Assessment section to record functional goals.

Also new to the second and third editions is an entire chapter devoted to charting wellness sessions. Manual therapy enhances wellness in addition to treating health conditions. Regardless of its intent, manual therapy is a health care service and therefore must be documented. However, extensive documentation using the SOAP format is not necessary in wellness care. In the second edition, I introduced a new format called the Wellness chart, appropriate for wellness care, sports venues, and spa environments.

xiv

HANDS HEAL:
COMMUNICATION,
DOCUMENTATION,
AND INSURANCE BILLING
FOR MANUAL THERAPISTS

Pedagogical Features and Resources

A vast array of stories, exercises, and quotations are included to enhance learning. In keeping with the native southwestern designs used in the first edition, I have assigned the following symbols to identify these categories:

Story Teller (Stories)—The story teller, weaving tales of the ancient ones, invites you to learn from those who came before us.

Bone Game (Exercises)—The dice, carved from the bones of animals, invite you to learn through play.

Wise One Speaks (Quotations)—The wise, old owl invites you to learn through the wisdom of others.

Throughout the book, important words appear in bold type and important phrases are italicized. The boldface terms make up the glossary. The italicized phrases represent what can be written on the SOAP charts.

In addition to these features, the third edition text is accompanied by a Resource CD-ROM containing the following useful study aids:

◆ Quiz Bank—The Quiz Bank provides questions that readers can use to review material from each chapter and self-check their progress and comprehension.
◆ Quick Reference Abbreviation List—This convenient reference will assist readers with learning and using abbreviations common in documentation.
◆ Forms—The CD includes all of the blank forms that appear in the book. These can be printed and used for class activities or in professional practice.

Teaching Resources

An Instructor Resource CD-ROM is available to instructors with this edition, and includes the following components:

◆ Instructor Manual—The Instructor Manual is organized into lessons that correspond with the chapters in the textbook. The lessons explore four categories of information: communication, documentation, insurance billing and ethics.
◆ PowerPoint Slides—The PowerPoint Slides provided on the CD are designed to assist instructors in presenting lecture material.
◆ Brownstone Test Generator—The Brownstone Test Generator contains a full bank of questions that instructors can use to create exams. The program allows instructors to add, delete, and otherwise customize the test questions to construct unique exams. The test bank includes questions that require the student to demonstrate knowledge and comprehension, as well as apply, analyze, synthesize, and evaluate information.
◆ Hands Heal Forms—The CD includes an array of blank forms that can be photocopied and distributed to students for use in class exercises.

The Instructor Resource Materials from the CD-ROM can also be accessed on *The Connection Web Site* at http://connection.lww.com/go/thompson3e.

I hope that you will find *Hands Heal: Communication, Documentation, and Insurance Billing for Manual Therapists* to be current, comprehensive, and critical to the integration of manual therapy into mainstream health care systems. It is my belief and intention that integration will positively influence the current health care environment.

User's Guide

Hands Heal: Communication, Documentation, and Insurance Billing for Manual Therapist, Third Edition gives you valuable guidance on taking client histories, setting functional goals, communicating with health care and legal professionals, documenting outcomes, billing insurance companies, and much more. This User's Guide shows you how to put the book's features to work for you.

CHAPTER OUTLINES

Each chapter opens with an outline that offers you a guide for material in the chapter.

BONE GAME BOXES

present activities and exercises that help you apply concepts and retain the material.

HIPAA INFORMATION

Crucial information on HIPAA regulations introduces you to privacy regulations.

STORY TELLER BOXES

share light-hearted anecdotes related to the content you just read.

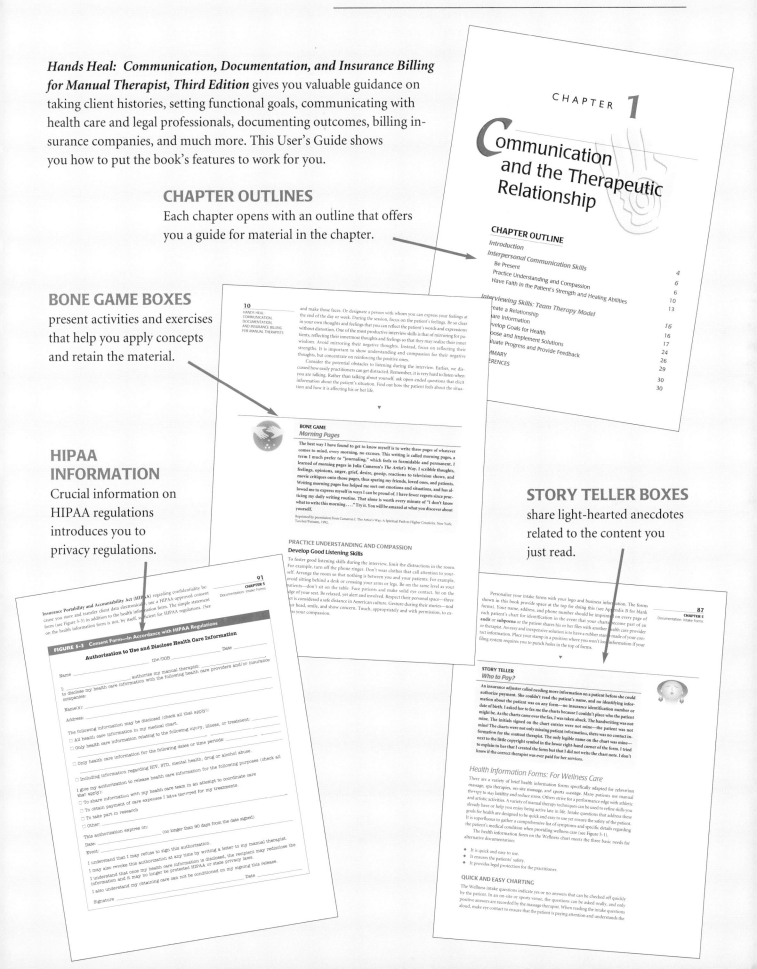

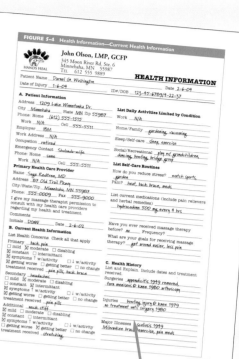
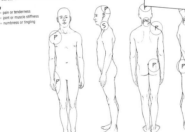

Acknowledgments

To all of you who generously shared your stories, appreciation, and feedback at conventions and workshops, thank you for providing much of the material for the second edition. Thank you Kerry Ann Plunkett, Eileen Stretch ND, and Alternáre Health Services for the opportunity to embrace the needs of managed care documentation. You planted the seed for the second edition. Diane Hettrick and Bob May ND, from Alternáre and Christine Carpenter from Regence helped shape the third edition.

A special thanks to Lori Bielinski and Deborah Senn, the Washington State Insurance Commissioner, for your dedication to complementary medicine and for setting national precedence in complementary and alternative health care integration; and the law firm of Adler◆Giersch PS for its commitment and service to manual therapists. Without its work, there would be little need for this book.

I offer my warmest respect and heartfelt thanks to the people who made this book possible: my guardian angels, Richard Adler and Lisanne Yuricich, who taught me what I know and gave me the opportunity to share it; my behind-the-scenes editor Alice Bloch, who makes words sing; the staff at LWW who raised the ante on professionalism and quality; and my reviewers whose brilliant insights shaped the final product. Huge thanks to Janice and Ananda at Ask Us! for reviewing the billing chapter; Duane Hobbs, the designer of the new forms; Lori and Janelle Otterholt for assistance with the glossary; Coleen Rene for the energy charting consult; Barb for surfin' the Net; and Terry for going over Chapter 6 just one more time. Thank you Sari Spieler and Clint Chandler for carrying a heavier portion of our workshop responsibilities while I was experiencing tunnel vision with this project. Annie Thoe, LMP, GCFP, and Anne Wardell, LAc, LMP, thanks for keeping my body healthy. I especially loved those sessions to unleash my mind and boost my creativity!

New to the third edition is my editing team from Hearthside Publishing: Anne Seitz and Diane Geesey. Thanks for your leadership and playful spirits. You both posess a rare gift: the ability to support and manage the person before the project. Thank you.

I am especially grateful to Richard Adler for editing both the second and third editions— I cannot thank you enough for sharing your wisdom. Also, to Duane for clearing my plate so I could be still and have creative thoughts and to Jackie Espejo Phillips for removing fear from my vocabulary. Without your support emotionally and financially, this would not have been possible.

Reviewers

The publisher and author gratefully acknowledge the many professionals who shared their expertise and assisted in developing this textbook, appropriately targeting our marketing efforts, creating useful ancillary products, and setting the stage for subsequent editions. These individuals include:

Joanne Braun, BSEd, LMT
Educator
Owner, Tranquil Touch Therapeutic Massage
Kinnelon, New Jersey

Nancy W. Dail, BA, LMT, NCTMB
Director, Downeast School of Massage
Waldoboro, Maine

Josh Herman, ATC-L, LMBT
Miller-Motte Technical College
Massage Therapy Instructor
Cary, North Carolina

Stephanie Kacena, LMT
Nationally Certified—Massage and Bodywork
Director of Operations, Carlson College of Massage Therapy
Stone City, Iowa

Mary Reis BA, LMT
Licensed Massage Therapist
Gainesville, Florida

Wendy L. Stone, MS, LMT
Chair, Pathology Department and
Practice Development Department,
Muscular Therapy Institute
Cambridge, Massachusetts

Tomi Lynn Wilson, LMT
Portland, Oregon

Contents

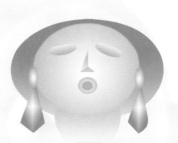

SECTION I

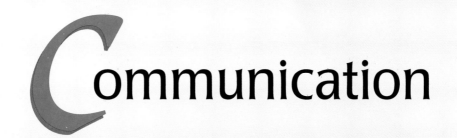

Communication

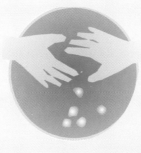

## CHAPTER 1

Communication and the Therapeutic Relationship

CHAPTER OUTLINE

*T*he Creator gathered all of creation and said, "I want to hide something from the humans until they are ready for it. It is the realization that they create their own reality."

The eagle said, "Give it to me, I will take it to the moon."

The Creator said, "No. One day they will go there and find it."

The salmon said, "I will hide it on the bottom of the ocean."

"No. They will go there, too."

The buffalo said, "I will bury it on the plains."

The Creator said, "They will cut into the skin of the earth and find it even there."

Then Grandmother Mole, who lives in the breast of Mother Earth and has no physical eyes but sees with spiritual eyes, said, "Put it inside them."

And the Creator said, "It is done."

(A story from a Sioux friend told to Gary Zukav, author of *The Dancing Wu Li Masters* and *Seat of the Soul.* Reprinted with permission from Zukav G. In search of the soul. Time 1997;12.)

Let's change one word in this poignant story and pretend the Creator said, "It is the realization that they create their own *health*." The change does little to affect the message, yet this new twist proposes a powerful and significant concept for health care providers and patients to consider: Individuals possess the ability to heal themselves. In reality, we exercise that ability every day when we make simple decisions about what to eat, or seek care when we need it, or survive against overwhelming odds. All of us possess a life force that is tenacious and enduring, undiminished until the moment of our death. That life force drives us toward health.[1]

Therefore, patients may be the best people to involve in the healing process. Patients have all the data, take all the risks, and implement much of the solution. When actively involved in their own healing, patients develop their self-confidence and sense of responsibility and become less dependent on their caregivers.[2] Our role as health care practitioners must expand to include providing our patients with opportunities for self-discovery, illuminating and expanding their unique strengths, tapping into their internal wisdom, and empowering them to heal themselves.

Introduction

In the past, the interview was used only to gather information about a patient's symptoms and health history. The medical model demanded that the expert—the physician—collect data that would lead to an accurate assessment of the patient's condition. Once a diagnosis was assigned, the standard of care for the patient's disease was administered.[3]

Today, allopathic and alternative health experts alike recognize the flaws inherent in the traditional approach. First, human beings are individuals and respond uniquely to identical treatments. Second, a growing body of evidence indicates that emotions are responsible, at least in part, for disease. Some researchers believe that 90 to 95% of all patients who visit physicians have physical symptoms that are directly caused by emotions.[4]

Consequently, the central focus of the interview process has shifted from collecting data to building relationships. Health care providers from all disciplines embrace the patient-practitioner relationship as their primary asset. One provider purports that the relationship *is* the therapy.[5] Some claim that trust is imperative for patient satisfaction and compliance; others assert that trust or lack of it affects the results of any care provided.

Cardiologist Herbert Benson writes, "Belief or faith—whether it's deep in the mind or heart or focused on some outside object, like a physician—can play a key role in generating a response in the body."[4]

Trust is the key component to building meaningful relationships. Once the bond of trust is formed, patients will confide in us, provide us with insight into their conditions, and lead us to solutions that fit their lifestyles. Trust is established when patients feel understood. Until patients believe that the practitioner really understands what they are trying to say, patients are unlikely to believe that the practitioner has their best interests at heart or can be of any use to them. In the book *Kitchen Table Wisdom* by Rachel Naomi Remen, Dean Ornish MD, puts it like this:

> Providing people with information—facts—is important but usually not sufficient to motivate them to make lasting changes in diet and lifestyle. If it were, no one would smoke. We need to work on a deeper level . . . to create a place safe enough for people to talk about what's really going on in their lives, to tell their stories, without fear of being judged, abandoned or criticized. Then, when people are really heard, are they likely to make lifestyle changes. (Reprinted with permission from Remen RN. *Kitchen Table Wisdom: Stories That Heal.* Riverhead Books: New York, 1996.)

This chapter first presents the communication skills manual therapists need for building relationships with their patients, and it includes exercises for developing those skills. It then describes the goals of interviewing patients and recommends approaches for reaching those goals. Entire books have been written on interpersonal communication skills and interviewing skills. This chapter introduces these two huge topics, but more importantly, it encourages you to explore these complex subjects further. Good communication skills are essential to the therapeutic relationship and to good recordkeeping. Some of these skills may sound simple, but they are much more difficult to incorporate effectively than they may appear. Practice by role playing with peers, performing the exercises in this book, attending workshops that will advance your communication skills, and reading books devoted to the subject. Invest as much time and energy in mastering communication as you devote to advancing your manual techniques. A suggested reading list is provided in Figure 1-1.

FIGURE 1-1   Resources for Communication Skills

1. *Kitchen Table Wisdom: Stories that Heal,* by Rachel Naomi Remen (Riverhead Books, New York, New York, 1996).

2. *Interviewing for Solutions,* by Peter DeJong and Insoo Kim Berg (Brooks/Cole, Pacific Grove, California, 1998).

3. *Messages: The Communications Skills Book, Second Edition,* by Patrick Fanning, Matthew McKay, and Martha Davis (New Harbinger Publications, Oakland, California, 1995).

4. *You and Me: The Skills of Communicating and Relating,* by Gerard Egan (Brooks/Cole, Monterey, California, 1977).

5. *The ABCs of Effective Feedback: A Guide for Caring Professionals,* by Irwin Rubin and Thomas Campbell (Jossey-Bass Publishers, San Francisco, California, 1997).

6. *People Skills: How to Assert Yourself, Listen to Others, and Resolve Conflict,* by Robert Bolton (Simon & Schuster, New York, New York, 1979).

7. *The Psychology of the Body,* by E. Greene and B. Goodrich-Dunn (Lippincott Williams & Wilkins, Baltimore, MD, 2004).

Interpersonal Communication Skills

A successful relationship with patients requires a variety of verbal and nonverbal communication skills. When you—the therapeutic professional—develop and use these skills, you lead patients to discover and accomplish their goals for health. You can enhance patient cooperation and motivation, not by overcoming patient resistance but by offering practical feedback that invites patients to focus on their strengths rather than on their pain. The interviewing skills introduced in this chapter will not only assist you in gathering information for a **treatment plan**, but will also help your patients change their attitudes and summon the strength and wisdom to heal on a deeper level.

Here are detailed examples of various communication techniques that promote successful relationships with your patients.

BE PRESENT

No person can fully comprehend another, but with practice, guidance, and self-awareness anyone can learn to talk with a patient. Talking may seem simple, but a great deal of skill is needed to be present with someone, especially a person in need. Illness or pain often makes a person feel vulnerable and weak, and they may become anxious about taking risks and sharing personal information. It has been estimated that without realizing it, people inject communication barriers—such as becoming argumentative, beating around the bush, or withdrawing—into their conversations more than 90% of the time when one or both parties has a problem to be dealt with or a need to be fulfilled.[2] A commitment to be present and available for your patients is the first step in manifesting trust and respect, which are the cornerstones of any productive relationship.

Being fully present for each patient can be nearly impossible at times. We, as therapists, can get distracted—for example, by the last patient who just suffered a tragedy, or the afternoon lecture we are rehearsing nervously in our mind, or the menu for tonight's dinner. We may habitually jump to conclusions and come up with a quick fix for a minor problem while the deeper concerns are yet to be uncovered. Or we may make quick and easy value judgments based solely on a patient's appearance or hear a familiar situation in the patient's words and filter the information through our own experience. Or we may show up with a personal agenda—the drive to succeed, a desire to contribute, an eagerness to practice new techniques or to try out new theories—and forget to honor our patients' role in their own health. We are human. These distractions are normal. The important thing is to make a commitment to being present. Notice when you are distracted and bring your attention back to the person in front of you.

More should be done than feigning interest in our patients' stories. Whenever we offer anything less than our authentic self, patients can see right through. Robert Bolton PhD, in his classic book *People Skills*, rates genuineness as the most important quality of communication and defines it as being open and honest, present and authentic. The keys to being genuine, as defined by Bolton, are self-awareness, self-acceptance, and self-expression. By cultivating these personal attributes, we will develop the skills necessary for being present and authentic with our patients.[2]

Here are some concrete tools and practical exercises for developing personal presence:

Self-Awareness

In today's fast-paced world, there is little time to sit still. We keep ourselves so busy that we often seek out experts to tell us who we are and what our purpose is in life. Self-help seminars and how-to books are numerous. We don't have time to explore our own ideas or to wait until the answers to our questions present themselves. The quick-fix attitude is everywhere.

On the other hand, self-awareness is not something found only on a mountain top or after years of meditation practice. It really can be found inside each of us—with a little practice. A simple way to develop our self-awareness is by listening to our inner voice.[2] If we are to trust in our patients' internal wisdom, we must learn to recognize our own. We must first acknowledge that we have a sense of inner direction, or intuition, and that we can trust it. Trust in our own intuition is strengthened with practice. We need to make time to listen to ourselves. We regularly tune out our internal voices or ignore them when they do surface by overworking, watching TV, or engaging in habits such as eating, drinking, exercise, and so on. Instead, we can get to know ourselves by spending a small amount of time each day being silent. With practice, we will begin to hear the voices inside us and distinguish where they are coming from. Some may be the voice of our mother or of past experience, but the voice that softens the belly when it speaks is the voice of our intuition. Our "gut instinct" is literally just that. In Chinese medicine, it is believed that the stomach is the original brain.

Practice using your intuition by placing your hand on your belly during your silent time and asking yourself yes or no questions. If your belly tightens, the answer is no; if it softens, the answer is yes.

▼

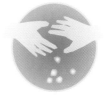

BONE GAME
Separate Self from Patients

Take five minutes between patient sessions to breathe, stay silent, and be with yourself. It may be helpful to sit in a quiet, dark room with no distractions. During this time, mentally separate from your last patient. You may need to run through the events of the last session and experience the feelings you may have chosen not to express in front of the patient. A medical intuitive told me that in order to separate from the previous patient, say silently or aloud, "I separate myself entirely—mentally, physically, spiritually, and emotionally—from Darnel. I call back all my energy, and I send him back all his energy."

When you have completed a session, check how you feel. Often, the lines blur between our patients' thoughts and feelings and our own. Be clear about who you are, separate from those you interact with throughout the day. Verify your feelings about the day, your work, and your health. Take a few deep breaths and feel the air move into your body. Notice how your body moves to accommodate the air as you breathe in and out. Imagine that the air moving through you is a life force, a warm light pushing life into every nook and cranny of your body. Experience your physical self and your emotional self.

Finally, prepare for the next patient by inviting your internal wisdom to surface during the session. The Upledger Institute, in the CranioSacral Therapy seminars, refers to internal wisdom or inner voices as your "inner physician." You may have other ways of referring to your intuition, in accordance with your belief system. If there is something you need help with, ask for specific guidance. Maybe you want the

(Continued)

BONE GAME   *(Continued)*

strength to refrain from judging Sara when she doesn't do her homework exercises, or the confidence to listen to your intuition when you see Clint tense up when he reports he is fine. Affirm your self-awareness skills by saying, "I am whole and separate from Sara. I practice with skill and provide care that honors Sara as a whole and separate human being. It is my heartfelt intent to be present with Sara, to offer her my understanding and compassion, and to facilitate her healing by tapping into her strength and internal wisdom."

Self-Acceptance

Self-acceptance is about recognizing all aspects of our character, embracing our humanness, and trusting that we are enough. Self-acceptance is not synonymous with self-approval. It is not about ego. It does not mean we have to feel good about our behavior when we are hurtful. Self-acceptance begins by simply recognizing that all of us contain parts we may consider negative or even frightening. When we do not accept the full range of our feelings and thoughts, we often ignore our inner voice.[2] Fear and denial prevent us from understanding and relating to our intuition. It is impossible to separate the good from the bad, to love one and hate the other. Rachel Naomi Remen MD, attended a seminar of Carl Rogers and reported him saying, "I realize there's something I do before I start a session. I let myself know that I am enough. Not perfect. Perfect wouldn't be enough. But that I am human, and that is enough."[6] When we begin to accept ourselves as being enough, we are able to be present for others.

An essential part of the individual healing process has to do with going within, into the shadow aspects—the aspects that, out of fear, we have denied, disowned, or suppressed. Shakti Gawain, in the book *Healers on Healing*, writes that the reason thoughts or feelings take a negative turn is because we do not accept them or allow them their natural expression.[6] Suppressed anger, for example, may manifest later as violence toward others or toward ourselves in the form of illness. If we can accept the good and the bad in ourselves, we will be better able to accept the positive and negative aspects of our patients. Start with yourself; kindness to others begins with kindness to yourself.

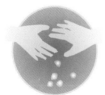

BONE GAME
Practice Acceptance

Exercise your ability to recognize a variety of human behaviors or characteristics in yourself.

Pick a day, preferably one with a full patient load. You may have a few patients who push your buttons. If so, pick a day when they have appointments scheduled. If you are in school, use conversations with your classmates for this exercise. The task is to observe the conversations with your patients and notice when your "judgment flag" waves, such as when the patient does or says something about which you form a negative opinion. Throughout the day, take time to consider these observations. It is possible to do this exercise and still be present for your patients. Make a mental note of the experience, or jot down a reminder word on a sticky note.

(Continued)

BONE GAME *(Continued)*

> Later that day, take a moment to review the situations that raised the judgment flag. Pull out all the sticky notes and lay them out before you. Give yourself permission to be honest and compassionate with yourself. Hold up the proverbial mirror and consider whether you have any of the traits you found fault with in your patients. Remember, a mirror should reflect a clear image, not a sermon.
>
> Repeat this exercise on another day, replacing the judgment flag with the times when you felt admiration for the person before you. Again, make mental or physical notes reminding yourself of the situations, and review them later in the day. Consider how you might find yourself in their stories.
>
> Practice several times to strengthen your ability to accept all aspects of yourself. You will then experience deeper compassion for others as well.

Self-Expression

Self-expressive people are aware of their innermost thoughts and feelings. They accept them, and, when appropriate, they shares their thoughts responsibly. In a patient–practitioner relationship, it is rarely appropriate for the manual therapist to divulge his or her personal thoughts or feelings. A rule of thumb is to share only the information that contributes to the healing relationship. Self-expression is not self-disclosure. It takes a practitioner with a developed sense of self-awareness and self-acceptance to know how to express the true self without revealing personal information.

For example, talking about yourself can distract the patient. Even though you may intend to create a true healing relationship, in which both heal and both are healed, clear roles must be maintained. The therapeutic relationship requires the practitioner to focus on the needs of the patient. Be whole and complete with your patients without relating your opinions or life events.

Self-expression can be relayed through a genuine interest in the patient. One of the basic premises in Dale Carnegie's *How to Win Friends and Influence People* is that friends are made when we become interested in others, not when we try to get others interested in us. He even goes so far as to say, "It is the individual who is not interested in his fellow men who has the greatest difficulties in life and provides the greatest injury to others."[7] Avoid imposing on your patients by making them feel they have to take care of you. For example, resist telling patients that your day got off to a rough start. That information may lead them to filter their own needs and not make your bad day worse. Allow them their own process and keep yours to yourself.

You can demonstrate your interest in patients by listening to them—with your whole body—and by watching their whole bodies and not just listening to their words. Many researchers claim that only a small portion of the understanding one gains from face-to-face interactions comes from words. The results of these studies vary slightly. For example, the importance of verbal information ranges from 7 to 35%, with the rest belonging to nonverbal communication.[2] Be conscious of your facial expressions. Surprise, alarm, worry, distaste, or annoyance will steal across one's face and should be avoided. Give credence to the expressions that steal across your patient's face.

The therapeutic relationship is not an appropriate context for talking about yourself, but that does not mean you should suppress your thoughts and feelings altogether. During the five minutes of quiet time between patients, feel those feelings, have those thoughts, and make those faces. Or designate a person with whom you can express your feelings at the end of the day or week. During the session, focus on the patient's feelings. Be so clear in your own thoughts and feelings that you can reflect the patient's words and expressions without distortion. One of the most productive interview skills is that of mirroring for patients, reflecting their innermost thoughts and feelings so that they may realize their inner wisdom. Avoid mirroring their negative thoughts. Instead, focus on reflecting their strengths. It is important to show understanding and compassion for their negative thoughts, but concentrate on reinforcing the positive ones.

Consider the potential obstacles to listening during the interview. Earlier, we discussed how easily practitioners can get distracted. Remember, it is very hard to listen when you are talking. Rather than talking about yourself, ask open-ended questions that elicit information about the patient's situation. Find out how the patient feels about the situation and how it is affecting his or her life.

▼

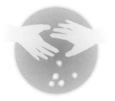

BONE GAME
Morning Pages

The best way I have found to get to know myself is to write three pages of whatever comes to mind, every morning, no excuses. This writing is called morning pages, a term I much prefer to "journaling," which feels so formidable and permanent. I learned of morning pages in Julia Cameron's *The Artist's Way*. I scribble thoughts, feelings, opinions, anger, grief, desire, gossip, reactions to television shows, and movie critiques onto those pages, thus sparing my friends, loved ones, and patients. Writing morning pages has helped me sort out emotions and situations, and has allowed me to express myself in ways I can be proud of. I have fewer regrets since practicing my daily writing routine. That alone is worth every minute of "I don't know what to write this morning . . . ." Try it. You will be amazed at what you discover about yourself.

Reprinted by permission from Cameron J. The Artist's Way: A Spiritual Path to Higher Creativity. New York: Tarcher/Putnam, 1992.

PRACTICE UNDERSTANDING AND COMPASSION
Develop Good Listening Skills

To foster good listening skills during the interview, limit the distractions in the room. For example, turn off the phone ringer. Don't wear clothes that call attention to yourself. Arrange the room so that nothing is between you and your patients: For example, avoid sitting behind a desk or crossing your arms or legs. Be on the same level as your patients—don't sit on the table. Face patients and make solid eye contact. Sit on the edge of your seat. Be relaxed, yet alert and involved. Respect their personal space—three feet is considered a safe distance in American culture. Gesture during their stories—nod your head, smile, and show concern. Touch, appropriately and with permission, to express your compassion.

Listen to the Words and Acknowledge the Feelings

Understanding patients involves grasping both the content and the process of patient communication. The content refers to what patients say; the process refers to how they say it, which includes their tone, body language, and facial expressions. As mentioned earlier, most information is communicated nonverbally. When we focus on the symptoms alone, we miss the patients' personal reactions to their condition; in essence, we miss the uniqueness of each individual. Information is all around us. Feelings are the energizing force that helps us sort our data and use them effectively to shape and implement relevant action steps.[2] Remember, when patients do not feel understood about the facts and the emotions they express, they will not trust the practitioner and the therapeutic relationship is at risk. To strengthen the relationship, we must explore the patient's feelings as we gather the data.

Although you should be attentive to your patients' feelings, do not analyze those feelings or attempt to cross over into a psychotherapeutic relationship until you are trained and licensed to do so. The goal is to understand how patients feel about their condition because their feelings can help or hinder the healing process. For example, research shows that excessive amounts of norepinephrine and epinephrine are secreted when a person is aggressive and anxious. The arteries thicken, and the excess hormones cause blood vessels to constrict. The gradual rise in blood pressure can cause hypertension, stroke, or heart failure.[6] Unless the patient's feelings—verbally or nonverbally expressed— are considered, understood, and reflected by the practitioner, recovery from disease can be an uphill battle.

Patients do not always express their feelings freely. In Western cultures, people tend to be private with their feelings. Often, experiences have trained patients to hide their personal feelings initially. Until your patients feel safe enough to express themselves, look for alternative ways to gather emotional information.

Body language is the best way to tap into the patient's feelings. Research shows that words are best at communicating facts, but body language is the primary means of emotional expression. The behavior of a person—facial expressions, postures, gestures, and other actions—is an uninterrupted stream of information and a constant source of clues to the feelings the person is experiencing.[2]

Reflecting and active listening are tools that can be used to acknowledge emotions you see in a patient's behavior, whether or not they are expressed verbally. **Reflecting** means repeating, paraphrasing, or summarizing the feelings the patient has expressed either verbally or nonverbally. **Active listening** involves paying attention to the speakers' tone, body language, and facial expressions and nonverbally demonstrating a sense of caring and respect. Use your intuition to read body language whenever patients do not name their emotion. Watch for facial expressions, postures, and gestures; listen to voice tone, pitch, and volume. If you are not sure what the expression means to the patient, consider what it might mean to you and reflect your interpretation for confirmation.

Until you feel comfortable reflecting, adopt the formula "You feel (name emotion) because (name event or condition)."[2] Practice this formula with your peers until it becomes natural. Use the formula to summarize the information the patient (peer) shares with you. For example, "You feel sad because pain prevents you from lifting your baby" or "You feel frustrated because you cannot concentrate on your homework with the headaches." Or even, "You feel happy because you were able to garden for an hour without back pain."

Sometimes, patients' body language reflects something different from their words. Check by saying, "You say you are happy that you were able to garden for an hour without pain, but you look as though you are sad that the back pain is still a problem and is preventing you from gardening for longer." Another example is, "Clint, I heard you tell me that you feel fine today, but I can't help noticing that you are wearing your shoulders like a pair of earrings. Is it possible that you are carrying some tension in your shoulders today?" A little humor, when used with discretion, can help to loosen up patients. Speak with compassion, not with prodding.

Exploring or reflecting feelings can be a useful tool for the following:

◆ Making the patient feel understood
◆ Helping the patient become more aware of her feelings
◆ Encouraging the patient to speak more about her feelings

While a patient is expressing personal feelings, use **silence** to explore the emotions further. Silence can uncover deep feelings. Don't complete the patient's sentences or fill pauses with more questions. If given time to think, patients will often sink a little more deeply into their thoughts and will express the feelings or problems that lie beneath the surface. Too often, therapists make the mistake of focusing on the first thing that comes up in the interview when the source of the problem is deeper. Your use of silence will add to patients' satisfaction with the therapeutic relationship and to their feeling of being deeply understood.

In the interview, explore the patient's entire relationship with her condition, including when and why she experiences it, how the condition affects her daily activities and emotions, and what she is doing to cope with it. **Following skills** are listening skills that can be used to discover how patients view their situation. **Door openers**—invitations to talk—can get things started. These can be as simple as, "You are here because of shoulder pain you experience while working on the computer. Tell me how you feel about this." Open-ended questions such as, "What do you notice when your shoulder starts to hurt and you have a deadline to meet?" can deepen the search. Reinforce the tools that work for patients by **complimenting** them on being active in their health care and responding with, "What a good idea, to stretch while sitting at your desk! It decreases the pain and helps you feel more energized." Lead them to explore additional ways of handling their stress and promoting physical healing with a question such as, "What could you do to remind yourself to stretch regularly even before the pain begins?"

See Through the Other's Eyes

Compassion is another key component to the relationship. We want the patient to feel understood but not judged. Compassion denotes respect for the patient's point of view. When developing relationships, see through the eyes of the other person—through his or her historical, cultural, and emotional filters. To do this, we must set aside our own belief systems, judgments, and expectations about the outcome of the relationship. Respect the patient's personal values and personal space and allow the patient to be her own person. You will still experience your biases and filters, but you will also demonstrate a commitment to understanding and compassion and can return your focus toward what is important to the person in front of you.

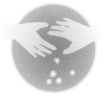

BONE GAME
Gain Perspective

Refer back to Bone Game: Practice Acceptance. After raising the proverbial mirror and considering the possibility that you may possess some of the same qualities as your patient, add the following piece to the exercise:

Evaluate each situation separately. Put yourself in the shoes of each patient. View the situation from the patient's perspective, with his or her history and values, and see whether you can understand the motivations behind his or her actions.

To be compassionate is to be fair, patient, kind, and consistent. It is unconditional love—concern for the well-being of others—regardless of your opinion of them. From a Buddhist perspective, compassion is equal to emptiness. Pema Chödrön describes compassion as being soft and gentle, clear and sharp, open and warm.[8] People who have a well-developed sense of self-acceptance and who have practiced kindness on themselves will have an easier time feeling and expressing compassion toward their patients.

HAVE FAITH IN THE PATIENT'S STRENGTH AND HEALING ABILITIES

In the opening story of Chapter 4, a patient named Sandee is having difficulty believing that her health is improving. Eventually, her manual therapist is able to illustrate Sandee's progress, convincing Sandee of specific improvements. Providing substantial proof of her progress was like flipping a switch inside Sandee's head. Suddenly, she had confidence in herself and in the therapy and was willing to work harder to achieve greater results. Patients' perceptions, meanings, and definitions shift over time and in interactions with others. As practitioners, we must recognize that how we think, feel, and act greatly influences how our patients' view their health.

According to research, people's perceptions of their own health can actually determine the quality of their health. People who feel hopeless about their situation or helpless to do anything about it generally have higher disease rates, are less able to fight infection and disease, and often will succumb to disease at a much higher rate.[4] Also, people who feel helpless have the same physiological response as people who *are* helpless: their heart rate slows, their blood pressure drops, the heart becomes prone to arrhythmia, the stomach pumps out less gastric secretion, and their urinary water and sodium decrease. The body secretes the stress hormone cortisol, which slows nervous system activity, decreases muscle tone, and suppresses immunity. The body behaves as though it is giving up.[4]

Encouraging clients to not give up—helping them believe that change is possible, even when they feel hopeless—is perhaps the most important thing manual therapists can do to help patients be successful in their efforts to heal. We must have faith in our patients, and in their ability to contribute to their own health.

The World Health Organization (WHO) defines health as "a state of complete well-being in all the aspects of one's life: physical, mental, social, and spiritual—not just the absence of disease."[4] The book *Mind/Body Health* provides a comprehensive list, shown here in Wise One Speaks: Qualities of Wellness. Use this list to develop ways to exhibit faith in your patients' strength and healing abilities and to influence the attitudes and emotions of

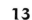

your patients to promote improved health. If our attitudes influence our patients' perceptions of their health, thereby affecting the outcome, we should make it a point to influence their health in a positive way. When the mental, emotional, and spiritual aspects of wellness are manifested, the physical aspects follow naturally.

▼

WISE ONE SPEAKS
Qualities of Wellness

- Sense of empowerment and personal control:
  - Control over one's responses, not necessarily one's environment
  - Integrity, the ability to live by one's deepest values
  - Feeling heard and respected
- Sense of connectedness and acceptance:
  - To one's deepest self
  - To other people
  - To earth and the cosmos
  - To all regarded as good, and to the sources of one's spiritual strength
- Sense of meaning and purpose:
  - Giving of self for a purpose of value; a caring sense of mission
  - Finding meaning and wisdom in here-and-now difficulties
  - Enjoying the process of growth
  - Having a vision of one's potential
- Hope:
  - Positive expectation
  - Ability to envision what one wants before it happens

Reprinted with permission from Hafen BQ, Karren KJ, Frandsen KJ, Smith NL. Mind/Body Health: The Effects of Attitudes, Emotions, and Relationships. 2nd Ed. Boston: Allyn & Bacon, 1996.

Sense of Empowerment and Personal Control

Ensuring that patients feel heard and valued—an important component of the sense of empowerment and personal control—is a skill worked on previously in this chapter. In order for patients to feel heard, we as therapists must demonstrate that we understand what they say and how they feel. A variety of listening and communicating skills to help us do that have been introduced. We can express our understanding by creating a nondistracting environment in which we use body language to show we are listening, ask patients about their feelings, and reflect what we hear and see. By accepting what patients say without judging or criticizing, we show that we value what they are telling us.

We can help patients live according to their values by listening for what is really meaningful to them and integrating their values into the treatment plan. If Darnel, for example, is deeply committed to playing with his granddaughter and to showing her affection, but his low back pain prevents the types of activities he is used to, we can help him discover play activities that will not increase his discomfort (and possibly strengthen his low back in the process).

Once patients begin implementing self-care routines that are aligned with their core values, the contribution they are making to their overall goals for health is reinforced. Compliment them on their ability to affect their health, and they will feel they have some control over their situation. Provide treatment options in your sessions and educate patients on the various benefits of each option. This allows them to choose their treatment and self-care. A sense of control regarding the outcome of the treatment contributes to the speed and quality of recovery and allows patients to take responsibility and act effectively on their own behalf.

Lack of control may have an even stronger negative influence on health than having a high level of stress. Hypertension, anxiety, and pain levels increase, and the immune system is compromised. People who don't believe they can control or change their situation or who don't believe they are capable of contributing to their healing, slacken their efforts or give up altogether. Whereas, those who have a strong sense of control and ability exert great effort to master the challenge. Little effort on our behalf is required to compliment people on their efforts and to point out their successes.

Sense of Connectedness and Acceptance

Reflecting patients' words and feelings often helps them more clearly understand their situation, what it means to them, and how it fits into their life, even though all you may have done is summarize what they said. The information may seem new to them when they hear it put together for the very first time. This sense of understanding and being understood can help people feel a connection to the world.

Accept your patients for who they are and support their own self-acceptance. Your respect for their values gives them space to be who they are when they are with you.

Be an example for your patients. Demonstrate consistency by showing your respect for others. Be tolerant and flexible. Celebrate diversity. If you are critical of others in front of your patients, they may assume you are critical of them behind their backs. Have a positive attitude about yourself, your connection to others, your work, your profession, and the things that are meaningful to you.

Sense of Meaning and Purpose

No one is more valuable to the patient than himself or herself, and nothing is more valuable than his or her health. One patient made millions from the stock market through employee stock options and fully acknowledges that all the money in the world is not a substitute for health. Each patient has only one body. Give your patients a sense of purpose by involving them in their healing process in a way that is satisfying and fulfilling.

Have your patients discuss the positives in their situation. When they believe something can be learned or accomplished from their pain, they are more able to muster up the courage to face it head-on.

Compliment your patients on their strength and wisdom and help them realize their unlimited potential to grow. Help your patients appreciate the process of growing and learning. They will have much to contribute to others after accomplishing the task at hand.

Hope

A positive expectation is the product of knowing what is possible and visualizing a positive outcome. When we help our patients understand how their condition is affecting them physiologically, and how the body works to heal itself, they can visualize successful healing and support the results. Dr. Rachel Naomi Remen uses visualization to combat terminal diseases. In her book, *Kitchen Table Wisdom,* she tells the story of a patient who used an image of catfish to enhance the function of his immune system and battle cancer. The patient visualized ". . . millions of catfish that never slept, moving through his body, vigilant, untiring, dedicated, and discriminating, patiently examining every cell, passing by the ones that were healthy, eating the ones that were cancerous, motivated by a pet's unconditional love and devotion."[1] Dr. Remen compared bottom-feeders eating what does not support the life of an aquarium to white blood cells attacking and destroying cancer cells to help her patient understand that his body was on his side. In the end, he was confident that the daily meditation contributed to his full recovery.

Hope is more than a positive expectation; it is the ability to fight against overwhelming odds and to laugh in the face of adversity. A fighting spirit has been shown to stimulate production of neuropeptides, which are chemical messengers that stimulate and mobilize the immune system. Humor dissipates stress and accentuates the positive. Laughter increases breath rate, circulation, and oxygen levels. Also, it relaxes muscle tension and breaks the pain-spasm-pain cycle—thus acting as a painkiller.

Physical health is only one aspect of wellness. Wellness includes mental acuity, a zest for living, and a tolerance for different ideas. Wellness brings with it empathy, compassion, and a sense of cohesiveness with the rest of humanity. Wellness encompasses a fighting spirit, an optimistic outlook, an attitude of hope. Take care of your patients' physical health, of course, but never omit the wholeness that is human. Whenever you can, maintain perspective, provide encouragement, boost patients' self-esteem, educate and provide options, prove that behavior can lead to positive outcomes, dispel doubts, encourage independence, and be flexible, consistent, positive, and responsive to your patients' needs. Do all this, and they will rise to the occasion and do much more for themselves.

Interviewing Skills: Team Therapy Model

In this book, a new paradigm for approaching interviews called the **Team Therapy Model** is proposed. As holistic practitioners, we cannot entirely embrace the medical model, which implies that the expert's perceptions about the patient's condition are more important than the patient's perceptions. As manual therapists, we provide treatment and, therefore, cannot wholly adopt the intervention-free model of solution-building. Some manual therapists use touch as an additional form of communication, rather than for corrective purposes, as with the Rosen Method. Most manual therapy professionals, however, apply manual techniques with curative intent, whether for relaxation, and stress reduction or to relieve pain and increase function. Therefore, a combination of the two models serves us best.

The primary goals of the Team Therapy Model approach to interviewing are:

1. Create a relationship
2. Share information
3. Develop goals for health
4. Choose and implement solutions
5. Evaluate progress and provide feedback

The rest of this chapter describes each goal and recommends methods for reaching it.

CREATE A RELATIONSHIP

Developing a deep and meaningful relationship that is productive for both patient and practitioner is the primary goal of the interview process. This goal requires the practitioner to be mindful of the relationship from beginning to end. Creating and preserving a meaningful relationship calls for our constant attention, understanding, compassion, and faith in the patient's personal strength and abilities. To foster such a relationship, practice the interpersonal communication skills described earlier in this chapter.

Countless opportunities exist for us to build productive relationships with our patients. The interview process is ongoing. It often begins before we meet the patient (often through brochures and phone conversations), and it extends beyond the time spent together. For example, the greeting on your answering machine can encourage or discourage the next step in initiating a relationship. For example, asking patients for permission to touch them and informing them of our intentions before massaging the chest may eliminate fear and open up potential for change, rather than resistance. Patients have described how, during times of pain or trauma, they heard their therapist's voice in their heads, instructing them to breathe, look, and listen for clues telling them how to take care of themselves. Relationships are developed before, during, and after every session, whether we are communicating actively or processing information indirectly. Make the most of these opportunities.

SHARE INFORMATION

Interviewing is an information-gathering process. Patients possess all the information you need, and you must simply create a trusting relationship in which information flows freely. Ask questions that lead to pertinent information and listen carefully to the replies. Every bit of information expressed by patients—verbal and nonverbal, symptoms and perceptions—leads to a deeper understanding of them and their health condition, as well as to potential solutions. Grasping the relationship among the patient, the condition, and the solution is the key to success.

According to Pema Chödrön, two primary obstacles to gathering information exist: thinking you already know the answer and being afraid to ask the question.[8] Proctoring countless practical examinations has shown me that it is human nature (or the product of watching television game shows) to leap to conclusions. We are so eager to solve the problem and to be the first to get the right answer that we don't take the time to thoroughly explore the possibilities or look beyond the obvious. We fall into what is most familiar to us. An examiner for a doctoral program in neurology explained that more than half the candidates failed the oral examinations, largely, he believed, because they didn't listen to everything the patient said and therefore didn't obtain adequate information. They were too apt to focus on a key phrase or word that pointed to a familiar dysfunction. Instead, they should pursue lines of questioning suggested by the patient's comments and gather additional information on which to base their conclusions.

▼

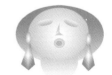

STORY TELLER
Explore Possibilities

I received a phone call from a chiropractor who was hosting a student apprenticeship program at her office. I was the faculty liaison. She called to complain that the student practitioner was treating all the patients as though they had rotator cuff injuries. Some patients did indeed have rotator cuff injuries, but others had thoracic outlet syndrome, carpal tunnel syndrome, or whiplash injuries. The student had recently studied rotator cuff injuries in a pathology and clinical treatment class. As a result, she was listening for familiar information and didn't bother to register other important information. Instead of exploring all possibilities, she jumped to the explanation that she had the most immediate information about: If the patient had shoulder pain, it must be caused by a rotator cuff injury.

Solving minor problems while ignoring deeper concerns is one of the biggest sources of inefficiency in industry, government, schools, and health care.[2] We leap to conclusions because we are eager to help or want to be right, are in a hurry, or have any number of other reasons or motivations. We are desperate to explain our experience, so we force-fit a few pieces of information into familiar scenarios and call it good, rather than searching for more details without the pressure of categorizing the data. Sometimes the process of asking questions and gathering information can be far more important than identifying a cause or pinpointing a dysfunction because it can lead patients to a better understanding of themselves, their relationship with their bodies, and their role in their own health.

Be more curious than afraid. Often, we avoid asking questions when we cannot control or anticipate the response. We are afraid of information we might not understand or feelings that could get out of hand. Someone's story might be more than we can handle, or we won't know what to do with the information once we know it. We fear the patient will think we are asking silly questions or being nosy. If the question arises in your mind, and a part of you believes the answer could contribute to the patient's health, trust your instinct and ask.

Other times, we avoid asking meaningful questions because we assume the patient's intentions are simple. If we work in an environment where relaxations massage is paramount, for example, we may assume that the only reason for the patient's visit is to relax or be pampered. We don't want to probe too deeply into their day celebrating Sue's birthday, so we avoid asking direct questions and automatically provide a routine session. A pointed question, such as, "Is there anything I should know about you that would help us reach your goals for health today?" could heighten the experience of your massage by inviting a deeper level of participation, which may ultimately lead to a session that satisfies specific health needs.

▼

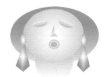

STORY TELLER
Be Curious

Do not let fear limit your ability to serve. I remember the first time a patient cried during a session. I handed her a tissue and considered stopping the work I was doing on her legs because it seemed too emotionally difficult for her. I was afraid to break the silence and ask her about it. Eventually, I summoned the courage to say, "I see that you are crying. Shall I stop what I am doing, or would you like me to continue?" She said, "Oh no, please continue. I am crying because I have never been touched in such a respectful and caring manner before." I almost missed out on the most moving comment anyone has ever made about my work.

Explore the data thoroughly and include the patient's thoughts, feelings, behaviors, and experiences. Reflect the content and the context of the patient's story. Affirm the patient's perceptions and your interpretations. Exploring and reflecting patient perceptions is the most important aspect of interviewing skills. When explored and understood, these perceptions help the therapist and patient alike make sense of health issues and can lead to a better understanding of the relationship among the patient, the patient's condition, and the successful treatment.

What questions are important to ask? It is difficult to determine whether information is helpful before you know what the information is and get a sense of how the patient feels about the information. Leading questions will follow a predetermined path—yours. Open-ended questions allow for individual expression and interpretation from the patient's point of view. Engage in conversation instead of asking an endless stream of questions. The conversation can begin with something as simple as, "Tell me about your health concerns," or "What are your goals for today's session?" Choose the significant details from the patient's story and listen for clues that provide a direction for additional open-ended questions.

Prevent people from rambling. Create purposeful dialogue by interrupting with brief reflections of helpful information. A long-winded story may have one vital piece of information that can be paraphrased back to the patient to break his chatter and to focus attention on providing deeper insight into the relevant detail.

Some patients have difficulty talking about their concerns or asking for what they want. Take your cues from the intake forms. Patients may find discussing their problems uncomfortable, but have no trouble putting the information on paper. The difficulty may lie in your choice of language or your focus on a particular condition. To let the patient lead you, ask, "What should I know today so we can meet your goals for health?" Compliment patients on what they have done for their own health—even showing up for the appointment. Compliments may help them open up.

Acquiring information from patients is an art. You will need to cultivate a flexible style to accommodate patients' differences in background, in knowledge about manual therapy, and in other health matters. It is important to use language that your patient understands and to use consistent terminology. As you ask your questions, define the specialized terms you use. Avoid either speaking down to patients or speaking over their heads.

The Pre-Interview

Patients initiate the relationship by gathering information about you and determining whether you are the right manual therapist for them. Make sure your external image—ads, brochures, office space, and the like—attracts the type of patient you are seeking. Identify your target clientele and speak directly to them in your marketing efforts and in the way you project yourself.

Once the patient takes the next step and contacts you directly, gather enough information before scheduling the appointment to determine whether you want to pursue the relationship. Find out why the patient is seeking care and get a few details about his or her health history, so you can decide whether you can and want to be of service or whether a referral is in order. Ascertain in advance whether you will need a doctor's prescription or consultation before treating the patient so that the first session will not be a waste of time for either one of you.

In advance of the first appointment, share any information you feel is important for preparing patients emotionally and physically for the session. Explain what they can expect during the session, what the fees are, and what to wear, for example. Invite prospective patients to ask questions about your experience, modalities, education, affiliations, and references to assure them that they have made the right decision and to put them at ease. Be prepared to mail information to them prior to the first session, such as your credentials, office policies, intake forms, directions, and so on. Avoid confusion and limit the potential for unmet expectations.

The Interview

Gather information that helps the patient relax, enhances the relationship, and opens the dialogue. Begin by asking how the patient prefers to be addressed—Ms. Freeman? Karen?—and tell her how you prefer to be called. Chat a little bit to make her comfortable and to get to know her a little bit. For example, you might begin with "It's a beautiful day today. Do you have plans to enjoy the weather?" Limit the sharing of personal information. For example, let them know you are looking forward to working in the garden, but don't delve into your plans for landscaping. Instead, place the focus on getting to know the patient.

Review how you work and what the patient can expect during the session. For example: "To begin with, I need to understand as much about your goals for health and your expectations of me as possible. In addition, it is helpful to explore how your past may be influencing today's concerns, so I may be asking you a lot of questions. All this can take a while, but I promise that at the end of the session, you will feel satisfied in the results from the therapy. In the future, a couple of minutes may be all that's needed to get me up to speed before we begin the therapy." Even if you explained things over the phone, information can be received differently when people are face-to-face. Watch patients' reactions to your information and be responsive to their needs.

Initial interviews can be extensive and time-consuming. It is advisable to schedule time for the interview in addition to the treatment session. **Insurance companies** may or may not pay for extended initial visits, depending on the **insurance plan** and the type of provider. You should know this in advance of scheduling the appointment. You may have to shorten the hands-on part of the initial session to allow for the extensive interview and to stay within the reimbursable timeframe. The information obtained in the interview is critical to conducting safe and effective treatment, and it increases efficiency in the long run. It is best to do a complete interview in the first session or two, rather than having information trickle in over time.

Patients may have health conditions that make it difficult to sit for extended periods of time. Others may get antsy. Be attentive and responsive to their spoken and unspoken needs. Intersperse movement assessment tests with the question-and-answer format. Patients may want to begin the hands-on part of the session immediately. Be flexible and gather information with your patient in sitting, standing, or lying positions. Make sure you have obtained adequate information before you begin treatment. Try juggling verbal questions with hands–on information gathering or relaxation techniques to keep the patient comfortable. Avoid beginning therapy before you have enough information to provide safe treatment.

▼

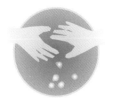

BONE GAME
Share Information During a Relaxing Foot Bath!

Initial interviews may extend beyond a half-hour for adequate information gathering. A foot bath is a creative way to keep your patients relaxed and the information flowing. If they think they are missing out on precious treatment time answering questions, they might tighten up the lips. A foot bath is a way to ensure that the patient is comfortable and feels that therapy has already begun.

To provide a foot bath in the initial interview, prepare two plastic dish tubs— one with hot water; one with cold. Before inviting the patient to select a tub, find out

(Continued)

BONE GAME *(Continued)*

whether any health conditions would preclude benefit from either water temperature. If no contraindications are present, invite the patient to choose one, alternate between them, or scoop water from one to the other until to obtain the preferred temperature. Tailor the foot bath by providing marbles to roll around underfoot or by adding essential oils. Have towels available within reach so the patient can remove his or her feet from the bath at any time.

Review the intake form, find out what the patient's goals and expectations are for the visit, and reflect the patient's general goals for health and priorities for treatment. Ask, "How can I help you?" or "Why are you here?" Hearing the patient speak adds to the written information on the form. It also apprises you of any inaccurate presumptions or unreasonable expectations and gives you an opportunity to change these instead of disappointing the patient. Setting reasonable goals is essential to a productive relationship, a subject that will be discussed at length in this book. Begin the discussion by listening and comprehending the patient's goals for health and for sessions with you. Later, move to shaping and developing the patient's goals with the purpose of tracking outcomes and promoting patient participation.

Explore the treatments the patient has tried and the techniques and modalities he is considering. Ask, "What worked or didn't work?" or "Do you have a sense of why the previous treatments did not work?" These questions will make your sessions more efficient, because you can use treatments the patient likes and believes are effective, rather than spinning your wheels with treatments that have already been proven ineffective.

Use the intake forms to begin a direct line of questioning regarding history and current conditions. Take note of your patient's priorities and focus on them. You may be interested in her respiratory history when she is intent on getting attention for a recent knee injury. Make the patient feel that his or her needs are being met before focusing on less urgent details.

▼

STORY TELLER
Memories Affect Healing

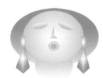

Explore relationships between current symptoms and previous history. Stimulate the patient's memory to connect previous events such as traumas, illnesses, repetitive movements, and the like that may have initiated the current condition. Little things may trigger important memories. For example, as a patient was watching a large family board an airplane, she noticed and identified with the eldest child's difficulty carrying a younger sibling. There were too many kids for the parents to take care of, so the older kids were helping with some of the younger ones. My patient, too, was the eldest in a large family. Her mother had died when she was young, and she shouldered a great deal of responsibility in caring for her younger siblings. That recent memory, combined with the interview question, "What kinds of things did you do as a child

(Continued)

STORY TELLER   *(Continued)*

that might have been stressful to your neck?" pulled it all together for her. She not only had a great deal of physical stress with her younger brothers and sisters clasping their hands around her neck to help her lift them, but she also carried the weight of the responsibility of trying to replace her mother. By recognizing the origin of the physical stress and acknowledging an emotional component, she reduced the occurrence of her neck spasms dramatically.

Explore the details of patients' health concerns. Prompt patients with consistent adjectives such as *mild*, *moderate*, and *severe* as you gather information. Using consistent terminology to describe, for example, the intensity of pain, will show progress more clearly over time. Comparing *moderate pain* with *mild pain* is easier than distinguishing between "hurts pretty bad" and "is kinda sore." The ability to prove progress is an important component of documenting information—measurable data leads to measurable results. Let them know the importance of using consistent terminology and paraphrase the details they provide until they are accustomed to the terminology. Soon, they will be reporting, "I had a constant, moderate headache that lasted for two days and interfered with my ability to concentrate at work."

Information regarding the patient's medications can be enlightening and helpful in creating a safe treatment plan. The list of medications on the intake form can be daunting at times. Keep a **Physician's Desk Reference (PDR)** handy to look up medications and their side effects. Better yet, ask the patient for information. Find out why he is taking the medication. You may uncover a condition not listed on the intake form. Ask about side effects. Manual therapy has the physiological effect of increasing circulation and may increase the metabolic breakdown of the medication.[9] Be alert to an onset or increase in those side effects. (For general principles regarding safe massage choices for patients on medications, refer to Persad RS. Massage Therapy and Medications: General Treatment Principles. Toronto, Ontario: Curies-Overzet, 2001.)

Hands-On Interview

The interview—asking questions, listening, and observing—segues into the hands-on interview—questioning the whole body, listening, observing, palpating, and testing. Make it a point to acknowledge that you are moving from hands–off information gathering to hands–on information gathering. The initial touch affects how the patient will respond to subsequent physical contact. He or she may relax into your touch or pull away or be open to treatment or resistant to it. Ask patients for permission to touch them prior to your first hands-on contact. This demonstrates respect and instills trust. It can make the difference between feeling poked and prodded, and being handled with compassion and caring. Tell patients where you are about to touch them and why you will be touching them there and ask for their consent before you follow through with the contact. You may need to do this for only a session or two. Once trust is solidified, you can obtain their permission to discontinue the consent questions.

Educate your patients throughout the hands-on interview. Prepare them to stand up, sit down, and walk this way before you put them through the paces. Let them know why you are palpating their neck especially if it is their back that hurts. Tell them your goals for each modality and invite them to visualize the results you intend. Inform them of your options and allow them to choose the techniques you will use.

The interview and the hands-on interview involve verbal and nonverbal communication, and they may present you with conflicting information. You may hear the patient say one thing, yet you may witness the opposite response in facial expressions or tension patterns. Reflect both findings when this happens, and invite the patient to make sense of the possible conflict. The patient may be unaware of the contradiction. Presenting your findings in a neutral or curious way invites the patient to work with you to resolve it. This promotes partnership and gives the patient a deeper understanding of herself rather than putting her on the defensive.

▼

STORY TELLER
Listen with Your Hands

Aisha came in for her monthly session after the holidays and was bubbling with stories of her festivities. After chatting for a moment I asked her, "What do I need to know to be of service to you today?" She replied that she was fine and couldn't think of anything to tell me. I struggled for a moment to release her respiratory diaphragm and asked her again. Again she replied that she couldn't think of anything. As she said that, her abdominal muscles tightened even more. I informed her that her belly was tighter than usual, but with her holiday glow, it sounded as though there was no stress in her family or social life. I asked her if anything unusual was going on at work. "The mayor is coming!" It was as though she was just remembering. She was in charge of a community service program and had spent the entire week preparing for the mayor's visit on Monday. Her stress level was over the top, and she put the site visit out of her mind to cope. Her body hadn't forgotten. She acknowledged that it was Friday, that there was nothing else to do, and that she felt prepared for the event. As she spoke about her week at work, her abdominal muscles softened and her diaphragm released. She admitted she could now relax, and she did.

Hands-on information gathering can take many forms, depending on the modalities used. You will use various techniques—palpation-assessing system integrity, postural analysis, motion testing, and the like—according to your individual specialty or training as a manual therapist. As you ask questions, the body responds as well as the voice. For example, in Upledger's CranioSacral training, practitioners are taught to listen for the truth in the body by asking questions, and feeling for changes in the craniosacral rhythm as the patient verbalizes answers. If the movement of the cerebral spinal fluid stops, the answer to the question is significant to the healing process. Develop your individual skills and gather adequate information for determining safe and effective treatment.

The hands-on interview is a mixture of information gathering, treatment, and evaluation. As new information presents itself, treatment shifts to comply. The effectiveness of the treatment application is immediately assessed, providing new data. The interview cycles continuously throughout the hands-on session. Be aware of this and don't reserve the information gathering for before and after only. If necessary, stop periodically throughout the hands-on session to record the information obtained. A Feldenkrais practitioner incorporates breaks into her sessions. Her invitation to rest for a few minutes gives her a chance to take notes without the client feeling that he or she is being ignored.

As you share the information you are gathering with your patient, try not to reflect only negative findings. Saying, "This is really tight" or "That feels very congested" over and over again can be discouraging. Instead of judging the patient's joint mobility, ask him to describe what he feels. For example, "How does your shoulder feel when I move it like this?" Asking the same question after you have applied treatment can help integrate the solution, making a mental connection to the physical change. "Now how does your shoulder feel when I move it? Notice what it feels like when you move it." Compliment the patient on his progress. Reinforce the work he contributes between sessions. "Your tissue feels great here. You must be very successful with your stretching routine."

Post-Interview

In the final stage of the interview process, summarize the information gathered throughout the session and confirm your findings with the patient. Ask the patient which treatment techniques and modalities and application locations felt productive and which ones were not so effective. Present your assessment of the patient's progress and response to the treatment. Compliment the patient on her participation during the session and verbalize your thanks for contributing to the outcome. By summarizing the information and drawing conclusions about the effectiveness of the treatment, you increase your patient's awareness of the value of the session, make her conscious of the benefits, and acknowledge her ability to contribute to the outcome.

DEVELOP GOALS FOR HEALTH

So far, the focus has been on building productive relationships with patients and uncovering information that aids in providing safe and effective treatments. To be truly effective in producing ongoing results, however, we must understand our patients' needs and identify goals that direct the treatment plan and illustrate progress over time. The goals should be specific, measurable outcomes that the patient and the practitioner strive to attain.

Health goals are hinted at early in the therapeutic relationship. During the initial consultation, patients describe the physical complaints and the desired results. Intake forms record their health concerns and goals for health. Throughout the interviews, the practitioner listens to the patients' needs, explores their symptoms, researches their history, and tries to understand the impact of the condition on their lives. This information empowers the practitioner to formulate goals to ensure that the patients' needs are met.

When developing goals with patients, explore the following questions: How do your patients define wellness? What are their expectations of you and of themselves? How can you contribute to their vision of their own health?

Define Patient Needs

First, focus on the needs of the patient. Often, we have agendas based on what we think is best. We may see things that need fixing and be eager to impress our patients with our ability to treat their conditions. We may pressure people into fixing problems they are not emotionally or physically prepared to address. Behavioral scientists have noted that the less a person is under pressure from others to change, the more likely change will occur.[2] Therefore, we should fully understand our patients' needs and support them to accomplish *their* goals for health—when and how they choose. We do not have the final say on what is best for our patients.

We must help patients articulate their needs. They may have well-formulated complaints but limited experience in transforming symptoms into goals. When needs become palpable, patients can identify significant, tangible goals. For example, Darnel complains of low back pain. He hopes the manual therapist will get rid of his pain. The goal—to eliminate the pain—can be intimidating and its pursuit frustrating for both the practitioner and the patient. It is difficult to measure changes in pain, and it is nearly impossible for the patient to experience progress—a decrease in pain—when the pain continues to be endured daily. Do not focus on pain when exploring the needs of the patient. Instead, focus on function—how pain limits the patient's ability to participate in daily activities. We are better able to comprehend the needs of our patients when we understand how their symptoms affect their quality of life.

Construct Measurable Goals Based in Activities of Daily Living

Once we discover how our patients' symptoms are affecting their daily routines, we can formulate **functional goals** (or measurable goals) for health. For example, Darnel cannot pick up his granddaughter Madi and give her hugs because of the pain in his low back. Both Darnel and Madi are negatively affected by the loss of intimacy. Rather than selecting a goal based on a symptom—to eliminate low back pain, which is difficult to measure and problematic to experience accurately—develop a goal based on a function, such as lifting Madi and hugging her, which is of great importance to Darnel and his granddaughter. Take a significant activity the patient is yearning to get back to and develop it into a well-defined goal that both you and he can strive to accomplish.

Functional goals are set by the patient, with assistance from the massage therapist, to address the specific needs of his or her everyday life with the purpose of leading to an effective treatment plan. Goals must be specific to an activity of daily living and be measurable and achievable in a reasonable amount of time. The patient and therapist can further define the goal by specifying the parameters for success. How often does the patient want to perform the activity? What is a reasonable timeframe for success? Will Darnel be satisfied when he can lift Madi five times a day but has to increase his pain medication as a result? A well-defined goal should reflect:

◆ Quantity, duration, or both—How much or for how long (duration)? What number of pounds to lift or stairs to climb three times a day or four hours a night (quantity)?
◆ Frequency—How often? Eight hours a day or five days a week?
◆ Quality—How are symptoms affected? Does the patient awake feeling moderately fatigued or does he experience mild pain?
◆ Time frame—When will goal be accomplished? Is it within two weeks or by the end of the month?

A functional, measurable goal for Darnel might be to lift and hug Madi three times a day, five days a week, and to feel no more than moderate pain in his low back, in a time frame of within 30 days.

Part of defining and developing goals with patients is to help them participate in life, look for alternative ways of living a quality life, and ultimately regain their ability to do the things they want to do. This is easily accomplished by setting short-term goals that they can achieve and by motivating them to stretch a little farther each week, to get closer and closer to their goals for health.

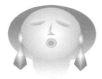

Functional Outcomes Prove Massage Efficacy

I gave a presentation at a symposium to 100 doctors on the integration of complementary and alternative medicine (CAM) and how to refer to massage therapy. A well-known researcher, Dr. Dan Cherkin, was scheduled to present his findings on the effectiveness of CAM care on chronic low back pain immediately after my talk. By way of introducing me, the moderator waived Dr. Cherkin's newly published research paper in the air, contending, "Can you believe these results? I'm sure you are as shocked as I am. Really, have you ever seen a SOAP chart from a massage therapist show that massage relieves pain anywhere?" Looking out over a crowd of physicians shaking their heads "no" was a humbling experience to say the least, but a telling one.

Unfortunately, the moderator was accurate in proclaiming that massage therapists' charts often do not adequately reflect the positive outcomes that result from our patient/practitioner relationships. I have reviewed thousands of SOAP charts from manual therapists as part of my work with insurance credentialing. It is rare that the charts reflect a cessation of pain. As a result, one could surmise that the treatment was ineffective. If, instead of focusing on the patient's pain, our charts recorded the patient's increased ability to perform daily activities, the 100 physicians at the symposium would have embraced the research results as affirming common knowledge.

The key to our credibility lies in charting functional outcomes. Drs. Cherkin and Eisenberg demonstrated this very issue in research results: Massage therapy resulted in a statistically and clinically significant improvement in the ability of patients to perform their daily activities when compared with self-care exercises ($P<.001$). Massage was also more effective than self-care exercises in decreasing pain ($P=.01$), but the benefits were less pronounced.[10] These results are easily understood when you consider one's threshold of pain. People feel compelled to follow their routines—bathe, dress, work, exercise, garden, and play—and tend to stop only when they reach a certain level of pain. If we rely solely on charting pain, we are likely to see a steady level of pain over time, even when the patient reports improvement. Whereas charts that record a patient's ability to perform daily activities may reflect considerable progress toward his or her goals for health. Translate patient complaints into functional limitations and set measurable goals based in activities of daily living, and you will be able to clearly demonstrate progress as a result of your manual therapy sessions.

CHOOSE AND IMPLEMENT SOLUTIONS

Solutions encompass all of the following:

◆ The patient's self-care routine and homework exercises
◆ The treatment provided by the manual therapist and other health care providers on the team
◆ Any belief, act, or intention that brings the patient closer to the health goals already set

The term "solutions" is used to encourage patient–centered treatment planning. Patients, their family members and friends, the spiritual figures they consult, and the health care team contribute to the patient's expression of health. The important point in choosing and implementing solutions is to consult the patients and encourage their participation in all aspects of treatment.

Discover the patient's strengths. Find out what she is already doing to take care of herself. Use questions about comfort, not pain, to discover the patient's abilities to heal. Focus on the positive whenever possible. Too often we dwell on pain. We ask patients to chart their pain on intake forms; we question patients about their pain during the interview; we ask, "Does this hurt?" when we touch them. Instead of asking how frequently they experienced pain today, ask about when they felt good. Use this discussion to explore their strengths. Find out what was going on around them when they felt good. Did they do something that triggered that good feeling? Help them see how they contributed to the good feeling. Compliment them on knowing what to do to feel better, reinforce that activity as a solution to their condition, and encourage its use. If we are to involve our patients in their healing process, we must tap into the resources already available to them.

▼

WISE ONE SPEAKS
Focus on the Positive

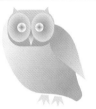

Consider this quote:

"When I focus on what's good today, I have a good day, and when I focus on what is bad today, I have a bad day. If I focus on the problem, the problem increases; if I focus on the answer, the answer increases."

Quotation attributed to Bill W. *Alcoholics Anonymous.*

Explore additional ways in which patients contribute to their own healing. Brainstorm solutions without clarifying, judging, or dismissing them. Be creative in the search and be open to different ideas. Share in the brainstorming by building on ideas the patient has presented. The goal is to create homework and self-care activities that the patient can successfully apply to improve his health. These discussions may take time in the beginning, but they will save time over the long run. The discussions promote self-awareness and reinforce the concept that the patient is capable of affecting his own well-being. The patient will learn from this experience and explore other solutions between sessions. He or she will be forthright in offering ideas throughout the therapeutic relationship, thus saving you the therapist from the process of trial and error. Failed attempts at homework assignments will be reduced because the homework will be the patient's idea. Treatment applications will be welcomed because they were discussed and agreed upon in advance. Show respect for your patients and consider their input in all decision making.

Educate your patients on the effectiveness of various solutions. They may have several ideas that they are willing to implement but lack particular knowledge about when to use one option over another and how each option works. If patients understand when to try a particular exercise and how that exercise helps them attain their goals, they may be motivated to try it more often. Solutions fall by the wayside when their value is not realized. Teach patients how the body's healing mechanism works, and demonstrate how their solutions affect their health. Invite them to imagine their body healing as they do their homework.

Narrow the list of possible solutions, and discuss the pros and cons of those remaining. A long list of solutions can overwhelm the patient. Select one or two to implement between now and the next session. Plan what, how, when, and where to do it. Remind the patient how it works. Demonstrate proper applications of solutions and correlate them with other activities. For example, teach Darnel proper lifting techniques to prevent reinjury and promote recovery. Invite him to practice his new-found lifting techniques with his granddaughter and apply the same techniques to lifting groceries and laundry.

Be vigilant in pursuing patient-centered solutions. Practitioner-imposed solutions are often unsuccessful. Too often, we classify patients as resistant or uncooperative when they do not follow through on assigned homework or self-care activities. Noncompliance is generally attributed to the patient's personal flaws or to some deep-seated pathology. In the medical model, the professional is rarely, if ever, held responsible for the mismanagement of the therapeutic relationship. If the patient shows progress, the practitioner can take the credit and feel competent, but the notion of patient resistance lays most of the blame for lack of progress on the patient and distances the practitioner from responsibility.[3] Steve de Shazer has proposed that what practitioners take to be signs of resistance are, instead, the unique ways in which patients chose to cooperate.[11] Keep in mind that it is your patients' choice to participate in their healing. Do not judge them if they are not successful in their efforts. Take responsibility. It is possible that you selected homework that doesn't fit their lifestyle instead of focusing on their own healing abilities.

Don't give homework to patients who are not committed to change. Giving them tasks to do would only show that you are not listening to them. Instead, ask them to pay attention to occurrences in their lives that tell them the condition can improve. Ask them to pay attention to the days that are better and notice what is different. Wait until patients are able to trust that their health can improve.

Encourage self-awareness before exploring solutions. Provide information and self-care education that heightens patients' awareness of their relationship with the condition. Help them listen and respond to the messages their bodies give them throughout the time between sessions. When patients are ready, teach them to pay attention to internal warning signs, such as tension in the shoulders, and to respond before their symptoms get out of hand.

Treatment Options

Treatment is a collaboration. When only one person in the therapeutic relationship is seen as the healer, fixing the problem may be possible, but healing is not. Although the patient may benefit in some ways, he or she will be stuck in a dependent relationship, with little opportunity to experience strength and growth. Each of us has a technique—perhaps several—that we use to treat our patients. It is important to remember that the technique does not heal; the relationship does. The treatment you provide simply facilitates the patient's own self-healing capabilities. Use the technique as another opportunity to listen to the patient, to understand her, and to help her find her way toward better health.

Typically, patients defer to the expert practitioner regarding treatment choices. They do not know the language of manual modalities or the full scope of what is available, they do not have experience in the variety of techniques, and they do not understand the pros and cons of the options before them. None of these facts justifies leaving patients out of the decision-making process. Whatever your treatment techniques, educate your patients on the advantages and disadvantages. Discuss the various places on their bodies that the techniques can be applied. Ask about their preferences to any style of treatment, the places you touch, or the order of application. Find out whether any technique does not sound appealing and should be avoided. Demonstrate the techniques if necessary. Be flexible. If the patient feels something isn't working at any time in the session, do something else.

Some patients want to respect your expertise and not get between you and your knowledge. When a patient says, "Just work your magic!" you may take this as a compliment, but don't stop there. Let them know you value their input. Give the patient a choice, no matter how simple. For example, "Shall we begin the session with you lying face up on the table or face down?" or "Do you prefer that work be done on your low back while you are prone or supine?" or, "Should I work on your neck to release the pain you feel in your hand?" Most patients are not accustomed to being asked for their input. It may take a little encouragement for them to discover that they really do have opinions and preferences. Always give patients the option to choose how, when, and where their treatment should be applied. Make sure you give them plenty of information on which to base their decisions.

Involve your patients during the treatment itself as well as during treatment selection. As you are working, invite them to notice how they feel before and after a treatment technique. For example, as you move a patient's shoulder, you might notice limitations in the available movement and that the quality of the movement is compromised. Rather than point out the limitations, ask what the patient notices. "How does this shoulder feel to you as I move it? Now move it yourself. How does that feel?" Apply the predetermined treatment and move the shoulder again. "Now how does your shoulder feel?" Show the patient how to perform the same or similar treatment techniques at home to get the same result. Don't make the treatments mysterious or magical. Share your expertise and knowledge, and empower your patients to heal themselves.

EVALUATE PROGRESS AND PROVIDE FEEDBACK

Communicate through all stages of the interview by evaluating the patient's progress and sharing feedback that can strengthen, modify, or correct the results. Progress hinges on all aspects of the therapeutic relationship: communication; trust; faith in the patient's strength and healing abilities; quality of touch; understanding the patient's needs; developing meaningful goals; providing education; and listening to the body, mind, and soul of the patient. If you intend to give quality service, you must evaluate each step of the healing process and elicit feedback from the patient continually.

Evaluate progress by summarizing your observations: what you hear, what you feel, what you see, what you interpret. You can present your summary to the patient immediately after your observation, during the post-interview, or at scheduled reevaluation periods, depending on how pertinent the information. For example, the patient's response to a treatment technique may be critical if it is the first time the technique has been used or the response was significant. Otherwise, wait until the end of the session to summarize the results. At the end of a series of sessions, evaluate the treatment plan together. Were the goals accomplished? Was the treatment style effective? Which techniques will you continue to use? Receive the feedback with an open mind and heart. Modify your treatment plan to accommodate the patient's preferences.

Use assessment techniques to reinforce the results of the session. Help the patient experience the changes in his body on many levels: physically, mentally, and emotionally. Often patients leave the session with little awareness of their progress. They may feel better but have no context to understand their experience or words to explain the sensations. Verbalize your findings and demonstrate the increased movement. Have them observe postural changes in the mirror and celebrate the progress. Compliment them on their ability to respond to the treatment and to integrate changes. Help them recognize their contribution to the results and reinforce the effects their homework will have on maintaining and furthering their progress.

Regularly schedule reevaluation sessions. Some patients are shy about giving feedback during the session. They may feel vulnerable on the table or they may enter a deep state of relaxation that makes it inappropriate to push for feedback. Setting aside time periodically for evaluation can provide a safety net for patients and will let them know you are committed to hearing their concerns and responding to their needs.

SUMMARY

Developing the therapeutic relationship is central to the interview process and is even more important than gathering information or accurately assessing the patient's condition. Trust, compassion, and understanding are the cornerstones of a productive relationship. Your ability to be fully present for your patients and to exhibit faith in their strength and healing abilities help lay these cornerstones in place. Without a strong bond, patients are reluctant to share their concerns and treatment planning becomes a guessing game.

Concentrate on building the therapeutic relationship while striving to achieve the goals of the interview. Your tasks include:

1. Create a relationship
2. Share information
3. Develop goals for health
4. Select and implement solutions
5. Evaluate progress and provide feedback

Communication is critical to achieving the goals of the interview. Employ the following verbal and nonverbal skills:

- Door-openers, open-ended questions
- Active listening: reflecting, paraphrasing, summarizing
- Complimenting
- Body language, including eye contact, posture, gestures
- Silence
- Touch

Develop and use communication skills. Lead patients to discover and accomplish goals for health. Maintain an open line of communication throughout the pre-interview, interview, hands-on interview, and post-interview. Ensure optimal results for the patient by eliciting feedback with the intent to strengthen, modify, and correct the treatment plan.

REFERENCES

1. Remen RN. Kitchen Table Wisdom: Stories That Heal. New York: Riverhead Books, 1996.
2. Bolton R. People Skills: How to Assert Yourself, Listen to Others, and Resolve Conflict. New York: Simon & Schuster, 1979.
3. DeJong P, Berg IK. Interviewing for Solutions. Pacific Grove, CA: Brooks/Cole, 1998.

4. Hafen BQ, Karren KJ, Frandsen KJ, Smith NL. Mind/Body Health: The Effects of Attitudes, Emotions, and Relationships. Boston, MA: Allyn & Bacon, 1996.

5. Taylor K. The Ethics of Caring: Honoring the Web of Life in Our Professional Healing Relationships. 2nd Ed. Santa Cruz, CA: Handford Mead, 1995.

6. Carlson R, Shield B. Healers on Healing. Los Angeles, CA: Tarcher Inc., 1989.

7. Carnegie D. How to Win Friends and Influence People. New York: Pocket Books, 1936.

8. Chödrön P. Start Where You Are: A Guide to Compassionate Living. Boston, MA: Shambhala, 1994.

9. Werner R. Pathology for Massage Therapists. Baltimore, MD: Lippincott Williams & Wilkins, 2002.

10. Cherkin DC, Eisenberg D, Sherman KJ, Barlow W, Kaptchuk TJ, Street J, Deyo RA. Randomized trial comparing traditional Chinese medical acupuncture, therapeutic massage, and self-care education for chronic low back pain. Arch Intern Med 2001;161:1081–1087.

11. de Shazer S. The death of resistance. Family Process. 1984;23.

## CHAPTER 2

Communication with the Health Care Team

CHAPTER OUTLINE

*F*requently, I am invited to speak with doctors and their staff on the benefits of manual therapy. During these discussions, doctors often complain: "I tried referring patients to massage therapists. I never heard back from them. Why should I refer to a therapist who does not apprise me of the patient's status?"

Manual therapists increasingly are being included on health care teams, and it is important to remember that communication helps to establish rapport, build trust, and create productive relationships.

Introduction

Team health care consists of a group of practitioners with a common goal: to provide complete and complementary care for the shared patient. Groups are defined by the patient, usually with the guidance of a doctor. Members of the group are selected according to the patient's needs and to each practitioner's ability to meet those needs. The group members form a team by consulting with one another, sharing information, and providing individualized care. Together, the patient and the practitioners complement and strengthen each one's efforts. The team approach is beneficial to the patient, the practitioners, and the patient's insurance company in many ways because it provides:

- Increased safety
- Increased productivity
- Increased efficiency
- Reduced duplication in treatment

Manual therapists are among the **complementary and alternative medicine (CAM)** practitioners commonly added to health care teams today. In the past, manual therapists had little motivation to seek medical referrals or to participate in team health care. Consumer demand, however, is changing that. Manual therapists are actively being solicited by consumers, **referring health care providers (HCPs)**, and medical specialists for their participation on health care teams. Consumers visit CAM practitioners nearly twice as often as they visit primary care physicians, and they are willing to pay out of pocket to do so. A study in 2003 showed that 32% of Americans had received care in the past five years from massage therapists. That number was up from 28% in 2002 and 17% in 1997. In addition, 62% of primary care physicians and family practitioners said they would strongly encourage their patients to pursue massage therapy as a complement to medical treatment.[1] It is essential that manual therapists learn to be productive members of the health care team.

Guidelines for Communication

Communication is expected in health care practices, with or without a team approach to healing. Insurance companies demand a paper trail that demonstrates **medical necessity**, **functional outcomes**, and cost efficiency. Referring HCPs feel the third-party pressure of justifying referrals and the responsibility for results. Reassure referring caregivers by providing them with the necessary paperwork—without being prompted—and demonstrate competency in documentation and report writing.

Keep correspondence simple and direct. Many doctors do not have time to decipher handwritten chart notes, to analyze test results, or to discuss issues over the phone. Correspond directly with the referring HCP through **initial reports** (brief letters that summarize important findings) and **progress reports** (brief letters that summarize details on patient progress). Send copies of relevant **SOAP charting** (acronym for Subjective, Objective, Assessment, Plan) and test results with the reports only when the referring HCP requests them.

Send copies of the reports to all members of the patient's health care team. Do not write additional reports specifically to the adjunctive therapists, but do send them copies of the original letter that you sent to the referring HCP. Do not be discouraged if you do not receive the same courtesy. Team health care is not universal. Specialists are expected to report back to the referring HCP, but the reverse is not standard. Set a good example of team communication and send reports to the entire team.

Follow these guidelines when communicating with the health care team:

◆ Type all correspondence on a word processor and print it on professional letterhead.
◆ Write in a narrative format in letter style.
◆ Use the patient's last name with Mr. or Ms.
◆ Avoid handwritten, fill-in-the-blank forms (save these for daily notetaking).
◆ Avoid abbreviations and symbols, such as ditto.
◆ Provide information clearly and promptly.
◆ Be brief; summarize details and state progress.
◆ Enclose copies of SOAP charts in addition to reports, if requested.
◆ Send duplicates or photocopies; file the originals.

Document verbal conversations and phone messages. Person-to-person meetings are rare, but they greatly enhance treatment planning. Voice mail allows information to be shared without calling back or interrupting the patient sessions. Take notes. Record date, time, names of participants, and content in the patient's chart. Follow the rule: "If it isn't written down, it didn't happen."

The patient's chart is also the place to file all patient-related correspondence with the health care team, including letters, reports, e-mails, faxes, phone calls, and meeting minutes. To document nonpaper correspondence, such as phone calls, or to track records requests, use the Correspondence form (see Appendix B: Blank Forms). If patient files are electronic, attach related correspondence files to the patient's electronic folder.

Standard Methods of Communication

Use familiar pathways and common language to establish communication and enhance relationships with referring HCPs. Standard methods of communication include:

◆ Introductory letters
◆ Prescriptions
◆ Initial reports
◆ SOAP charts
◆ Progress reports

Communication with the health care team should establish rapport and accessibility, convey professionalism, and create a conduit for requesting information and exchanging data.

Initial correspondence educates others on the benefits of your treatments and explains how to use your services effectively. Once contact is established, a prescription will identify treatment preferences and provide billing information. If necessary, call the referring HCP to clarify contraindications and cautions for treatment. After the patient's first visit, an initial report will state your plans for treatment. Write progress reports every 30 days to update the team on the patient's progress and to suggest changes in the **treatment plan**. Make sure reports are based on and substantiated by information recorded in the SOAP notes.

INTRODUCTORY LETTERS

Introduce yourself to other health care providers in your area. Many referrals are casual and often do not name a specific practitioner or style of manual therapy. Physicians, naturopaths, chiropractors, and others who are well-educated on the various types of massage, bodywork, and movement therapies are better able to serve their patients by providing individualized referrals. Encourage direct referrals by establishing a relationship with HCPs in advance. Send a letter introducing yourself (see Figure 2-1) and enclose brochures explaining your services and information on your references, credentials, and professional affiliations. Include articles that demonstrate the benefits of your techniques. Offer to meet at their office or talk on the phone.

Begin by writing to your patient's HCPs. Mention that you share a patient—with your patient's permission, of course. A built-in recommendation from him or her often puts a doctor at ease. Contact providers in your community or neighborhood. Target caregivers whose clientele is similar to yours. For example, if you specialize in chronic pain, contact the chronic pain clinic in your area. If you are fluent in sign language, write to providers who have patients in need of that service.

An introductory letter includes the following:

◆ Credentials and certifications
◆ Experience with similar referrals
◆ Commitment statement assuring that you support the HCP's treatment plan and will communicate regularly
◆ Specialties
◆ Request for referrals based on your specialties
◆ Education and advanced training
◆ Professional affiliations and references

In the first paragraph of the letter, introduce yourself and state your credentials and intent.

Hello. I am a certified Polarity Therapist. You and I share a patient—Kate Nelson. I wish to take this opportunity to introduce myself and tell you about my work. I enjoy working with other health care providers, and I am committed to providing quality care. I hope we will work together.

In the second paragraph, state your experience working with similar HCPs. The intent is to demonstrate interest in them, create trust, and convey confidence.

I understand that you are fluent in sign language and have many patients with hearing disabilities. I, too, am fluent in sign language and have deaf and hard-of-hearing patients. I am experienced in participating in team health care, communicating regularly, and supporting referring caregivers' treatment plans. Enclosed are samples of my documentation and report writing style. I am looking for doctors to refer to and receive referrals from.

Next, describe your specialties, modalities, and treatment philosophy. Ask for referrals specific to your area of expertise.

FIGURE 2-1 **Letter of Introduction**

Naomi Wachtel
567 Sunnydale Dr.
Flat Irons, CO   80302
TEL   303 555 8866   •   FAX   303 555 8867   •   EMAIL   wachtel@email.com

---

Dr. Shawn Hall
1234 Main Street
Flat Irons, CO 80302

Dear Dr. Hall:

Hello! I am new in your area and would like to introduce myself. I am a licensed massage therapist certified in lymphatic drainage. I recently opened an office down the street from you and am looking for a doctor specializing in chronic pain whom I can refer to and possibly receive referrals from.

I am experienced in working with chronic pain referrals. I am accustomed to the needs of chronic pain patients and the level of documentation and communication required to participate on the health care team. Enclosed are copies of SOAP charts and progress reports of a recent chronic pain case, and a letter of reference from the referring physician.

I understand the complications of chronic pain syndrome and am trained to work with the passive congestion of phase two inflammation—a typical component of the condition which hinders healing. I have received advanced training in lymphatic drainage which has been proven effective in resolving the inflammatory issues of chronic pain syndrome. Manual lymphatic drainage has been safe and effective in cases in which long-term use of NSAIDS has failed or is contraindicated. Enclosed are a few articles that detail specific findings.

Enclosed are brochures designed to inform patients about the benefits of manual lymphatic drainage. These brochures explain what to expect from a lymph drainage session. Detailed in the brochures are my services, hours, and fees, and directions to my clinic. If my services are of interest to you, please hand these brochures to your patients.

If possible, I would like to schedule 5 minutes of your time to meet you and find out more about your services. I would like to pick up some of your brochures to pass out to my patients, and answer any questions you may have. I will call within the next week to schedule an appointment with you.

Thank you for your time and consideration. I look forward to meeting you.

Yours in health,

Naomi Wachtel, LMT

As a Polarity Therapist, I palpate points and patterns in the patient's energy anatomy to assist in the flow of healing energy in the patient's body. I teach a series of self-help exercise techniques to promote self-awareness and create relaxation and balance.[2] I specialize in facilitating healing in patients preparing for and recovering from surgery. Enclosed is an article describing the benefits of presurgery and post-surgery energy treatment. I also enjoy working with individuals who seek a natural, effective way to reduce stress and increase wellness. Please think of me when referring these types of patients for manual therapy.

Include your educational background, years of experience, and professional affiliations. Enclose copies of one or two of the following: therapy license, certifications, professional memberships, Code of Ethics or Standards of Practice.

I have been a certified Polarity Therapist and a member of the American Polarity Therapy Association for five years. My precertificate and postcertificate training includes more than 500 hours of class time and 250 hours of supervised clinical time. I studied anatomy, physiology, kinesiology, and Polarity theory and practice, and I have clocked more than 1,000 hours of patient sessions. Enclosed is a copy of my Polarity Therapy certification and Code of Ethics.

End the letter with a request for referrals and provide the necessary information to facilitate referrals, including fees, hours, location, services, and contact information.

If you feel that I may be of assistance to any of your patients, please pass along my name. I am interested in working with you to serve them. Enclosed are several brochures explaining my treatment style and details of service. Please make these available to patients who could benefit from my work.

Once you have contacted the HCPs you are interested in working with, call to schedule a brief appointment. Five minutes is enough to make an impression and to establish a physical connection. Place a smiling face and a firm handshake behind your letter and brochures. Always remember to ask how you can best serve the caregiver—don't focus entirely on yourself. Start the conversation by inquiring about the caregiver's practice. Then, ask how you might best fit in and serve. Go to the meeting stocked with additional brochures and prescription pads. Explain how to use the prescriptions (detailed in the next section) and reiterate your request for patients who fit your specialty. This is an effective marketing technique to ensure that your name comes to mind first when your type of patient shows up. Of course, let the practitioner know that you are able to treat less specialized cases, but if you are perfect for one or two patients, the ball will be in motion and more referrals will follow.

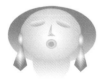

STORY TELLER
Marketing

Lucas, the owner of a large massage clinic, has a unique way of introducing himself and his therapists to chiropractic offices in his neighborhood. The entire massage team takes on-site chairs and healthy box lunches to the chiropractor's office during a prearranged lunch hour. Everyone on the chiropractic staff gets a chance to ask questions and experience 5 to 10 minutes of each therapists' work. Even the busiest doctors find a moment to peek in on the fun their staff is having. Once the doctors have been rubbed and grubbed, Lucas can engage them in a relaxed conversation and make a lasting impression.

PRESCRIPTIONS

Prescriptions are formal referrals for adjunctive services, and they communicate information from the patient's primary HCP to the manual therapist (see Appendix B: Blank Forms.) Prescriptions mandate medical necessity and define treatment parameters.

Sometimes, referrals come in the form of a suggestion. An HCP may say, "Try massage for your shoulder pain . . ." or "Have you thought about getting chiropractic care for your back pain?" General referrals such as these are often oral and may or may not include a recommendation for a specific treatment technique or a specific practitioner.

Prescriptions, on the other hand, are very specific. The referral outlines instructions to be followed and is often directed to a particular specialist. Timelines and frequencies are stated, and specific treatment goals and treatment areas are defined. Here's an example of a prescription:

> 10 sessions of neuromuscular therapy with Rafael Hernandez. Complete treatment by June 23. Treat the neck and shoulders to reduce pain and restore function. Address other direct and indirect symptoms resulting from carpel tunnel syndrome—including posture, inflammation, and muscle tension—and treat related structures. Treatment should include hot/cold packs and stretching exercises as needed.

To expedite referrals, create your own prescription form[3] and send pads of them to HCPs (see Figure 2-2). Their use guarantees that you will have the information you need to provide safe treatment and facilitate insurance reimbursement. If a patient has serious health problems or a condition that manual therapy may exacerbate, a prescription provides critical information and peace of mind. A prescription gives permission to treat the condition and sets guidelines for safety.

A prescription is also necessary whenever you or your patient seek reimbursement from an insurance company for medical services. Insurance only covers treatment that is deemed **reasonable and necessary**. A prescription states that the treatment—in this case, manual therapy—is medically necessary for the patient's condition. The prescription includes the patient's diagnosis, which is also necessary for insurance reimbursement. Manual therapists without diagnostic capabilities are able to use the diagnostic codes necessary for bill processing when the diagnosis is recorded on the prescription and is on file in the patient's chart. Keep in mind, however, that a prescription does not authorize insurance coverage, but it is necessary for facilitating reimbursement of authorized services (see Chapter 8 for information on insurance billing).

If a patient schedules an appointment based on an oral referral, and later, you determine that a prescription is necessary, contact the referring HCP and request the information you need to ensure proper care and to facilitate reimbursement. An oral referral for general services or a prescription that simply states "massage" is insufficient documentation for insurance reimbursement. In the event of an oral referral or an incomplete prescription, prompt the referring HCP to write a prescription, state the diagnosis and ICD-9 codes, and direct the frequency and duration of treatment. To expedite a response from a busy HCP, fill in the pertinent details on the prescription form and fax it over to his or her office with a request for approval and a signature.

Suggest a treatment plan to referring HCPs who are unfamiliar with manual therapy or your style of work. If the HCP writes a prescription for a treatment plan that is inconsistent with your treatment style, discuss the issue with the HCP. The doctor may suggest treatment twice a week for four weeks, and you may wish to change the frequency to three times a week for the first week, twice a week for two weeks, and once during the last week. Rather than contradicting the prescription, request a change. Most referring HCPs are

FIGURE 2-2 Sample Prescription

John Olson, LMP, GCFP
345 Moon River Rd. Ste. 6
Minnehaha, MN   55987
TEL   612 555 9889

HANDS HEAL

PRESCRIPTION

Patient Name _Darnel G. Washington_   Date _2-30-04_

Date of Injury _1-6-04_   ID#/DOB _123-45-6789_

A. Diagnosis

(Include ICD-9 codes that specifically
address Manual Therapy Treatment)

Scoliosis   754.2

Spasm   728.85

Neck Pain   723.1

Thoracic Pain   724.1

Condition is related to

☒ Auto Accident
☐ Work Injury
☐ Illness
☒ Other: _concomittant scoliosis recurrance_

B. Medically Necessary Treatment: Implement Plan as Prescribed Below

Application (Primary & Secondary)

☐ Head _whiplash_
☐ Neck _whiplash_
☐ Chest _scoliosis_
☐ Shoulders _2°—as needed_
☐ Abdomen _2°—as needed_
☐ Back _scoliosis_
☐ Lowback/Hips _whiplash_
☐ Upper extremities _2°—as needed_
☐ Lower extremities _2°—as needed_
☒ All of the above
☐ Other: _____

Frequency & Duration

☒ 1× wk for _6_ wks
☐ 2× wk for _____ wks
☐ 3× wk for _____ wks
☐ 2× month for _____ months
☐ 1× month for _____ months

Specific Instructions/Precautions:
as needed

Treatment Type

☒ Manual Therapy
☒ Hot/Cold Packs
☒ Self-Care/Exercises
☐ Other _____

Treatment Goals

☐ Decrease Pain
☐ Decrease Inflammation
☐ Decrease Muscle Tension/Spasms
☐ Decrease Compensatory Patterns
☐ Increase Mobility
☐ Increase Strength
☐ Restore Function
☐ Restore Posture
☐ Patient Education
☒ All of the Above
☐ Other _____

C. Referring Health Care Provider (HCP)

Contact Information

HCP Name _Sage Redtree MD_
Address _87 Old Trail PKWY_
City _Minnehaha_ State _MN_ Zip _55987_
Phone _555-0009_
Fax _555-9000_
Email _____

Reporting—I will send an initial report after
the first visit and a progress report after
every 6–8 sessions. Please check how you
would like to receive this information:

☒ Fax   ☐ Mail   ☐ Email
☒ Send Copies of Chart Notes with each report

HCP Signature: _Sage Redtree MD_   Date _2-30-04_

Revised and reprinted with permission, Adler ♦ Giersch, PS

amenable when the request is substantiated. To amend a prescription, initial and date the changes and write "Authorized per phone: Dr. Lutack ND."

Prescriptions for manual therapy are an indication of medical necessity and must contain the following:

◆ Patient's diagnosis, including ICD-9 codes
◆ Treatment application
◆ Frequency and duration of treatment

Manual therapists who cannot diagnose or prescribe treatment rely on referring HCPs to provide both the diagnoses and the corresponding ICD-9 codes. When a patient is self-referred and there is no prescription, a manual therapist without diagnostic scope (in some cases) can use ICD-9 codes that are considered "symptom" codes (see Appendix E for a list of symptom codes). Verify specific regulations regarding self-referrals with each insurance company before submitting ICD-9 codes that have not been provided by a referring HCP.

The prescription should state diagnoses that pertain to the manual therapists' treatment. For example, a cervical subluxation may not be treatable within the scope of practice of a massage therapist; however, it may be appropriate to treat a spasm in the paracervical musculature. Confirm that the prescription contains ICD-9 codes applicable to your treatment. If not, make suggestions and call in or fax the changes to the HCP's office for authorization.

Make sure the prescription specifies all areas where treatment should be applied. If the diagnosis only indicates that the neck, for example, is involved in the whiplash injury, treatment to the back and arms may be considered unnecessary and may not be covered by insurance. As a holistic practitioner, you may find it impossible to treat whiplash without treating pain in the back and arms, which often accompanies whiplash injuries. The referring HCP must authorize treatment to indirect areas of concern.

The frequency and duration of treatment must be specified, such as once a week for six weeks or twice a month for three months. Many HCPs will defer to the manual therapists' expertise. All nondiagnostic practitioners must state their preferences to the HCP and record (on the prescription form) the specific number and frequency of sessions authorized.

In addition to the diagnosis and basic treatment plan, prescriptions may include further instructions, such as:

◆ Types of treatment
◆ Treatment goals
◆ Cautions and contraindications

Prescriptions often indicate general treatment approaches, which may include massage therapy, soft tissue manipulation, or movement education. Others may identify specific techniques, such as lymphatic drainage, craniosacral therapy, or manual traction. Avoid requesting authorization for specific techniques. Manual therapists rely on a variety of techniques to elicit the desired response in a patient, and many referring HCPs do not know the difference between, for example, muscle energy technique and strain/counterstrain. Prescribing specific techniques limits the practitioner to the techniques identified and may not be reimbursable by the insurance company. If, for example, trigger point therapy is prescribed, the cost of drainage techniques may not be reimbursed. Offer general treatment options on the prescription form or none at all.

Request permission to instruct the patient in self-care exercises. This is helpful in states where rules are vague concerning the manual therapist's **scope of practice**. Although insurance companies encourage teaching the patients stretching and strengthening exercises, some manual therapy professions compete for the right to own this scope of practice. Stay within your governing law and ask referring HCPs to use this section of the prescription to authorize the instruction of patients in self-care exercises in which you are trained.

If you seek additional instruction for your treatment plan from the referring HCP, provide a checklist on the prescription form for treatment goals rather than specific techniques. Include goals such as decreasing pain or increasing range of motion. This approach authorizes the use of any techniques within the practitioner's training and scope to accomplish the specified goals.

It is always helpful to request information from the referring HCP about cautions and contraindications to treatment. The referring HCP may have information that will assist you in providing safe and effective care.

Use the prescription to determine the referring HCP's preferred style and frequency of communication. For example, find out whether she prefers to receive copies of the SOAP charts with each report and whether she wants the reports faxed, e-mailed, or mailed to her office. If the referral is oral, send an introductory letter to find out how the doctor would like to receive your reports.

INITIAL REPORT

The initial report thanks the HCP for the referral, offers a brief summary of the patient's presenting complaints and your assessments, and informs the HCP of your goals and treatment plan. The HCP is usually familiar with the patient's condition, so limit the information to key data. The most important information is the treatment plan—what you want to accomplish in the next 30 days and how you and the patient will work together to achieve the goals (see Figure 2-3).

The initial report is a summary of the **initial SOAP notes** written in paragraph form. The initial report contains:

◆ Initial treatment date
◆ Functional goals
◆ Treatment plan
◆ Commitment to report back by a set date

To support your treatment plan and the functional goals, include a brief summary of the patient's presenting symptoms, functional limitations, and pertinent objective data. It is not necessary to list all of your findings. Include compelling data that is both quantitative and qualitative. For example, you might write that Ms. Hostetter is unable to cook because of severe pain and fatigue in her shoulders, back, and neck . . . or that Mr. Tu reports moderate headaches that affect his ability to concentrate at work, lasting 2 to 3 days, occurring weekly. Omit lists of tight muscles or findings that are vague or cannot be substantiated. The focus of the report should be on the treatment plan:

◆ Functional goals (based in activities of daily living)
◆ Treatment goals (based in objective data)
◆ Treatment techniques and modalities
◆ Treatment application

A functional goal states in measurable terms the activity to which the patient wishes to return (see Chapter 6 for in-depth information on setting goals and charting outcomes). Include a time frame, such as 30 days, by the end of which the patient will have achieved the goal. For example, you might write that Ms. Hostetter will be able to stand for 30 minutes while cooking, repeatedly lifting and extending up to 25 pounds over a stove and tossing food, three days a week, with moderate pain and fatigue, within 30 days. Functional goals demonstrate progress in terms the patient can comprehend on an experiential level.

Treatment goals provide the parameters by which the practitioner will measure the patient's success, such as decrease muscle spams, increase range of motion, or reduce inflammation. All parameters must be measurable in quantifiable or qualifiable terms, such as mild, moderate, or severe; or 0 to 10; or normal, good, fair, poor.

Treatment techniques and modalities listed should address the needs of the goals. Include the areas of application. Example: Lymphatic drainage will be applied to the neck to reduce pain and inflammation and strain/counterstrain to the shoulders and spine to decrease

---

FIGURE 2-3 Initial Report with Treatment

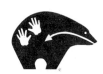

Helena LaLuna, CR
123 Sun Moon and Stars Drive
Capitol Hill, WA   98119
TEL   206 555 4446   •   FAX   206 555 4447   •   EMAIL   laluna@email.com

Manda Rae Yuricich, DC

4041 Bell Town Way, Ste. 200

Capitol Hill, WA 98119

Thank you, Dr. Yuricich, for referring Ms. Hostetter to my office. Our first appointment was on April 4, 2001. The results of the sessions are as follows:

Functional goals: Ms. Hostetter would like to return to work as a chef as soon as possible. To facilitate that, our initial goal is to have her cooking for 30 minutes per day, 3 days per week, with moderate pain and fatigue within 30 days. Currently, she is unable to cook due to severe pain and muscle spasms in her neck, shoulders and back.

Together, we will resolve those findings and accomplish those goals with the following treatment plan: myofascial release for 10 sessions, addressing her shoulder, neck, back and sacral soft tissue injuries, ice packs to reduce the inflammation, and homework exercises to facilitate self-care.

I will report back to you by May 5. Please contact me if you have questions, comments, or feedback.

Yours in health,

Helena LaLuna, CR

muscle spasms and increase range of motion. State how the patient will participate in accomplishing the goals. For example, you might write that Ms. Hostetter will continue to apply ice packs to the neck over a protected area for 10 to 12 minutes twice daily.

Recommend a set number of sessions you believe is necessary for accomplishing the goals. Example: Ms. Hostetter will receive six one-hour sessions, two per week for the next two weeks, then one a week for the remaining two weeks. I will report on her progress at the end of the series of sessions.

If the referral did not result in an appointment with the patient, write a simple report explaining the reason. Example: The patient neglected to attend the scheduled appointment, or I am currently unavailable for new patients (see Figure 2-4).

FIGURE 2-4 **Initial Report Without Treatment**

Naomi Wachtel
567 Sunnydale Dr.
Flat Irons, CO   80302
TEL   303 555 8866   •   FAX   303 555 8867   •   EMAIL   wachtel@email.com

Dear _Dr. Hall:_____:

Thank you for referring _Jackie Shenge_____ to my office. Your patient and I were unable to connect for the following reason(s):

_____ The patient did not schedule an appointment.

_____ The patient did not attend the scheduled appointment.

_____ I am not scheduling new patients at this time. I anticipate my schedule to open back up again _____.

___X___ I am unable to benefit the patient for the following reason(s):

Her condition necessitates intraoral techniques outside my scope of practice. I recommend

referring to Sari Goldsmith, LMT, who also has a license in dental hygiene and specializes in

craniofacial pain syndromes. Her number is (303)555-5434.

_____

Thank you for the referral. I hope to work with you again in the future.

Yours in health,

Naomi Wachtel, LMT

Provided is a standard report form for referrals that do not result in appointments (see Appendix B: Blank Forms). It is necessary to inform the referring HCP of the status of the referral. The intent is to be courteous without investing time in a relationship that is not producing income, yet at the same time, leaves the door open for future referrals. This is one instance in which a handwritten, fill-in-the-blank form is appropriate. This can be done quickly and easily by checking off the applicable reason from a list of possibilities explaining why the referral has not resulted in a therapeutic relationship.

If the initial report is your first correspondence with the referring HCP, include a modified introductory letter and several brochures. The referral may have come your way because the patient already has a relationship with you, your reputation precedes you, or the patient selected your name from a list of providers. Take the opportunity to educate the referring HCP on your services, the benefits of your techniques, and how to refer to you in the future.

PROGRESS REPORT

Progress reports summarize the patient's progress over a period of time. The period may be 30 days, 6 to 8 sessions, or the length of the prescription, whichever coincides best with the treatment plan. Progress reports are critical for keeping the HCP informed of the success of the referral (see Figure 2-5). Do not delay in sending progress reports and never wait until they are requested. An omission in reporting can result in a loss of referrals. Progress reports consist of:

◆ Current functional outcomes
◆ Status of the patient
◆ Plan for care

If you are recommending ongoing patient care, include:

◆ New functional goals
◆ Updated treatment plan

Progress reports focus on functional outcomes—the patient's increased ability to participate in daily activities. It is not necessary to repeat information stated in the initial report or in previous progress reports. Focus only on the patient's progress and, if necessary, any requests for authorization of additional treatment. The improvement in the patient's health is noted by comparing the current report to the previous reports. Each consecutive progress report builds on the last, making it unnecessary to repeat the patient's initial condition.

Initial reports state a functional goal, and progress reports give an accounting of the status of that goal. If the goal has been accomplished in its entirety, it is stated as an outcome—Ms. Hostetter has accomplished the initial goal of being able to stand for 30 minutes while cooking, repeatedly lifting and extending up to 25 pounds over a stove and tossing food, three days a week, with moderate pain and fatigue. At times, the patient and practitioner are only partially successful in accomplishing the functional goal. In those circumstances, the outcome is stated as accomplished, and the new functional goal becomes a modification of the previous goal.

In some cases, functional goals and outcomes are not applicable and treatment goals are the only measures of success. Report measurable changes in symptoms and objective findings whenever functional limitations were minimal or nonexistent and functional goals were not set. For example: Mr. Tu's headache pain has changed from moderate to mild and occurs weekly, lasting for 2 to 3 hours rather than 2 to 3 days as previously stated.

State the current status of the patient in each report. Here are some common statements explaining the patient's status:

- ◆ Patient has achieved identified goals
- ◆ Patient has not achieved identified goals
- ◆ Plateau in patient's progress

FIGURE 2-5 Progress Report

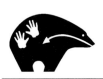

Helena LaLuna, CR
123 Sun Moon and Stars Drive
Capitol Hill, WA   98119
TEL   206 555 4446   •   FAX   206 555 4447   •   EMAIL   laluna@email.com

---

4041 Bell Town Way, Ste. 200   5-12-04
Capitol Hill, WA 98119

Patient: Zamora Hostetter

DOI: 3-31-04

Claim #: C98-7654321

Dear Dr. Yuricich:

Thank you for referring Ms. Hostetter to my office for manual therapy. After 10 sessions of myofascial release, Ms Hostetter has achieved her initial goal. She is able to stand and cook for 30 minutes, while repeatedly lifting and extending up to 25 pounds over a stove and tossing food, 3 days a week, with moderate pain and fatigue.

To facilitate Ms. Hostetter's to return to work, ongoing care is requested. We must extend her cooking time to 90 minutes, 3 days a week, and include 3 hours of additional time at work preparing food. However, Ms Hostetter is able to sit down at work and take frequent breaks during her preparation time. With 3 additional sessions of myofascial release, we should be able to reach the new goal of cooking for 90 minutes, while repeatedly lifting and extending up to 25 pounds over a stove and tossing food, 3 days a week, with mild pain and moderate fatigue. Ms. Hostetter will attend session weekly for 3 weeks, receive additional self-care instructions including alternating hot and cold pack applications, and participate in home exercises and to stretch and strengthen injured areas during this time.

Please inform me of your decision to continue Ms. Hostetter's manual therapy. I look forward to working with you in the future.

Yours in health,

Helena LaLuna, CR

State the current plan of care. Care may be complete or additional care may be necessary. Suggest changes in the treatment plan, referrals to another type of practitioner, or assistance with self-care education. You may have reached the limits of your abilities and can suggest additional care that will take the patient beyond a plateau. The patient may not have reached his or her long term goals or returned to preinjury status and may request ongoing care from you. Common care plans include one or more of the following:

◆ Care is complete:

–Patient has reached the limits of the referral

–Patient met the goals under the referral limits

–Anticipate that patient will reach long-term goals independently

◆ Additional care is necessary:

–Ongoing care is requested

–A change in the treatment plan is suggested

–A referral is recommended

◆ Patient to return to referring physician

If the patient could benefit from ongoing care, state the new goals for treatment. Propose an updated treatment plan by explaining how the goals will be accomplished. Identify the treatment techniques that will be used and explain why they are necessary, specify the treatment frequency and duration necessary for accomplishing the goals, and describe how the patient will contribute to the plan.

Send progress reports to adjunctive therapists and to referring HCPs. Keep all members of the health care team apprised of the patient's progress.

All the information in a progress report comes from the SOAP charts, but occasionally, referring HCPs need more than a brief summary to create their reports and treatment plans. Send copies of the SOAP notes when they are requested.

SUMMARY

Communication is expected between referring caregivers and adjunctive therapists. Use familiar pathways and common language to establish relationships with the members of the health care team and to share information. Be brief and professional with your communications.

Establish communication with caregivers by sending letters and brochures introducing yourself and outlining your services. Create prescription pads to streamline referrals. Once you have received a referral from a HCP, send an initial report describing the status of the patient. Every 30 days, or at the end of every prescription, send a progress report. Use the information recorded on the patient's daily SOAP notes to write the reports.

Progress reports include:

◆ Current functional outcomes or summary of current subjective and objective progress
◆ Status of the patient
◆ Plan for care

If a request for ongoing care is needed, include the following:

◆ New functional goals
◆ Updated treatment plan

REFERENCES

1. Opinion Research Corporation International. Hands On: The Newsletter of the American Massage Therapy Association November/December 2003.

2. Polarity Therapy brochure. American Polarity Therapy Association. For information call 800-359-5620.

3. Adler RH, Giersch P. Whiplash, Spinal Trauma, and the Personal Injury Case. Seattle, WA: Adler◆Giersch, 2005.

CHAPTER 3

Communication with the Legal Team

CHAPTER OUTLINE

*U*ncle Darnel was in a car crash on the way to a hockey game. He was riding in the passenger seat, chatting with his nephew, when a large pickup truck rear-ended them. Initially, there were no serious injuries, just some fender damage. The guys were eager to get to the game and were ready to leave after exchanging phone numbers when a police officer pulled up to assist. She asked each of them a few questions. As it turned out, the driver of the pickup truck was uninsured and a report needed to be filed.

At first, Darnel was not in pain, just a little shaken up, and he and his nephew were able to attend the hockey game after all the paperwork was completed. Later that evening, however, he developed a headache, as well as stiffness and soreness in his back and neck. A few weeks later, his back pain was getting worse. Darnel finally went to his family physician, who prescribed anti-inflammatories and referred him to a manual therapist. After a month of manual therapy, the neck symptoms were clearing up but the back pain was not. John, the manual therapist, and Darnel were both concerned, so Darnel returned to the doctor. The doctor ordered x-rays, which confirmed what they all suspected—spinal degeneration. Darnel had a history of scoliosis, but with regular exercise, he had been successful in halting the degenerative process early on and had been pain-free until the car crash. Now, he was in constant pain, and his spinal degeneration had accelerated.

Unfortunately, the scoliosis was not Darnel's only worry. There were financial complications as well. Darnel's private health insurance did not cover manual therapy. The at-fault party had no insurance. Neither the nephew's nor Darnel's car insurance carrier was coming forward to pay the bills. Which one was responsible? Did Darnel have a choice about whom to bill, based on quality of coverage? John wondered whether he could treat the scoliosis and bill the car insurance for the treatments. Darnel was beginning to worry that he was going to be stuck with the medical bills. He was ready to quit therapy, even though the treatments eased his pain and helped him stay active.

John knew just enough about personal injury law from experiences with other patients to know that Darnel needed some professional help. Before the next session, they sat down together and discussed the financial problems. John wanted to help Darnel relieve his financial worries so Darnel could focus on getting well. First, they had to determine whose insurance would pay the medical bills and what type of coverage was available. Second, they needed assurance that the insurance carrier would pay for the scoliosis treatments because the collision caused the flare-up of Darnel's symptoms. John suggested that Darnel consult with an attorney specializing in personal injury law about access to health care and for advice about his financial concerns.

Darnel met with Charma Storro, JD and was immediately relieved. Under the laws of the state where the accident occurred, the nephew's car insurance was the primary insurance carrier responsible for Darnel's medical bills. The nephew's policy included **Personal Injury Protection (PIP) coverage**, so Darnel's medical bills should be paid reasonably promptly. The insurance company's staff would be able to track down the at-fault driver of the pickup truck from the police report and would handle all communication with him. The attorney instructed the insurance company to put two different adjusters on the case to ensure fair representation for Darnel—one to handle PIP matters and the other to handle issues related to the uninsured motorist claim. Because Darnel's physician had treated him throughout his adult life, he had solid documentation that his scoliosis was asymptomatic before the crash and that the flare-up was related to the collision. As a result, the treatment for the scoliosis flare-up was covered under the PIP policy.

John noticed a difference in Darnel's health when the stress of managing the claim was removed. Darnel was able to turn over the worry to the experts and focus on getting well.

Introduction

Every manual therapist must have basic knowledge of personal injury law, including an understanding of the rights and obligations of the practitioner and the patient, in order to avoid burdening themselves and their patients with unnecessary risk and stress. Patient records can be subpoenaed or testimony required years after treatment has ended, even if the patient never mentioned a motor vehicle collision (MVC). It is imperative, therefore, to keep good records on *all* patients and to understand your role with the legal team in order to act responsibly in the therapeutic relationship.

The legal team consists of an attorney hired by a person who has suffered injuries as a result of carelessness or recklessness by another person or business. The attorney's staff may include other attorneys, paralegals, investigators, and support personnel. The legal team and the health care team form the first line of protection between the victim and often debilitating physical and financial losses that can be the medical and legal consequences of physical injury, emotional injury, or both.

MVCs include collisions between cars, cars and motorcycles, and cars and pedestrians. Work injuries that result in short-term injury or long-term disability may also call for legal intervention, as may slipping, falling, or tripping at a private residence or a commercial location. For example, Alice suffered a ruptured disk while fighting a fire and was forced into early retirement, Lisa was helping her dad clean the gutters when she tumbled off the roof and broke both feet, and Steven was watching a baseball game at a sports bar when a ceiling tile fell on his head and gave him whiplash. All these injuries may have resulted from someone's negligence. The legal team will gather and preserve evidence to prove liability; will understand and defend the patient's rights; and will negotiate compensation for physical injury, loss of income, pain and suffering, health care expenses, and future health care needs.

The manual therapist is a natural and important part of the medical-legal team. The manual therapist contributes to the team by keeping good patient records, communicating regularly, and understanding personal injury law (see Chapter 6 for in-depth information on recordkeeping).

The Role of the Legal Team in Personal Injury Cases

Some patients suffering from personal injury can receive health care benefits even when no fault can be established or when the car or home insurance policy includes Personal Injury Protection or **Medical Payments (Med-Pay) coverage**. For example, if Darnel had driven his car into a telephone pole after falling asleep at the wheel, he would still be eligible for medical benefits up to the limits of his PIP or Med-Pay insurance coverage, provided the services were deemed reasonable, necessary, and related to the collision. In other words, health care expenses are covered regardless of who caused the trauma. If Darnel had PIP coverage, he might also be eligible for lost wages and household services, in addition to medical coverage. Each state has laws, regulations, and rules establishing the mandatory minimum coverage that owners of vehicles must carry. It is critical for each health care professional to have a thorough working knowledge of his or her state's automobile insurance requirements.

Legal representation may be unnecessary if the injuries are minor, the car repairs are cosmetic, and the insurance company is paying the bills promptly (even when negligence can be established).

Some patients understand the benefits of legal counsel in personal injury cases and retain representation when a situation arises that requires it. Others will at least obtain a legal consultation to better understand the issues, rights, and duties of all the parties and insurers. Whether hiring an attorney or just consulting with one, follow the guidelines in this chapter to communicate with the legal team.

Other patients are unaware of the benefits of legal representation, and they struggle unnecessarily with their insurance carriers or with the insurer of the at-fault party. Perhaps the insurance adjuster is not forthcoming about the coverage available or the injuries are complicated and the patient needs assistance in proving that the injuries resulted from the incident. Patients are often unaware of their rights regarding insurance coverage and personal injury law, and many health care providers shy away from answering legal questions or addressing legal concerns. If the interests of the patient would be served by professional legal consultation, then the manual therapist should say so. Example: An insurance carrier terminates care even though the patient continues to suffer from flare-ups and coverage is still available, significant physical injury exists and long-term disability is imminent, major health care expenses have been incurred, or applicable **statutory time limits** are fast approaching for filing a claim, to name just a few. Even though manual therapists cannot dispense legal advice, it is important to discuss the need for legal consultation rather than remain silent while the patient's rights slip away or the patient's financial and health care interests worsen. Fair resolution of a legal claim often provides resources for health care and bears significantly on the patient's physical and emotional well-being.

Here are common scenarios in which patients could benefit from consulting an attorney experienced in personal injury and insurance law:

- The insurance carrier refuses to pay the medical bills or discontinues coverage.
- Liability is contested.
- **Proximate cause** is challenged because:

    –The patient delays seeking initial treatment (implying that the injury is minor and does not need treatment)
    –The patient's onset of symptoms are delayed (implying that the injury was not caused by the trauma)
    –Gaps of time exist between incident and treatment (implying that the patient failed to mitigate his or her injuries by not getting the treatment needed).

- Physical injuries are moderate or severe.
- Physical injuries are having an impact on the patient's ability to return to his or her usual work.
- Physical injuries are having an impact on the patient's earning potential.
- **Pre-existing conditions** flare up after the accident.
- Additional accidents occur before previous injuries are resolved.
- The insurance company schedules an **insurance medical exam** (**IME**), also known as an independent medical exam (although "independent" is often a misnomer), selects the doctor, and pays for the examination of the insured.
- The at-fault party has no insurance, and the patient needs to present an uninsured motorist claim to his own insurer.
- The accident involved minor visible property damage, yet it resulted in injury. It is common for insurance carriers to argue that a person cannot be injured when the visible car damage is minimal.

The attorney and legal team can address issues and provide services to your patient regarding:

1. Evidence—legal team reviews, retains, and preserves evidence regarding liability and biomechanics of the incident.
2. Statute of limitations—legal team provides insight and advice in addressing state-mandated time limits pertaining to the filing of claims and lawsuits and can assist in settling the claim or in filing the lawsuit. In Oregon, as an example, the time limit for filing an injury claim is two years. In Washington, the limit is three years.
3. Stress—legal team can monitor the payment of bills, collect evidence, obtain records and reports, and deal with the insurance company, thereby helping to reduce the patient's stress and the often daily burdens of keeping up with these tasks.
4. Negotiations—legal team negotiates and represents the patient's interests (patients have little or no negotiating power with the insurer) with claims representatives who are also trained, experienced negotiators and understand that patients cannot file lawsuits without an attorney—not to mention their loyalty and duty to the insurance company—and who often try to settle the claim at the lowest amount possible.
5. Knowledge—legal team brings in-depth awareness of personal injury and insurance laws and advocates for the patient's rights to make sure the insurer complies with **good faith provisions** of the law and, if not, can take legal action to remedy the situation.
6. Protection of patient when an IME is requested—legal team may be able to negotiate with the insurer for the selection of a truly independent medical examiner. Moreover, if the insurance company insists on the IME with a doctor of the company's choosing, then the attorney can accompany the patient to the IME or retain another person to serve as the attorney's observer.
7. Compensation—legal team works to ensure that the patient receives reasonable and fair compensation for injuries and losses (without an attorney, patients may be harassed, intimidated, or pressured into accepting unreasonable or unfair settlements and forfeiting their rights).
8. Contingency fee arrangement—legal team receives no payment for time expended if there is no recovery from the settlement or lawsuit.

Be prepared to respond to patients whose circumstances require a legal consultation from an attorney who specializes in personal injury law *and* who understands the benefits of manual therapy. To help the patient and the practitioner, the attorney retained should be knowledgeable and supportive of the manual therapist's role in the patient's care, should encourage compliance with the practitioner's treatment plan, and should not try to compromise or reduce the therapist's bill once the case concludes. Become familiar with the attorneys in your area who specialize in personal injury law and are pro-manual therapy. Find out which attorneys work as a team with health care providers and support **complementary and alternative medicine (CAM)**. Also, find out which ones frequently ask manual therapists to discount their bills or who refuse to sign letters that guarantee payment from the settlement. Know your allies and work with them.

Look for the following qualities in a personal injury legal team:

1. Understands the manual therapist's role in rehabilitation of injuries and ensures the patient's right to CAM care
2. Encourages compliance with the referring HCP's prescription for manual therapy

3. Assists in communication about the patient's case with all members of the health care team

4. Readily knows whether insurance coverage is available, how much PIP coverage is available, when PIP coverage will expire, and whom to bill

5. Advises the practitioner if there is secondary insurance coverage through the patient's health care plan (when PIP is not available or has been exhausted) and provides accurate information about whom to bill (see Figure 3-2 for a sample of an Insurance Status request form)

6. Intervenes when the insurance company is not complying with laws, regulations, or the terms of the insurance policy, such as not making reasonable and prompt payment of bills

7. Answers the practitioner's questions about deferring payment and waiting for settlement in the event that PIP, Med-Pay, or secondary insurance is not available or has been exhausted

8. Honors the patient's written commitment to be responsible for the manual therapist's bill at the conclusion of the personal injury case (see Figure 3-5 for a sample of a Guarantee of Payment for Medical Services contract)

9. Challenges the legality of an insurer's request for a medical opinion about the necessity of manual therapy, and in the case of an IME, attempts to ensure that the examination is independent

10. Assists in educating the patient about the effectiveness of manual therapy

Communication With the Patient's (Plaintiff's) Attorney
ESTABLISH RELATIONSHIP

Send a letter to your patient's attorney introducing yourself and your practice (Figure 3-1). Include an Insurance Status request form (Figure 3-2). For a blank sample of this form, see Appendix B at the end of this book. Ask the attorney to complete the form and fill in information about the patient's insurance coverage. The attorney will have the most accurate and current information on whom to bill and on whether PIP coverage is in effect and how much PIP money is available. Having this information is critical if you are sending bills directly to the insurance company and the patient has agreed to defer insurance payments to you. If the PIP money has been exhausted on hospital stays, lost wages, household services, or other medical services, you will need to bill the patient directly or decide whether to defer payment until a settlement has been reached. The attorney can answer your questions, ensuring that the patient's access to health care remains open.

In your letter, inform the attorney that you will be in touch monthly to send copies of the bills and update statements. If you bill the insurance company directly, send statements to the patient's attorney as well. This way the attorney can monitor PIP availability and track expenses, and your bill and balance will be known throughout the case. Your statements will also keep the legal team and the patient apprised of the insurance company's payment record. The patient can see how the insurance company is handling the claim and can intervene when bills are not being paid. The attorney can step in for your patient when the insurance company does not make payments in a timely fashion.

End the letter by asking the attorney how you can support the patient's case. Find out how the attorney wishes to receive information—by fax, e-mail, or regular mail, for example. Does the attorney want information in addition to the medical bills and statements? Some attorneys want copies of the patient's SOAP charts and progress reports sent to them monthly. Others will wait until immediately before settlement to ask for the patient's file. (Remember: Patient records are confidential. All requests for patient information must be in writing and must include the patient's written authorization, even requests from the patient's own attorney.) Most attorneys will tell you that keeping accurate, reliable, and relevant chart notes is the best thing you can do to support the patient and the legal team.

The next section provides information on handling requests for medical records.

FIGURE 3-1   Introductory Letter

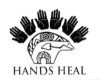

HANDS HEAL

John Olson, LMP, GCFP
345 Moon River Rd. Ste. 6
Minnehaha, MN   55987
TEL   612 555 9889   •   FAX   612 555 9887   •   EMAIL   olsen@email.com

---

B. Charma Storro, JD

5 Hive Lane

Minnehaha, MN 55987

(612)555-2337

Dear Ms. Storro:

I am treating your client, Darnel Washington, for injuries sustained in a motor vehicle collision on January 6, 2001. I look forward to working with you on this personal injury case. I have enclosed one of my brochures and I am available by phone and e-mail if you have any questions about my work or my practice.

I have been unable to confirm which car insurance carrier to bill for Mr. Washington's treatments. Please advise me of the applicable insurance company, the name of the adjuster assigned to the case, and the claim number. Please include information regarding insurance coverage: is there PIP coverage? Med Pay? Health insurance? Uninsured Motorist coverage? If so, how much is currently available?

Enclosed is a form for your use. If Mr. Washington does not have PIP or Med Pay coverage available, I will forward two copies of a Guarantee of Payment for Health Services for you to sign. Please keep one for your records and return the other to me in the envelope provided.

I will update you monthly with copies of the patient's billing statements. Is there any other information you would like me to send in addition to the monthly statements? Do you prefer that I send you the information by fax, mail, or e-mail?

Yours in health,

John Olson, LMP, GCFP

FIGURE 3-2 Insurance Status Request Form

John Olson, LMP, GCFP
345 Moon River Rd. Ste. 6
Minnehaha, MN   55987
Tel   612 555 9889

INSURANCE STATUS— PERSONAL INJURY

Patient Name ___Darnel G. Washington___   Date __2-15-04__

Date of Injury ___1-6-04___   ID#/DOB __123-45-6789__

A. Reporting to Attorney
Which information would you like to receive monthly and how do you prefer to receive information:
☐ copies of billing   ☐ fax
☐ monthly statements   ☐ mail
☐ SOAP charts   ☐ email
☐ Progress reports   ☐ upon request

B. Primary Insurance Coverage   Effective dates: from _____ to _____
Please provide the following information regarding your client's/my patient's insurance status:
Insured _____
Insurance ID# _____
Insurance Carrier _____
Billing Address _____
City _____ State _____ Zip _____
Adjuster _____
Phone _____ Fax _____
PIP policy amount $ _____
Dates of coverage _____
PIP available $ _____
Med Pay policy amount $ _____
Dates of coverage _____
Med Pay available $ _____

C. Secondary Insurance Coverage   ☐ N/A   ☐ Effective date: _____
Insured _____
Insurance ID# _____
Insurance Carrier _____
Billing Address _____
City _____ State _____ Zip _____
Adjuster _____
Phone _____ Fax _____
PIP policy amount $ _____
Dates of coverage _____
PIP available $ _____
Med Pay policy amount $ _____
Dates of coverage _____
Med Pay available $ _____
If secondary coverage is through the patients' private health insurance, is manual therapy a covered benefit: ☐ Yes   ☐ No   ☐ Don't Know

D. Third Party Insurance Coverage   ☐ N/A   ☐ Effective date: _____
Insured _____
Insurance ID# _____
Insurance Carrier _____
Billing Address _____
City _____ State _____ Zip _____
Adjuster _____
Phone _____ Fax _____
Liability policy amount $ _____
Dates of coverage _____
Liability available $ _____
Uninsured/underinsured Motorist (UIM)$ _____
Policy Amount $ _____
UIM available $ _____

Maintaining Client Files

Make sure your recordkeeping is complete, accurate, and well-organized. A complete manual therapist's file will include:

◆ SOAP notes of every treatment date, including extensive SOAP charting of examinations and reexaminations (and brief SOAP notes for daily treatment sessions)
◆ Correct treatment date clearly stated on every SOAP note, corresponding accurately with the treatment date billed
◆ Prescriptions covering every treatment date, verifying treatment as medically necessary
◆ Supportive documentation, including SOAPs, intake forms, and pain questionnaires, and all information written in progress and narrative reports
◆ Correspondence with the health care team, such as progress reports, requests for medical records, copies of other providers' progress reports, and notes from phone calls
◆ Legend of abbreviations and symbols

Strengthen your medical records against common attacks by insurers. Currently, insurers are using the definition of proximate cause to deny payment. As stated in Washington Pattern Jury Instructions 15:01: "The term proximate cause means a cause which is a direct sequence (unbroken by any new independent cause) produces the injury complained of and without which such injury would not have happened." In other words, only the present trauma is directly and solely responsible for the patient's injury and nothing else happened to influence the result. Often, a delay in seeking treatment, a delay in the onset of symptoms, or gaps in treatment may be used as evidence that the injury is not as symptomatic as claimed or that a pre-existing condition or a subsequent trauma is responsible for the patient's condition, thereby relieving the insurer of the responsibility of payment. The medical-legal-insurance context draws a distinction between asymptomatic or dormant conditions versus symptomatic or active pre-existing conditions. An injury that "lights up" an asymptomatic or dormant condition requires the responsible party or insurer to cover all reasonable and necessary treatment expenses. However, an injury that "aggravates" a symptomatic or active condition requires the responsible party or insurer to cover only those expenses attributed to the aggravation of the condition.

Explain delays in the onset of symptoms and all gaps or delays in treatment. If treatment was not sought immediately after the injury, ask the patient to reflect on the reasons why and record their answers in your notes. An insurer could claim that another incident occurred during the time between the MVC and the initial treatment session. Often, it is possible that the patient waited to see whether the symptoms would dissipate, or the patient diligently tried self-remedies (such as rest, heat pads, or over-the-counter pain medications) and, weeks later, gave up and sought care. Also, patients who are unsure about their insurance coverage may try to tough it out because they cannot afford to pay for treatment out of pocket.

Similarly, a patient might take a break from treatment because he or she becomes concerned about mounting medical expenses. Others might discontinue care out of fear of losing their job because of time taken off for medical appointments, or they become overwhelmed by multiple treatments. An insurer might purport that the gaps in treatment are an indication of a new, independent event resulting in renewed care. Rule out intervening trauma and document the patient's worsening condition without treatment.

If the patient's onset of symptoms is delayed, chart possible functional or physiological explanations, such as the patient was on bed rest and it wasn't until he returned to work that the symptoms flared or inflammation prevented full range of motion, then with a reduction in inflammation and an increase in mobility, the patient began experiencing pain with activity. Be proactive by staying informed of insurance strategies for denying payment and recording information in the patient's chart that effectively responds to them.

Requests for Medical Records

The attorney will request the patient's entire medical file at some point in the personal injury case. Everything in the file should be sent, not just SOAP charts and progress reports. Include all intake forms and consent forms, requests from doctors and insurance companies—every piece of paper in the file.

Requests for medical records are made in writing and include the patient's signature authorizing the release of the patient's records to a specific party. *Never* share confidential patient information over the phone unless you have a current and valid legal authorization signed by your patient to release information to the caller. Always wait before sending documents until you have a written request with the patient's signature authorizing the release of medical records. After you receive the request and authorization, send copies of the patient's file. Sometimes, the request may specify whether the entire file is requested or simply the SOAP charts and progress reports.

A release form is valid for a set period of time, depending on state law, after which a new release form must be signed to authorize the additional release of medical information. Check the release form for the expiration date and make sure you have a valid one on file before sending out copies of the patient's confidential file.

The attorney may ask the patient to sign a release form that contains a clause negating all previous release forms (see Figure 3-3). For example, Darnel signed a release form on January 12, authorizing his insurance company to receive copies of his medical records. On March 22, he retained an attorney to represent him and signed an exclusive medical release form voiding the insurance company's release form. Only the attorney's release forms are now valid. Be aware of any exclusive release clauses and honor them.

NARRATIVE REPORTS

The attorney may request **narrative reports** from the patient's health care providers that summarize the patient's injuries, treatment, and progress from beginning to end. These support the attorney in substantiating the patient's personal injury case. Ultimately, the attorney needs narrative reports from health care providers that contain a diagnosis, examination findings, test results, and a prognosis that establish significant injury, validate the medical treatments received, and, if necessary, demonstrate residual effects, disability, or the need for ongoing care. Manual therapists without **primary care status** have less to offer in a narrative report than do the referring HCPS because of their inability to diagnose or provide a prognosis. However, if the role of the manual therapist is primary in the patient's recovery, a narrative may be requested, but will be modified to include only information found in the treatment notes and progress reports (see Figure 3-4).

It has been my experience that attorneys rely more on manual therapists' SOAP charts and progress reports than on narrative reports to substantiate a personal injury case. Good documentation decreases the need for narrative reports from manual therapists, and, when necessary, a good narrative report decreases the need for testimony at depositions or trials.

FIGURE 3-3 Exclusive Release of Medical Records

PATIENT'S RELEASE OF HEALTH CARE INFORMATION

Patient's Name _Darnel G. Washington_

Social Security Number _123-45-6789_   Date of Birth _4-22-37_

I hereby instruct my providers to provide full and complete information to _B. Charma Storro, JD_ and to accept this authorization form and release the protected information requested without requiring any additional authorizations. I specifically waive any "minimally necessary" limitations of HIPAA.

Health Care Provider/Facility _John Olson, LMP, GCFP_
is hereby authorized to release health care information, including intake forms, chart notes, reports, correspondence, billing statements, and other written information to my attorneys, employees, and designated agents of my attorneys, to wit:

Attorney's Name _B. Charma Storro, JD_   Phone _(612) 555-2337_

Address _5 Hive Lane_

City _Minnehaha_   State _MN_   Zip _55987_

This request and authorization applies to:

_✓_ Health care information relating to the following treatment, condition, or dates of treatment: _MVC 1-6-04_

___ All health care information:

___ Other: _____

How the Information will be used: Said information shall be used for any and all purposes for _B. Charma Storro, JD_ to pursue payment of care expenses and in providing legal services to me in conjunction with my case. Following said disclosure the information may no longer be subject to HIPAA protection, as it may be subject to re-disclosure that is unprotected absent specific laws protecting specific sensitive information.

Revocation of Prior Authorization: All medical authorizations by the patient or patient's authorized representatives given before the date of this release for any reason whatsoever are hereby revoked.

Unlawful Disclosure Prohibited: State and Federal prohibits any healthcare provider from releasing any healthcare information about a patient to another person without the consent of the patient. You are requested to disclose no such information to any insurance adjuster or any other person without written authority from me which is printed on the letterhead of my attorney.

Effect of Photocopy: A photocopy of this release shall have the same force and effect as a signed original.

Authorization expires 90 days from date of signature. Thereafter, no authorization exists unless an updated release is provided by: _B. Charma Storro, JD_

I understand that I have the right to revoke this release for any information not yet provided to _B. Charma Storro, JD_ by providing notice of revocation in writing to the above named care provider. I also understand that I have the right to refuse to authorize disclosure at all.

Darnel G. Washington   _2-15-05_
Signature of Patient or Patient's Authorized Representative   Date

FIGURE 3-4 Narrative Report

John Olson, LMP, GCFP
345 Moon River Rd. Ste. 6
Minnehaha, MN   55987

HANDS HEAL   TEL   612 555 9889   •   FAX   612 555 9887   •   EMAIL   olsen@email.com

January 20, 2005

Patient: Darnel G. Washington

DOI: 1-6-04

Claim Number: 123-45-6789

Date of Exam: 1-20-05

Mr. Washington was first seen in my office on 2-6-04 for manual therapy treatment to injuries sustained in a motor vehicle accident on 1-6-04. He was referred by Dr. Sage Redtree, MD, with an initial diagnosis of spinal sprain-strain in the neck, mid-back and low back areas, and headaches. Within 2 months of the accident, Dr. Redtree diagnosed Mr. Washington with a flare-up of scoliosis with accelerated spinal degeneration.

Mr. Washington stated: he was a passenger in a Honda Accord and was rear-ended by a Ford F250 pick-up truck. The Honda was stopping for a yellow light, and the Ford was speeding up to go through the intersection. It was a cold and snowy January afternoon and the roads were slick. The car was pushed across the intersection but did not come in contact with any other vehicles or objects. Mr. Washington was turned to his left in his seat to chat with the driver at the time of impact. His head was thrown from side to side.

Initial Subjective Data:

On 2-6-04, Mr. Washington complained of mild neck pain and stiffness, moderate mid-back pain and stiffness, mild low back stiffness, and a moderate headache. The symptoms were constant since the evening of the accident, and increased in severity with all attempts to to lift his granddaughter, garden with his wife, or sit for over 30 minutes playing bridge with the club he presides over.

Initial Objective Findings:

I palpated moderate muscle spasms in the right sternocleidomastoid and scalene muscles, left trapezius and rhomboids, and right quadratus lumborum. Trigger points were elicited with light digital pressure in the paraspinal muscles, intercostals, and diaphragm. Muscle tension was mild to moderate throughout the spinal postural muscles. Cervical range of motion was moderately limited with active flexion and extension, and passive lateral flexion bilateraly. Inflammation was palpable in the cervical and thoracic regions: redness, heat, swelling, and loss of function; pain and inflammation seemed to be preventing full range of motion. Mr. Washington's posture showed a moderate left shoulder elevation with internal rotation, mild right hip elevation, mild "hump" or kyphosis in the mid-back, mild curvature of the thoracic spine, and a mild forward head position. He was weight-bearing moderately more on the right, his leg swing mildly closed on the right and arm swing moderately closed on the left when I observed his gait.

Initial Functional Goals:

Mr. Washington is the primary caregiver for his granddaughter during the day. Because of her age, he needed to pick her up to put her into the high chair at meals, and into the car seat, and to put her to bed at nap time. At the beginning of treatment, he was unable to lift or carry her because of pain and stiffness. His initial goal was to be able to lift her 10 times a day with mild pain and fatigue.

FIGURE 3-4 (Continued)

After the scoliosis flared up, his activity level dropped considerably. Simple activities such as getting dressed and driving a car became too painful without assistance or frequent rest periods. His goal was to wash himself, dress himself, and walk around the block every day.

A year later, he was able to accomplish his initial goal.

Current Subjective Data:

Mr. Washington has infrequent and mild episodes of pain and stiffness with mild activity, which increase to moderate episodes of pain and stiffness lasting for several hours if he exceeds the following: 5 minutes of carrying his granddaughter, 1 hour of gardening, and 2 hours of sitting.

Current Objective Data:

Mr. Washington's kyphosis and spinal curvature are more pronounced than they were initially. The muscles around the scoliosis are constantly and moderately tight. His muscles in the mid-back area spasm only with activities in excess of the limitations described above, the rest of the spasms have resolved. The trigger points have resolved except around the scoliosis, the headaches are gone, and his cervical range of motion is normal. His gait is excellent and his posture is compromised only by the scoliosis.

Treatment:

Initially, I used full body lymphatic drainage techniques to reduce the swelling and pain, increase mobility, and strengthen the immune system. Soon I began incorporating movement reeducation techniques to find ways that allowed Mr. Washington to move and perform daily activities, such as sitting, standing, and lifting, with more comfort and ease. Initially, the treatment frequency was weekly, increasing to bi-weekly with the exacerbation of scoliosis. After one year of treatment, the frequency returned to weekly, then bimonthly as progress permitted. There was one gap in treatment, due to an extended vacation, during which time Mr. Washington increased his self-care activities.

Progress Summary:

Within six sessions, the neck pain and stiffness, headaches, and low back stiffness were infrequent and mild. Unfortunately, the mid-back pain and stiffness worsened for several months and were debilitating. After several months, the treatments slowly and steadily diminished the pain and increased Mr. Washington's ability to return to a modified level of activity, but it was more than a year before Mr. Washington's scoliosis stabilized and he could return to his normal activities.

Mr. Washington is able to lift his granddaughter as needed, but can carry her for only 5 minutes at a time. He is able to garden for up to 1 hour, and can sit at a bridge table for 2 hours, after which time the pain kicks in.

Patient Status:

Mr. Washington participates in a daily stretching and strengthening routine, and comes in monthly for group movement classes to maintain his daily activity level. We have attempted to discontinue his treatments and rely solely on his self-care routine; however, after 45–50 days without treatment, his ability to function is compromised and his pain increases to moderate and frequent.

In summary, Mr. Washington responded positively to treatments and adapted to a higher level of self-care responsibilities. Please call if you have questions.

Yours in health,

John Olson, LMP, GCFP

Thorough documentation that is contemporaneous with treatment minimizes work in the future and is a tremendous asset and support to the legal team and your patient.

In the event that a narrative report is requested, be prepared to write one that reflects accurately and completely the patient's course of treatment. Because a narrative is written for attorneys and insurers and not for health care providers, use common language and avoid using Latin or formal names for conditions. For example, use the term *headache* instead of *cephalgia*. Explain everything in ways that can be understood by any layperson. Make sure the report includes all pertinent information and is to the point and not excessive. Present the information impartially—do not exaggerate or advocate for the patient. Do not use the narrative as a platform to promote your style of therapy. A narrative report should state the facts of the case clearly from the point of view of an expert. A narrative report includes:

◆ Initial treatment date
◆ All *initial* subjective and objective findings that pertain to the condition
◆ All *current* subjective and objective findings that pertain to the condition
◆ A summary of the treatment plan for the course of treatments, including:
  –Treatment goals that substantiate the treatment as reasonable and necessary
  –Manual therapy techniques and modalities
  –Locations on the body to which treatment was applied
  –Treatment frequency and duration of sessions
  –Thanges in the treatment plan and why, such as gaps in treatment
◆ A summary of progress that includes:
  –Subjective changes
  –Objective changes
  –Functional outcomes
◆ The status of the patient that describes:
  –Whether or not the patient's care has ended (if it has ended, include the final date of treatment; if it has not, give a projected date of completion)
  –Whether or not the patient has reached pre-injury status
  –Whether or not a course of self-care for the future is needed (if it is needed, provide one)

Narrative reports differ from progress reports in several ways:

◆ Narratives summarize the entire personal injury case from beginning to end. Progress reports summarize progress month by month.
◆ Narrative reports include data from all four sections of the SOAP chart: Subjective, Objective, Assessment, and Plan. Progress reports only report progress—information found in the Assessment section.
◆ Narrative reports are written for the attorney and reviewed by the insurers, are several pages in length, and are provided for a fee (a customary practice). Progress reports are written for the referring HCP, are a few paragraphs in length, and are complimentary.

Guarantee of Payment for Health Care Services

If there is no PIP coverage or the PIP money has been exhausted and you agree to defer payment until a settlement has been reached, obtain a signed authorization from the patient granting permission for your services to be paid directly from the proceeds of the settlement or judgment (Figure 3-5). After the patient signs two copies of the contract, submit both

FIGURE 3-5 Guarantee of Payment for Health Care Services

CONTRACTUAL GUARANTEE OF PAYMENT FOR MEDICAL SERVICES

I hereby authorize and direct you, my attorney, to pay directly to my health care provider(s), _John Olson_, the total dollar amount owing for health care services, including applicable interest charges, provided for injuries arising from the motor vehicle accident on _1-6-04_. I hereby authorize my attorney and the involved insurance companies to withhold sums from any settlement, judgment, or verdict as may be necessary to adequately protect my health care provider(s) and their office. I hereby further consent to a lien being filed on my case by said health care provider(s) and their office against any and all proceeds of my settlement, judgment, or verdict which may be paid to you, my attorney, or myself as the result of the injuries for which I have been treated.

I agree never to rescind this document and that any attempt at recession will not be honored by my attorney. I hereby instruct that in the event another attorney is substituted in this matter, the new attorney shall honor this Contractual Guarantee of Payment for Health Care Services as inherent in the settlement and enforceable upon the case as if it were executed by him/her.

I fully understand that I am directly and fully responsible to said health care provider(s) or their office for all health care bills submitted by them for services rendered to me. Further, this agreement is made solely for said health care providers' additional protection and in consideration of their forbearance on payment. I also understand that such payment is not contingent on any settlement, judgment, or verdict by which I may eventually recover damages.

I specifically request my attorney to acknowledge this letter by signing below and returning it to the office of said health care provider(s). I have been advised that if my attorney does not wish to cooperate in protecting the health care providers' interest, the health care provider(s) will not await payment, but will require me to make payments on a current basis.

Date _1-3-05_ Patient's Signature _Darnel G. Washington_

Patient's Social Security Number or Driver's License Number _123-45-6789_

The undersigned, being attorney of record for the above patient, does hereby agree to observe all the terms of the above, and agrees to withhold such sums from any settlement, judgment, or verdict as may be necessary to adequately protect said health care provider(s) named above.

Date _1-6-05_ Attorney's Signature _B. Charma Storro, JD_

Please date, sign, and return one original to
John Olson, LMP, GCFP
345 Moon River Rd. Ste. 6
Minnehaha, MN 55987
_(612) 555-9889_
fax (612) 555-8998

THANK YOU.

Revised and reprinted with permission, Adler♦Giersch, PS

copies to the attorney and request his or her signature on both. One copy will be kept on file; the other will be returned to you. This contract is sometimes called an **Attorney Lien**, but is more appropriately referred to as an attorney contract or Letter of Guarantee (see Appendix B: Blank Forms).

A contractual guarantee of payment is not necessary if the insurance company is making regular payments, but it is highly encouraged otherwise. The contract, when signed by the patient and attorney, guarantees that you will be paid. Also, it ensures that you will receive payment in full upon settlement, rather than having to collect the money yourself from the patient.

▼

STORY TELLER
Guarantee Payment Upon Settlement

A patient of mine spent her settlement funds on a vacation. She spent the money that was supposed to pay her medical bills. She eventually paid $100 per month until the bill was retired, but it was three years from the last date of service before I was paid in full. A letter of guarantee, signed by the attorney, would have prevented this delay in payment.

Include a clause restricting the patient from revoking the contractual guarantee once it is signed and stating that the contract follows attorneys in the event the patient decides to change attorneys later in the case.

The same contract that guarantees payment directly from the settlement can prevent attorneys from reducing your bill. State in the contract that payment for health care services will cover the total balance due at the end of treatment. Include a statement that the payment of interest is owed to you (if you are charging interest) and that the patient has received written notification of the interest charges at the beginning of treatment. (Notification of interest fees can be printed on your fee schedule.) See Chapter 5 for additional information on fee schedules. If the attorney signs the contract, the only way the bill can be reduced without your express permission is if your bill is found to be unreasonable, unnecessary, or unrelated to the injuries in question, as determined by a judge, jury, or arbitrator. An experienced personal injury attorney who supports CAM care will make sure that the settlement is adequate for all the patient's medical expenses.

Communication With the Liability Insurance Company Attorney for the At-Fault Party
MEDICAL RECORDS

The insurance company and the attorney for the at-fault party are not entitled to the patient's records unless (1) the patient signs a medical authorization giving them permission or (2) a lawsuit is filed and you receive a subpoena or stipulation (signed by all parties) requiring you to provide the records. Many cases settle successfully before a lawsuit is filed, without the insurance attorney ever reviewing the patient's medical information. If settlement negotiations fail and a lawsuit is filed, the attorney for the at-fault party begins preparing for the case by gathering medical information from the patient's health care providers. No direct contact is permitted between the health care providers and the at-fault party's legal team, except to schedule a formal deposition. Requests for medical records by the insurer's attorney is often made through private record collection firms. There are two common types of requests for medical records. One, known as a **stipulation**, contains the consent of both the patient and the patient's attorney authorizing the release. The other is a **subpoena**, a compulsory demand for access to records.

Before sending medical records to the defense counsel, check the request for signatures and call the patient's attorney to verify that the records can be sent.

DEPOSITION TESTIMONY

The opposing counsel begins formal preparations for a lawsuit by requesting the patient's medical records and scheduling depositions. All health care providers who treated the patient are potential witnesses and can be deposed. As a health care provider and member of the patient's health care team, you possess important information about the patient's injuries and treatment. To substantiate the patient's injuries and to explain his or her need for treatment, your expert testimony may be necessary.

A **deposition** involves the taking of your testimony under oath. It is conducted out of court, and the location can vary. For example, in Massachusetts, depositions take place in the opposing counsel's office; in Washington state, they generally take place in your office. You will be asked questions by the opposing attorney and, in some cases, by your patient's attorney. The meeting will be recorded by an official court reporter who will record every word of every question and answer. The primary difference between a deposition and a trial is that in a deposition, there is no judge or jury.

The opposing counsel will depose you to assess what you know and do not know regarding the case. He or she will ask specific questions in order to analyze your abilities as a health care witness and to test your credibility. In a deposition, the attorney will be looking for evidence of any or all of the following:

- Delay in initial treatment
- Delay in the onset of symptoms
- Gaps in treatment
- Patient noncompliance
- Patient history that differs from that given by other providers
- Pre-existing conditions
- Subsequent injuries
- Inconsistencies in patient's reporting of symptoms
- Mistakes in billing
- Poor recordkeeping
- Unprofessional conduct

The patient's attorney will prepare you for the deposition. He or she will go over with you in advance about specific questions from the insurer's attorney that may be anticipated. Discuss the weak and strong points of the case before the deposition, so that you feel confident answering the attorney's questions. Use the preparation time as an opportunity to teach the patient's attorney about your work. Some of the information may be useful during the questioning. Review all your notes, so you can speak confidently about the patient's case. If relevant for the deposition, read the reports of the other practitioners on the patient's medical team so that you are familiar with all aspects of the patient's treatment.

Follow these guidelines when giving a deposition:

1. Tell the truth.
2. Never lose your temper.
3. Don't be afraid of the attorneys.
4. Speak slowly and clearly.
5. If you don't understand the question, ask that it be repeated or explained.
6. Answer all questions directly, giving concise answers. If you can answer simply "yes" or "no," do so and stop.
7. Do not provide information beyond that which is sought in a specific question. Never volunteer any information beyond that required to qualify the answer as needed.
8. Stick to the facts and testify only to that which you personally know.
9. Describe your patient's injuries clearly and simply, without magnifying them. You are a health care professional, not the patient's advocate.
10. Testify only to basic facts, not your opinions or estimates, unless you are asked and believe that you are informed and qualified to give such opinions.
11. If you do not know an answer, admit it. Do not think that you have to have an answer for every question asked.
12. Resist requests to interpret or draw conclusions from the records of another health care provider.
13. Do not be drawn into arguing with the insurer's lawyer.
14. If the patient's attorney objects to a question, stop talking. You will be instructed when or when not to continue with your answer.
15. Demonstrate competence, fairness, and honesty.

TRIAL TESTIMONY

If settlement attempts are unsuccessful after a deposition, the case will go to trial or arbitration. Trial or arbitration testimony is similar to that of a deposition except that it is done in a courtroom in front of a judge, jury, or arbitrator. Manual therapists are rarely called to testify because of their inability to offer a diagnosis or prognosis. Usually, the referring HCP or other specialist is called by the patient's attorney to testify and to explain treatment approaches, such as the referral for manual therapy. Make testifying on your behalf easy for the referring HCP. Provide documentation that he or she can use to explain, interpret, and defend with confidence the reasonableness and necessity of your treatment.

Follow these guidelines when you are subpoenaed to testify at trial:

1. Review your testimony from the deposition. Be consistent. Review the guidelines for giving deposition testimony (listed earlier in this chapter).
2. Educate! Everyone in the courtroom can learn a lot from you. Don't hesitate to explain, demonstrate, give examples, or cite authorities.
3. Define and explain every technical term you use. If jurors do not understand, they will tune you out.
4. Use visual aids when possible. Models, diagrams, slides, and transparencies make strong impressions.
5. Listen to the questions, wait, organize the answers in your head, then speak. Do not try to out-strategize the attorney or anticipate the questions.
6. Face the examiner when answering questions. Do not play to the jury.

7. Balance support for the patient with the impartiality of an expert witness. Don't be an advocate. Leave that to the patient's attorney.

8. Be familiar with your records. Avoid thumbing through the file.

9. Stay within your area of expertise.

10. Don't respond to hypotheticals, such as "If the patient could perform a certain activity, would this change your opinion?"

11. Hold to your position and don't equivocate.

12. Be authentic, spontaneous, and professional.

Payment for Services

The patient's attorney is responsible for paying the practitioner for services related to the preparation and prosecution of the patient's personal injury case. For example, the attorney, on behalf of the patient, is responsible for covering the practitioner's expenses associated with prosecuting the case, including:

◆ Copying fees
◆ Narrative reports
◆ Consultations and preparation time for depositions and trials
◆ Testimony at depositions and trials, including travel time

Ultimately, the patient will reimburse the attorney for the expenses at the end of the case. Fees for services vary among individuals. Take special consideration to ensure that you are compensated for your time and that your charges are reasonable. Although the attorney pays you directly for litigation services, the patient eventually will pay for all expenses of the case. Here are some guidelines for determining fees for litigation services:

◆ Medical records—Some states regulate access to medical records and set maximum charges allowed for the copying of those records. This often includes a flat fee for clerical searching and handling and a per-page fee. Know the regulations for your state and follow them.

◆ Narrative reports—The value of the report is based on its clarity and content. A report is worth more if it provides a diagnosis, conclusive evidence (such as x-ray results), and a prognosis that substantiates the case. Research the charges of referring HCPs and other manual therapists in your area to estimate the value of your reports. Check for state regulations that capitate fees for reports.

◆ Consultation and testimony—The hourly rate for consultation and testimony often reflects the practitioner's hourly rates for health care services, because the time you spend being consulted, being deposed or testifying in court is time spent away from your practice. If your maximum patient load equals five hours of billable time, you may consider estimating your fee for testimony based on your daily rate.

Prepayment for these services is the norm. Submit an invoice stating the fees for your services and request payment in advance of providing the service. Use the CPT code 99075 for billing medical testimony. Be prompt with mailing the information upon receipt of the payment.

SUMMARY

Traumatic injury has medical and legal consequences. The legal team can be a valuable asset to the patient and manual therapist. Fair resolution of a legal claim often provides resources for care and improves the patient's well-being. Attorneys can:

◆ Gather evidence
◆ Reduce the patient's stress
◆ Negotiate on behalf of the patient
◆ Advocate for the patient's rights
◆ Protect the patient when an IME is requested
◆ Ensure that the patient receives reasonable compensation
◆ Provide immediate access to legal representation under a contingency fee arrangement, meaning that the legal team will not expect to be paid for its services if no compensation is recovered from the settlement or lawsuit
◆ File a lawsuit within a specified time frame governed by state law

Establish a relationship with the patient's attorney who has valuable information about the patient's insurance carrier, the type of coverage, and the risks involved in deferring payment. Be prepared to request a Guarantee of Payment from the patient and the attorney if the patient does not have insurance coverage that will pay for medical expenses before the claim is settled.

Keep the legal team apprised of the patient's treatment bills and the insurance company's payment record. Maintain complete, accurate, and well-organized treatment records to support the patient and the legal team in the personal injury case. Make sure the patient's file contains:

◆ SOAPs for every treatment date
◆ Prescriptions covering every treatment date
◆ Backup documentation for all information in progress and narrative reports
◆ Copies of all correspondence with the health care team
◆ Legend of abbreviations and symbols

The patient's attorney may request medical records or additional reports, such as a narrative report, on the patient's entire course of treatment. Check for valid authorization before releasing medical records to the insurance carriers or to attorneys. Look for proper dates and signatures and check other releases for exclusive clauses.

If a settlement cannot be reached, pretrial activities begin. The opposing counsel begins formal preparations by requesting medical records and scheduling depositions. The patient's attorney will prepare you for this type of testimony. Make sure that your treatment notes are in order and that you present yourself professionally, confidently, and honestly.

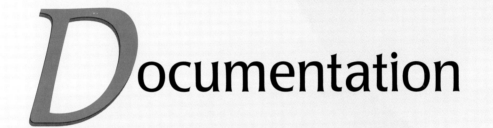

SECTION **II**

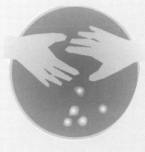

Documentation

CHAPTER 4

Why Document?

CHAPTER OUTLINE

*S*andee was a middle-aged woman with a history of chronic pain that was becoming a way of life for her. She had tried drug therapies and even surgery to rid herself of debilitating back pain, but the pain seemed to be getting worse rather than better. On the advice of a friend, Sandee began to explore manual therapy. She tried out a few therapists and started seeing Holly, a licensed massage therapist who specialized in chronic pain conditions. Holly thought things were going well, but then Sandee approached her for a referral—she wanted the name of another therapist who might better be able to rid her of pain.

Holly was familiar with this kind of frustration and told Sandee that, of course she knew several good manual therapists in the area. She gently asked Sandee to have a seat so they could go over Sandee's file and discuss her goals and results together. Holly wanted to clearly understand Sandee's goals for health so she could adequately select a therapist to match Sandee's specific needs.

As Sandee sat down, Holly laid out 10 pages in front of her—10 pictures with Sandee's own handwriting on them. As with all her patients before each session, Holly asked Sandee to draw the location of the pain on a page showing human figures. Seeing all of the pictures together, Sandee now found it impossible to deny the changes that had taken place. She could hardly take her eyes off the drawings. Her hand shook in amazement as she retraced the circles of pain she had drawn on the figures. On her first visit, Sandee had drawn a big circle around the entire low back and hips, a circle larger than the figure itself, and on a pain scale of 1 to 10 had numbered nine. Each picture that followed showed the circle of pain shrinking in size and the intensity of the pain diminishing in number. Today's figure showed a circle tightly drawn around the sacrum and marked with the number four.

Softly, Holly asked what living with her condition had been like over the years. Sandee explained that because she woke up every day in pain and went to bed every day in pain, she was frustrated. She felt that her condition was unchanged. She had gone from doctor to doctor, trying various treatments. Once again, she found herself repeating the same pattern of going from therapist to therapist, seeking an end to the pain. She had never experienced a cessation of pain and therefore concluded that there was no change in her condition.

Sandee had not recognized the subtle, progressive shifts in her pain. Looking at those pictures, however, she began to accept her healing and to acknowledge the increase in time spent in her garden and the new-found energy to take her grandson to the park. She smiled at Holly and chose to continue care.

Introduction

Documentation is critical, necessary, and expected, but fun? Not exactly. None of us entered the hands-on healing arts because we loved paperwork. All manual therapists have stories of the patient whose life was changed as a result of their work together. Our work is about relationships and interactions with people—that's what fuels our fire. Neither **Wellness charting** nor **SOAP** (Subjective, Objective, Assessment, Plan) **charting** deliver the same emotional satisfaction.

Yet, there may be a way for the paperwork to contribute to the success of those healing relationships as well as preventing paperwork from getting in the way of healing relationships. If so, we might be motivated to put more energy into the task.

Who Should Document?

Every manual therapist should document *every* manual therapy session. All licensed health care providers are required by law to document patient visits. Insurance provider contracts require documentation, professional organizations publish practice standards that mandate documentation, and malpractice insurers strongly urge therapists to produce documentation of every patient visit. Yet, documentation is a skill and a habit that not all manual therapists have developed. Some manual therapists have not felt the need to document their sessions because they are not licensed health care providers. Massage therapists were not considered health care providers until fairly recently. Even today this inclusion is not universal, as evidenced by the lack of consistent licensure in every state. In addition, many manual therapists feel it necessary to chart only those patients who are referred by a physician or whose insurance company is reimbursing them for the sessions. At sporting events, health fairs, and in spas, charting can seem cumbersome. Historically, consumers generally paid cash for their treatment sessions and came without physician referrals, and thus massage therapists, among others, were accountable to no one but their patients. As a result, charting massage clients became less common, especially for one-time, palliative, or relaxation massage sessions.

Our patients perceive us as health care providers, regardless of whether state laws or insurance company policies do. As people are recognizing the benefits of massage, bodywork, and movement therapies, they are receiving manual therapy regularly for the treatment of physical, emotional, and spiritual ailments, as well as for wellness and preventative care. In a consumer survey conducted in August of 2003, 52% of those polled viewed the role of massage therapists as health care providers, up from 36% in 2002.[1] We are responsible for the health of others, and we must act accordingly. Manual therapy is a powerful healing tool, and we are accountable for the outcomes. Good documentation serves as a shield when a patient claims wrongdoing, and it is a part of our providing safe and effective treatment. Documentation is a necessary skill to implement and to master in our practices.

Why Document?

A common misconception among manual therapists, whether or not they are seasoned paper pushers, is that they chart for someone else. We are driven by the belief that we have to document or we will not get paid; therefore, we chart only those who are insurance patients. Maybe we chart for fear of being sued, or we drum up a report from memory to maintain the referral flow when a doctor requests a patient's file. On the other hand, we may be discouraged from charting because of pressure put on us by our employer. The spa manager, for example, may believe that there is no time for customers to fill out an intake form or no space to store patient files. We tend to chart for the many eyes that may see our records, including insurance adjusters, lawyers, and doctors. Perhaps we should begin to chart for our patients.

Therapists have plenty of reasons not to document. Sometimes, we don't want to bother our patients with too many forms to fill out, especially when they arrive late for their appointments. Sometimes, we interpret a patient's squirms during the interview to mean, "Hurry up and get me on the table," so we cut short our questioning. At other times, we rush through the assessments because we think the only part of the session that the patient values is the hands-on part. Or we skip the closing interview to avoid disrupting the mood and spoiling the work we've just done.

The reasons to chart far outweigh the reasons not to chart. We chart because we care about the safety of our patients and we want to provide the best service possible. To avoid medical complications, we have to begin with a health history. To ensure that we are using the most effective treatment interventions, we need to track patients' responses to the various techniques and modalities we are employing. It is difficult to encourage patients to keep up their homework exercises when we can't remember what we asked them to do. And without written proof, it is sometimes difficult to convince them of their progress.

Ideally, serving our patients is the ultimate motivation for documentation. We document to gather and record information that ensures safe treatment and effective care, educates the patient, and clearly states the treatment results so that the patient acknowledges the benefits of the treatment.

The financial and legal motivations are in addition to the primary reason to document our patients' condition. We should maintain written records on all our patients, regardless of treatment goals or payment method. To tame the paper tiger, let's look through the eyes of all the different parties invested in our documentation.

THE PATIENT

Professionalism

Some patients may consider manual therapies "alternative," meaning riskier or less evidence-based than other, more traditional allopathic medical practices. With the integration of complementary therapies into mainstream health care, some people are seeking the care of practitioners they have never before considered. The acts of filling out health history forms, performing assessment tests, and answering questions while the practitioner takes notes can link wary patients to the familiar traditional therapies. This common thread can instill confidence and provide a professional atmosphere, reassuring the patient that you are a health care specialist providing safe and effective health care, sports injury treatment or performance enhancement, or wellness care.

Trust

Manual therapy is intimate. Often, patients remove their clothes and lie on a table with only a sheet covering them. When they are lying face down, they are not able to see us enter the room or move around, and they may feel vulnerable. Even when they don't remove their clothes, we may be touching them in places few people outside of their immediate family touch. Filling out health questionnaires may provide them with a sense of confidence and a feeling that their concerns are our concerns. Interviews focused on gathering and giving information may ease their minds about how and why we will touch them. The act of taking notes demonstrates that what happens in the session is being documented. All of these things may contribute to building a solid relationship between health care professional and patient before we ever put our hands on the person. When we demonstrate concern for the patient's health and take a professional approach, in part through notetaking, we may build a strong bond of trust that can contribute to a successful treatment outcome. The hands-on part of the session may not be the only part that has value after all.

Historical Record

A patient's file is a historical record of wellness and health challenges over time, tracking health patterns and documenting treatment approaches. This is a valuable resource from the patient's perspective for many reasons. Patients may move or change providers and may need to get their new therapists up to speed to avoid wasting time or money. Other health care providers may seek clues in our charts regarding progressive illnesses—information that ultimately could help the patient toward recovery. Patient files may provide the proof necessary to validate ongoing reimbursable treatment for awakening dormant, pre-existing conditions or aggravating active conditions by recent motor vehicle collisions (MVC), allowing patients to get the care they need and deserve without bearing the financial burden.

Safety

Patients need to feel safe in our hands. Repeatedly asking for the same information week after week does not do much to instill a feeling of safety. A written record serves as a database or repository of pertinent information. In completing a thorough health history, patients are assured that the practitioner has access to information that will assist in determining the treatments that are safe and appropriate for them. Nothing is left to memory, and patients do not have to repeat information every session to be assured that precautions will be taken.

Proof of Progress

As in Sandee's story, it is difficult to maintain an accurate perspective of one's condition when one lives with daily pain. An ongoing and periodic account of one's experience and expression of health is critical as a supplement to subjective memory. Daily charting can serve as a witness to the patient's pain and progress.

Quality Assurance and Value

When progress is evident and goals are being met, patients are better able to rest assured that their money is being spent well. Manual therapy is one form of health care that people have traditionally paid for out of pocket.[2] (A testament to positive outcomes!) This means we are competing with the groceries, mortgage payments, and childcare. Typically, for people to feel good about how they spend their money, the end product must outweigh the expense, or the need must be based in survival. Proper documentation can express our goal-oriented approach and be a record of the physical results, thus proving the value. Even emotional and spiritual results have a measurable physical expression. If we are not able to demonstrate long-term, positive results, we may expect our patients to seek better value for their time and money somewhere else.

Education

Documentation performed in the presence of the patient can be an educational experience. The intended result is to encourage patients to participate more fully in their treatment. By participating in the documentation process, they may experience the results on a deeper level, understand what contributes to positive results, and become motivated to progress more quickly. Often, they learn from seeing what you write down and can understand what is working and what isn't and why, including what your plan is for the future. They know that you will hold them accountable for their homework because you wrote it down and will check in with them about it habitually. Involving patients in the treatment process, which includes charting, gets them participating actively and committing to the final outcome. This educational experience can instill a sense of confidence in their own abilities to care for themselves and to control their experience of their situation, which ultimately is the best outcome we can provide for our patients.

THE PRACTITIONER

Financial Security

Patient charts that demonstrate positive outcomes can be financially advantageous. Whether you are self-employed or work in a clinic, patient flow depends primarily on your ability to form productive, healing relationships with your patients. Successful results lead to repeat patients and solid referrals. Documented evidence of your effectiveness in assisting patients helps them keep a positive perspective if they ever lose sight of their progress when, for example, they can't see beyond their immediate pain. It also demonstrates subjective and objective outcomes of your care to referring caregivers who have greater access to your charts than to your healing hands. Documentation is often the referring health care provider's (HCP's) only resource for proof of those successful patient relationships. Moreover, not providing updated reports to referring providers goes against documentation protocol.

The fundamental difference between charting for cash patients and charting for insurance patients is that insurance companies can refuse payment when no documentation exists or they can reverse or deny payment or even terminate treatment based on your documentation.[3] To any manual therapist who depends on insurance reimbursement for income, having documentation is essential for financial security. And not just any documentation—the contract between the insurance company and the insured or the preferred providers requires that treatment be **reasonable and necessary**. This means that your documentation must demonstrate a need for your care in addressing the patient's presenting condition and that the treatment provided must produce documented, measurable results.[3] For example: State Farm's automobile PIP insurance policy states specifically that the treatment must be "essential in achieving maximum medical improvement."[3] We may be asked to present documentary evidence before payment, or the companies may elect to perform periodic audits of patient files. In any case, it is in the best interest of all practicing manual therapists to protect their financial investment by performing their charting appropriately.

Many patients who have been injured in an incident or motor vehicle collision because of someone else's negligence may or may not have an attorney representing them. The outcome of the case may determine who pays the bills and how much money is available to cover those bills. Attorneys typically must prove that the patient was injured by the incident in order to legitimize the need for financial remuneration. They look to medical documentation for this proof. Your documentation can support the patient's case and contribute to the financial award—thus being a support to you in receiving full payment at the time of settlement.

Legal Assurance

In litigation cases, documentation assists in securing payment for your professional services. In the case of a malpractice suit, documentation may save you more than money. Malpractice suits are rarely filed against massage therapists,[4] but in the unfortunate event you are named as a defendant in one, your job and reputation may also be on the line. Applicants for clinical positions or for preferred provider status on insurance lists can be rejected on the basis of complaints filed.

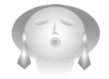

STORY TELLER
Winning and Losing

In my experience with a malpractice suit, thorough documentation showed that the symptoms the patient accused my colleague's treatment of causing had existed months before care was provided at my clinic. Good documentation on behalf of my colleague and the patient's physicians contributed to a positive result for us.

Here is a completely different situation, one in which the lack of documentation produced a detrimental result. I received a phone call asking for support in a malpractice suit. A person filed for damages as a result of an on-site massage at a health fair. The catch was that the person had never received a massage at the booth. However, no documentation existed to prove it—no sign-in sheet, no signed medical release form, and no treatment notes on any recipient at the booth. A favorable outcome for the manual therapist and the company that ran the booth seemed unlikely.

Without written records, few opportunities exist for manual therapists to fight such claims. Protect yourself with documentation.

Professional Image

Hands-on healing has been in existence for thousands of years. Unfortunately, in our history, massage was sometimes associated with sex for money. Perhaps no other health care profession has had to deal with this kind of stigma, at least to the same degree. Other manual therapy professions have had to deal with claims of quackery because scientific evidence of curative ability may have been lacking. With all this working against us, it behooves all professionals in our field to apply certain professional practices stringently. The **scope of practice** or standard of practice for all health care professions requires providers to document. To gain or maintain credibility as a health care profession, all manual therapists must document all treatment sessions. Practitioners who do not consider their services "treatment" may consider the possibility that any session that has a health benefit, such as improving posture, reducing muscular effort, or increasing circulation, is considered a treatment.

Communication With the Health Care Team

The team approach to health care relies on communication for its success. Information is rarely conveyed in person. Most communication, including referrals, progress reports, and the like, is in written form. Other members of the team evaluate your effectiveness by reading your documentation, not by experiencing your touch or hearing patient testimonials. The charts and reports must adequately reflect the patient outcomes, or ongoing referrals may not ensue. Regular, brief written communications demonstrate your professionalism and high standards and substantiate your effectiveness. Referring HCPs are more willing to work with manual therapists who follow familiar lines of communication. Consider this to be the least expensive form of marketing available to you.

Historical Record

Patient charts serve as a memory database, relieving you of the responsibility to remember all the details of each case. Thus, charts free you up to think ahead rather than backward.

For example: Instead of struggling to remember whether the right foot or the left foot had the broken metatarsal or whether the strain/counterstrain technique or the muscle energy technique (MET) produced the quickest result, you can simply reapply the MET to the right foot, reassess, and move on to another stage of the treatment session.

Safety

A universal vow of health care providers is to do no harm. We are in this profession because we want to help others. We need to educate ourselves appropriately about our presenting clients, and we need to discover adequate information about them to assist in making safe decisions about massage. A health history can provide information about past or current illnesses that potentially are aggravated by some modalities. We can track the patient's response to treatments through the daily SOAP charts and reduce the risk of overtreatment. Documentation gives us access to patient information that helps us do our job with reasonable skill and safety.

Efficiency

People on the paying end of health care generally insist on the most effective care available for the least amount of money.[5] To be efficient in the available time, you need to know what has been effective in the past. Health history can provide information about treatments used for past conditions and give insight into their effectiveness. Keep a running log of the techniques and modalities you have used and the patients' responses to those. Wellness charts and SOAP charts record treatments and track the results. This information aids in creating individualized, effective treatment plans. Each session builds on the last, for increased effectiveness and efficiency.

SOAP charting provides a system for tracking the treatments that are effective and the condition and patient for whom they are provided. This allows you to make decisions that streamline the care you are giving on an individual basis and across the board. You may wish to study the results you have achieved with a given technique or for a particular condition. Reviewing many patient files allows you to use your own caseload as research and to evaluate your own effectiveness as a practitioner.

Clear Boundaries

Patient charts may also serve as a reminder to separate your experience from that of the patient. Transference and countertransference are as real in manual therapy as in psychotherapy. The lines between the patient's experience and the practitioner's experience can become blurred. It is not uncommon, for example, to take on the frustration of the patient and make it your own. Use your charts as a reminder of both your successes and your patient's progress. Evaluate plateaus in treatment and keep your self-esteem intact.

However, do not confuse ego with self-esteem. It is possible that the patient's frustration is warranted. Some HCPs, as an example, may take responsibility for the patient's successes and blame the patient for the failures. A full assessment of the patient's experience is necessary. Start with good listening skills. Acknowledge the patient's experience as real for them, check in with yourself, and examine your role in their experience, and when appropriate, share your experience of the situation. Highlight the data collected or explore new options for treatment that could produce different results. It is helpful to review the patient's files before each treatment session, to establish your own feelings based on the data collected and prevent being drawn into the patient's feelings.

The Team Approach

Every person is unique, even in his or her expression of trauma and disease, and has individual triggers for a condition, as well as unique manifestations and different combinations of common symptoms. Because of this, it is rare for any one treatment to cure a given condition for all patients. Applications of a standard of care can produce varying results. Not every person with stage II lung cancer who receives chemotherapy and radiation ends up with the same prognosis. Some people die, some fully recover, and some experience a recurrence of the disease. Life stresses, attitudes and beliefs, and general constitution, to name a few, contribute to the unique expression of a patient's situation. We must treat the whole person and consider all options.

A team approach to treatment can lead to the discovery of the most efficacious care for each person. It is in the patient's best interest for each member of the team to work together, and the team relies on communication for its success. In many situations, direct communication is rare. If we are to function as a team, documentation is essential.

Communication

Communication among members of the health care team may promote complementary treatment plans, ensuring that treatments are not duplicated and that practitioners support one another's efforts and build upon one another's results. The patient may experience the power of the team and feel confident that the combined efforts will produce successful results.

When the patient moves and wishes to continue treatment in a new location, our charts may assist the next manual therapist in maintaining the progress. It is important for adjunctive therapists to be able to rely on us and continue the patient's progress without wasting effort. If you go on vacation and someone takes over your patients, a well-stated treatment plan can assist your replacement in a successful continuation of care. Solid documentation can ensure the success of the health care team, regardless of who is or will be added to it.

Education

Traditional allopaths may not be well versed in the manual therapies. More and more, however, physicians are eager to educate themselves on **complementary and alternative medicine (CAM)** or **complementary and alternative health care (CAHC)** therapies. This was prompted by the Eisenberg Study, which stated that "in 1990 Americans made an estimated 425 million visits to providers of unconventional therapy. This number exceeds the number of visits to all U.S. primary care physicians (388 million)."[2] In the follow-up National Survey, Trends in Alternative Medicine Use in the United States, 1990–1997, Eisenberg claims "a 47.3% increase in total visits to alternative medicine practitioners, from 427 million in 1990 to 629 million in 1997, thereby exceeding total visits to all U.S. primary care physicians."[6] The manual therapists' documentation is a direct and immediate source for educating referring HCPs on how to employ our skills, when to refer to us, and why they benefit from working with us.

Relationship and Referrals

Written communication is standard and anticipated. There is a system in place for building relationships in health care. As with all specialists, manual therapists are expected to send the referring HCP an initial report after the first session with the patient and a progress report every 30 days thereafter. It is common courtesy and a standard in medical documentation to report back to the referring caregiver about your findings and treatment plan. Without it, an HCP may be hesitant to maintain the relationship.

Responsibility and Liability

Everyone on the team has the patient's best interests in mind, but few bear as much responsibility for the patient's health as the referring HCP. Referring HCPs are accountable both to patients and insurance companies for the productivity of the specialists to whom they refer. A referring HCP may be held responsible for the actions of another practitioner in the event of a malpractice suit. The presence of familiar documentation can alleviate the weight of that responsibility. Chart every session, send progress reports, and thank HCPs for referrals. When you support referring HCPs' need for documentation, they will support you with referrals.

THE INSURANCE TEAM

Responsibility for Payment

Insurance personnel are accountable to two parties: the insurance company as its employees and the insured for honoring the terms of the insurance policy. They must provide for the insured within the bounds of their policy and nothing more. Several issues are considered when they are determining whether a medical service is the financial responsibility of the insurance company. Your documentation may be used by insurance personnel to help make this determination.

Insurance contracts with the insured and the providers require documentation to support and justify the services provided. Medical reviewers use manual therapists' charts to determine responsibility for payment. Document the necessary information and protect yourself and your patients financially.

Proof of Services

Insurance personnel look for evidence that the services being billed for were actually provided. It is not enough to have the patient's name in your appointment calendar. Treatment notes will suffice and must reflect the same date as the billing form. Services itemized on the billing statement must be recorded in the treatment notes. For example: If you billed for hot and cold packs, your treatment notes should reflect that an ice pack was applied to the neck for 10 minutes.

Medical Necessity

Services provided must be medically necessary to qualify for insurance reimbursement.[7] Documentation can demonstrate medical necessity. Patient files must show that the services provided were consistent with the patient's symptoms and diagnosis. For example, reimbursement could be denied if a referral with a diagnosis of lumbosacral strain-sprain was received and the treatment notes reflect that the patient was treated for tennis elbow.

Insurance personnel rely on the manual therapist's documentation to verify that the techniques and modalities used improved the health of the patient. Functional outcomes demonstrate improvement in the patient's quality of life. Progress may be slight or significant, but it needs to be measurable over time and documented to validate the legal and insurance standard of reasonable and necessary care.

Safe and Economical

Finally, care must be safe and economical. Manual therapy has few reported complications, but proving that manual therapy is economical can be difficult. Insurance carriers have standards for determining whether fees are **usual, customary, and regular (UCR)**. But more importantly, carriers want to know whether manual therapy services are more cost effective than other equally effective services. The cost of treatment is calculated as total dollars spent, but rarely are the manual therapy dollars spent compared to the surgery dollars saved, for example. Insurance representatives at a CAM committee meeting in Washington State, stated clearly that manual therapy dollars are considered to be in addition to other dollars spent, not instead of. "Everyone can benefit from a good rub, but why should the insurance company pay for it? Prove that the surgery won't be necessary in the future, once the palliative care has worn off," they chided. Although scientific research on manual therapy is sparse, pilot studies suggest that "massage therapy has established a significant beachhead as a vital treatment for general health as well as injury from trauma."[8] Until further research is available, the onus is on the manual therapist to prove effectiveness in as few sessions as possible and to provide the case study statistics necessary for convincing the insurance companies that manual therapy produces long-term results with reasonable financial investment. Use documentation to improve efficiency, by tracking functional outcomes and challenging yourself to be more efficient with your treatments.

▼

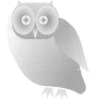

WISE ONE SPEAKS
Therapeutic Massage Provides Long-Lasting Benefits

According to a recent study: "Outcomes observed for massage and acupuncture at ten weeks remained relatively unchanged at one year. Massage was superior to acupuncture in its effect on symptoms (P=.002) and function (P=.051). . . [and] use of medications (primarily nonsteroidal anti-inflammatory drugs) remained lower in the massage group than in both other groups (adjusted P<.05)." During the year after randomization, the number of provider visits, number of filled pain medication prescriptions, and costs of related outpatient services were about 40% lower in the massage group than in other groups.*

* From Cherkin DC, Eisenberg D, Sherman KJ, et al. Randomized trial comparing traditional Chinese medical acupuncture, therapeutic massage, and self-care education for chronic low back pain, published by the American Medical Association in the Archives of Internal Medicine in 2001. Reprinted with permission.

THE LEGAL TEAM
Winning a Personal Injury Case

Lawyers need evidence. Medical documentation is the primary source of evidence validating a personal injury case.[9] Clear and complete documents contribute to the solidness of the case. Typically, personal injury attorneys work on a contingency fee, meaning they are paid a set percentage upon conclusion of a case. Lawyers and their clients have a financial interest in the manual therapist's documentation.

Proof of Significant Injury

Lawyers look to our records for evidence that the patient suffered "bodily injury" as a result of the collision. For the bodily injury to be relevant to the case, documentation must illustrate the patient's pain, location, severity, and frequency. Just as important is the ability of our paperwork to show how the injury has affected activities of daily living. Medical records are necessary to substantiate injuries resulting from the collision.

In addition to proving that the injury is significant and that it warrants treatment, the treatment provided must be proven reasonable and necessary before it will be included in the settlement. With your treatment records, the attorney can justify treatment that is effective in promoting a change in the condition.

Insufficient documentation can lead to requests for narrative reports or testimony at depositions or in court to clarify or defend the care provided. These are costly additions to the patient's out-of-pocket expenses. Recalling details of treatment can be difficult when you are in a stressful, unfamiliar environment, such as a courtroom, or in a deposition with a video camera positioned mere feet away.

Winning a Malpractice Case

To defend a malpractice case against a manual therapist effectively, the attorney must prove that the treatment was within the therapist's scope of practice and was provided with reasonable skill and safety. Once again, medical documentation is the primary source of evidence to substantiate the case. Solid documentation resolves claims and lawsuits. Lack of documentation weakens the evidence and can have a negative impact on the timely resolution and ultimate outcome of a case.

THE PROFESSION

Positive Image

Manual therapy organizations are invested in the public perception of their profession. A number of associations provide a professional affiliation; promote education, ethics, and standards; and work as a group to provide public education and increase public awareness. These benefits are highly regarded by members and consumers alike. Documentation is often among the standards discussed, defined, and required.

Manual therapy professions value relationships with the health care community. The public may view integration into traditional health care as a stamp of approval that legitimizes the work. Increased public exposure increases the number of people receiving manual therapy. The number of new manual therapists entering the profession will grow as a result, and membership in professional associations will increase accordingly.

Research

Research data supporting the efficacy and cost effectiveness of manual therapy validates its use as a viable treatment option and promotes public access. No one likes to take risks with another person's health. Insurance companies and physicians rely on research results to help them make informed decisions regarding health care services. With good data, manual therapy becomes increasingly available to all who can benefit from hands-on healing. Traditional methods of research are difficult to apply to manual therapy. Case studies provide qualitative information and are a popular method for drugless therapies. Case study research is only as good as the therapist's documentation.

SUMMARY

Manual therapists who practice documentation display professionalism and high standards, and they communicate easily with other health care professionals. Documentation is vital to case study research, which provides statistics supporting health care integration and increased public access.

Manual therapists benefit in a variety of ways when documenting patient relationships. Documentation makes good business sense because charting the patient's condition protects our investment of time and services, and provides evidence of the necessity of care and the effectiveness of the treatment provided, thus ensuring payment. Having adequate documentation means legal difficulties may be avoided and the patient's injury treated successfully. Patient charts can be used as a communication tool with referring providers, proving patient progress and the effectiveness of treatment and encouraging future referrals. Communication through documentation establishes rapport within the health care team, promotes a team approach to treatment, and ensures that your patient is well cared for when transition becomes necessary.

Manual therapy patients also benefit from our documentation efforts. We recognize that, in their eyes, thorough charting demonstrates our professionalism and high standards, provides written proof of their own progress and the value of their time and resources, documents the efficacy of treatment (which encourages confidence in their treatment choices), and provides an awareness that they can contribute to a higher quality of life for themselves.

Insurance companies look to our documentation for proof that services were provided, were consistent with the patient's condition and the referring diagnosis, and were medically necessary. The patient files should show that the services improved the patient's quality of life and involved the most effective modalities for the least amount of money.

The legal team depends on medical documentation to win personal injury and malpractice cases. It's as simple as that.

REFERENCES

1. Caravan Survey. Public Attitudes Toward Massage Study. Opinion Research Corporation International. August, 2002.
2. Eisenberg D, Kessler RC, Foster C, et al. Unconventional medicine in the United States, prevalence, costs, and patterns of use. N Engl J Med 1993;328.
3. Adler RH, Whiplash, Spinal Trauma, and the Chiropractic Personal Injury Case. Seattle: Adler◆Giersch, PS: 2005.
4. Interview, Marlys Sperger, Executive Director, American Massage Therapy Association, 2000.
5. HMO Washington Participating Health Care Provider Agreement, 1996.
6. Eisenberg D, Davis RB, Ettner SL, et al. Trends in alternative medicine use in the United States, 1990–1997. JAMA 1998;280:18.
7. Regence BlueShield Practitioner and Organizational Manual, UM-2, 2004.
8. Adler RH. Massage Therapy and Immune Response. Perspectives, Spring 2004:1–2.
9. Adler RH. Medical-Legal Aspects of Soft Tissue Injuries, Handling Motor Vehicle Accidents. Deerfield: Callaghan and Co., 1990.

CHAPTER 5

Documentation: Intake Forms

CHAPTER OUTLINE

*D*avid was a good student. He performed his duties in student clinic professionally and sincerely. One day, after a 30-minute massage on an elderly patient's neck and shoulders, the patient looked up suddenly and said, "I forgot to tell you, I have blood clots in my neck." As David learned early in school, thrombosis is a contraindication for massage—blood clots could become dislodged and move toward the brain, resulting in a stroke. Luckily, the woman was not harmed by the session, and David learned a poignant lesson about the importance of taking a thorough health history.

Introduction

Intake forms are the first step in gathering information from the patient. They ask general questions about personal identification, contact information, health history, and current conditions. This chapter introduces a variety of intake forms:

◆ Health information forms
◆ Fees and policies forms
◆ Health reports
◆ Pain questionnaires
◆ Injury information forms
◆ Billing information forms

All of these forms are completed before the initial session, and some are completed periodically to evaluate progress. Some forms are for all patients to fill out; others are only for patients whose medical conditions warrant additional information. This chapter explains the purpose of each form and provides assistance in determining the appropriate application of each form for your practice and your patients.

Intake forms are easy to use, and they don't require one-on-one attention from the manual therapist. They are self-explanatory and can be filled out by the patient before the initial session begins without cutting into precious treatment time. It is a good idea to review the forms with the patient after the forms have been completed. This helps ensure that they are filled out accurately and provides an opportunity to add pertinent details. For example: If an attorney or physician has a question regarding the patient's responses on a form, it is critical that you know the responses are correct and complete.

Once you have reviewed the forms, you are well-equipped to ask specific, personalized questions based on the information provided. These in-depth interviews are important in developing a better understanding of the individuals with whom you are working and in learning about each person's unique concerns and goals for health. Think of the forms and the ensuing interviews as stepping stones to building healing relationships.

Intake forms serve an additional purpose for patients who are relying on insurance for payment. Recordkeeping needs to meet two goals for insurance reimbursement. First, there must be justification of care on the specific day the patient is receiving treatment. Second, there must be justification for the patient's overall treatment plan.[1] To justify care, documentation must demonstrate that the medical condition was significant and must record the patient's symptoms and functional limitations. To justify the treatment plan, the documentation must demonstrate that the treatment being provided is reasonable and necessary. In other words, the treatment is justified if it has a positive effect on reducing the symptoms and returning the patient to his or her normal activities of daily living. The intake forms presented in this chapter will help you record this important information.

Personalize your intake forms with your logo and business information. The forms shown in this book provide space at the top for doing this (see Appendix B for blank forms). Your name, address, and phone number should be imprinted on every page of each patient's chart for identification in the event that your charts become part of an **audit** or **subpoena** or the patient shares his or her files with another health care provider or therapist. An easy and inexpensive solution is to have a rubber stamp made of your contact information. Place your stamp in a position where you won't lose information if your filing system requires you to punch holes in the top of forms.

▼

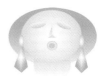

STORY TELLER
Who to Pay?

An insurance adjuster called needing more information on a patient before she could authorize payment. She couldn't read the patient's name, and no identifying information about the patient was on any form—no insurance identification number or date of birth. I asked her to fax me the charts because I couldn't place who the patient might be. As the charts came over the fax, I was taken aback. The handwriting was not mine. The initials signed on the chart entries were not mine—the patient was not mine! The charts were not only missing patient information, there was no contact information for the manual therapist. The only legible name on the chart was mine—next to the little copyright symbol in the lower right-hand corner of the form. I tried to explain to her that I created the form but that I did not write the chart note. I don't know if the correct therapist was ever paid for her services.

Health Information Forms: For Wellness Care

There are a variety of brief health information forms specifically adapted for relaxation massage, spa therapies, on-site massage, and sports massage. Many patients use manual therapy to stay healthy and reduce stress. Others strive for a performance edge with athletic and artistic activities. A variety of manual therapy techniques can be used to refine skills you already have or help you enjoy being active late in life. Intake questions that address these goals for health are designed to be quick and easy to use yet ensure the safety of the patient. It is superfluous to gather a comprehensive list of symptoms and specific details regarding the patient's medical condition when providing wellness care (see Figure 5-1).

The health information form on the Wellness chart meets the three basic needs for alternative documentation:

- ◆ It is quick and easy to use.
- ◆ It ensures the patients' safety.
- ◆ It provides legal protection for the practitioner.

QUICK AND EASY CHARTING

The Wellness intake questions indicate yes or no answers that can be checked off quickly by the patient. In an on-site or sports venue, the questions can be asked orally, and only positive answers are recorded by the massage therapist. When reading the intake questions aloud, make eye contact to ensure that the patient is paying attention and understands the questions being asked. The questions are brief but critical, especially at a sporting event when it is necessary to determine whether first aid is more appropriate than massage.

PATIENT SAFETY

Intake questions are designed to ensure the safety of the patient. Wellness charts have very few intake questions, but the questions are designed to get right to health issues. Any yes answer to an intake question may require additional information to rule out potential harm. The manual therapist must be able to identify health situations that contraindicate treatment or require precautionary measures when providing treatment. For example, inflammation may indicate infection, which contraindicates circulatory massage. Numbness contraindicates deep pressure touch. Some symptoms contraindicate locally but not systemically, some techniques are contraindicated but not others.[2] Know how to respond to positive answers to intake questions.

Adapt the intake questions to discover possible contraindications specific to your work environment. For example, the intake questions for a sporting event cover signs and symptoms of shock—the primary contraindication for treatment after physical stress. Intake questions for a spa environment emphasize allergies to scents, oils, and other products used during aromatherapy and herbal wraps. Include information-gathering questions specific to the treatment provided, such as a question about allergies to honey.

LEGAL PROTECTION

Protect yourself in the rare event of a malpractice case by demonstrating that health screening was considered and treatment was appropriate. To do this, have the patient fill out, sign, and date a health questionnaire. If the practitioner completes the form for the

---

FIGURE 5-1 Wellness Chart—Health Information with Personalized Header

Naomi Wachtel
567 Sunnydale Dr.
Flat Irons, CO   80302
TEL   303 555 8866

WELLNESS CHART

Name _Lin Pak_____   ID#/DOB _5-31-63_____   Date _7-27-04_____

Phone _(303) 555-0033 x 253_____   Address _IBM 3rd Floor_____

1. What are your goals for health, and how may I assist you in achieving your goals? _Limit_____
   longterm complications of diabetes through relaxation and stress reduction.

2. List typical daily activities—work, exercise, home. _I sit a lot at work and watch movies_
   ____at home

3. Are you currently experiencing any of the following? If yes, please explain.
   pain, tenderness   ☒ No ☐ Yes: _____   stiffness ☒ No ☐ Yes: _____

patient, require the patient to initial the entries. Show that you checked for possible health complications and provided safe treatment.

▼

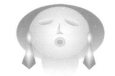

STORY TELLER
Review Health History Before Treating

Always look over the health history before proceeding with the treatment. A malpractice case was filed in which a client accused an on-site massage therapist of harming him. Before the session, the therapist handed the intake form to the client. The client read the form and handed it back to the practitioner without completing it. The massage therapist proceeded with the treatment without realizing that the client had not signed off on the statement of health. As it turned out, the person had one of the conditions listed on the form as a contraindication and alleged that he was injured as a result of the treatment provided. Take steps to protect yourself and follow through with them.

Health Information Forms: For Curative Care
CONTENT

A health information form is designed for patients with medical conditions, such as whiplash, sports injuries, and carpal tunnel syndrome, and records five basic kinds of information:

◆ Personal identification and contact information
◆ Current health information
◆ Goals for health
◆ History of injuries, illnesses, and surgeries
◆ Contract for care

Questions in the five categories may vary according to the specialty of the practitioner. For example, an acupuncturist may include detailed questions regarding the person's diet in the section for current health status. A massage therapist may request more specific information on musculoskeletal dysfunction in the health history section. All basic categories pertain to all patients, regardless of their reasons for the visit (see Appendix B for blank forms).

Personal Identification and Contact Information

The patient's name, date of birth, and a date should appear on every piece of paper in the patient's file. The name connects the data to a living, breathing person, and can be used to organize the files. Date of birth differentiates two individuals who have the same name. The date places the information in time, an important reference for tracking the progress of the condition. If multiple entries are made on a single page, each entry should be dated.

Cases involving insurance reimbursement often require the patient's name, claim number assigned to the case, and the date of injury (DOI), when applicable, on every form sent to the insurance company. Use the same header on all forms—name, date of birth, date, insurance identification number, and DOI. If the insurance identification number and the DOI do not apply to the case, you may simply leave the spaces blank. If you omit these identifiers from the header, you risk omitting necessary information and causing a delay in insurance payment. (Note: Wellness charts are not appropriate for charting curative treatment and, therefore, will not include the date of injury or insurance identification number in the header.)

Record all possible contact numbers on the health information form. Know how to reach your patient in a timely fashion in case appointments need to be changed or issues need to be discussed. Sometimes, you may need to get information to the patient before a session. The patient's address is also useful for marketing. Send birthday cards, referral thank-you cards, and discount coupons to stay in touch and show you care. Protect the patient's confidentiality—don't leave messages that disclose details of the appointment and don't sign your name in a way that indicates the current relationship.

Be prepared in the unlikely event of an emergency. Have the patient list a contact person who can be reached immediately in case of a sudden illness or accident. Know how to contact the patient's primary health care provider (HCP). Health complications may require additional information or treatment consent. In addition, you may want to apprise other members of the health care team of the patient's progress. Make sure you have phone, fax, and address information for all team members. Later, confirm how they wish to receive information.

On the health information form, request permission from your patient to consult with the other HCPs on the patient's team. This simple permission request is sufficient for most purposes (see Figure 5-2). Asking permission is courteous, and it models open communication with the health care team. It is also a legal requirement according to some state and federal laws. Some state laws waive the requirement for written permission when sharing health care information between referring HCPs and specialists. Even if this is the case, patients will appreciate being asked. If you are required to comply with the **Health**

FIGURE 5-2 Health Information—Permission to Consult with Health Care Provider

Primary Health Care Provider

Name Manda Rae Yuricich, DC

Address 4041 Bell Town Wy, Ste 200

City/State/Zip Capitol Hill WA 98119

Phone: 555-3535   Fax 555-4646

I give my manual therapist permission to consult with D.C. & P.T.
regarding my health and treatment.

Comments re: work injury only

Initials ZH   Date 4-4-01

Insurance Portability and Accountability Act (HIPAA) regarding confidentiality because you store and transfer client data electronically, use a HIPAA-approved consent form (see Figure 5-3) in addition to the health information form. The simple statement on the health information form is not, by itself, sufficient for HIPAA regulations. (See

---

FIGURE 5-3   Consent Form—In Accordance with HIPAA Regulations

Authorization to Use and Disclose Health Care Information

Name _____ ID#/DOB _____ Date _____

I: _____, authorize my manual therapist: _____,
to disclose my health care information with the following health care providers and/or insurance companies:

Name(s): _____

Address: _____

The following information may be disclosed (check all that apply):

☐ All health care information in my medical chart.

☐ Only health care information relating to the following injury, illness, or treatment: _____

_____

☐ Only health care information for the following dates or time periods: _____

_____

☐ Including information regarding HIV, STD, mental health, drug or alcohol abuse.

I give my authorization to release health care information for the following purposes (check all that apply):

☐ To share information with my health care team in an attempt to coordinate care

☐ To obtain payment of care expenses I have incurred for my treatments.

☐ To take part in research

☐ Other: _____

This authorization expires on:

Date: _____ (no longer than 90 days from the date signed)

Event: _____

I understand that I may refuse to sign this authorization.

I may also revoke this authorization at any time by writing a letter to my manual therapist.

I understand that once my health care information is disclosed, the recipient may redisclose the information and it may no longer be protected HIPAA or state privacy laws.

I also understand my obtaining care can not be conditioned on my signing this release.

Signature _____ Date _____

Chapter 8 for more information regarding HIPAA compliance or visit http://www.aspe.hhs.gov/ admnsimp/index.shtml.)

Even when patients are not referred by a HCP, they may have a condition that warrants a consultation with their primary HCP. It is important to get written permission from these patients for a variety of reasons (for example, their physician may not know they are receiving massage therapy and they may want the chance to tell the doctors first). Some patients may have shared information with you that they do not want discussed. Let them know *what* information you will be sharing, with *whom*, and *why*.

Current Health Information

This section of the form asks the patient to list, prioritize, and classify current health concerns and to identify ways in which those conditions are affecting daily life (see Figure 5-4). The goal is to learn why individual patients are seeking treatment, so you can address their needs and contribute to their goals for health. Specific questions help patients clarify their reasons for seeking manual therapy. Unmet expectations are often the product of unspoken desires. Leave little room for interpretation and be clear about goals for the session.

Information in this section is useful for insurance cases to prove significant injury and thereby justify treatment. Symptoms and their effect on normal activities as stated by the patient are considered by insurance adjusters and peer reviewers to validate care. Subjective documentation—information the patient reports—is critical. Intake forms record historical subjective information—everything prior to the initial treatment.

In addition to recording the patient's concerns, this form asks what treatment the patient has received for these conditions in the past and what self-care strategies they have employed. Use this information to formulate a treatment plan. You can eliminate ineffective techniques, avoid those that other practitioners on the health care team are using, and use or encourage solutions the patient finds helpful. Consider the patient's goals for the session, and together with your ideas for a treatment approach, discuss the various options in the interview.

If the patient's condition is recent and the patient has not yet received treatment for this complaint, look to the general health history for information regarding a treatment approach. Something in the patient's history may have contributed to his current health, or the treatment sought for other conditions may provide information that shapes what could be a successful treatment plan for the unique individual before you. You can get a sense of the patient's preferences toward treatment based on the type of self-care he or she has incorporated into his daily care routine, such as conventional or alternative, participatory or passive.

Health History

This section consists of two parts: (A) a chart listing surgeries, accidents, and major illnesses and (B) a checklist of symptoms and conditions. The chart allows the patient to identify major health crises and provides quick referencing for the practitioner (see Figure 5-5A). The checklist provides important information regarding all systems of the body, enabling you to pinpoint conditions that may require special precautions

FIGURE 5-4 Health Information—Current Health Information

John Olson, LMP, GCFP

345 Moon River Rd. Ste. 6
Minnehaha, MN   55987
TEL   612 555 9889

HANDS HEAL

HEALTH INFORMATION

Patient Name _Darnel G. Washington_   Date _2-6-04_

Date of Injury _1-6-04_   ID#/DOB _123-45-6789/4-22-37_

A. Patient Information

Address _1209 Lake Winnetonka Dr._

City _Minnehaha_   State _MN_ Zip _55987_

Phone: Home _(612) 555-1515_

   Work _N/A_   Cell _555-5511_

Employer _IBM_

Work Address _N/A_

Occupation _retired_

Emergency Contact _Shalonda—wife_

Phone: Home _same_

   Work _N/A_   Cell _555-5511_

Primary Health Care Provider

Name _Sage Redtree, MD_

Address _87 Old Trail Pkwy_

City/State/Zip _Minnehaha, MN 55987_

Phone: _555-0009_   Fax _555-9000_

I give my massage therapist permission to consult with my health care providers regarding my health and treatment.

Comments _____

Initials _DGW_   Date _2-6-02_

B. Current Health Information

List Health Concerns Check all that apply

Primary _back pain_
☐ mild ☒ moderate ☐ disabling
☒ constant ☐ intermittant
☒ symptoms ↑ w/activity   ☐ ↓ w/activity
☒ getting worse ☐ getting better ☐ no change
treatment received _pain pills, back brace_

Secondary _headaches_
☐ mild ☒ moderate ☐ disabling
☐ constant ☒ intermittant
☒ symptoms ↑ w/activity   ☐ ↓ w/activity
☒ getting worse ☐ getting better ☐ no change
treatment received _pain pills_

Additional _neck stiff_
☒ mild ☐ moderate ☐ disabling
☒ constant ☐ intermittant
☒ symptoms ↑ w/activity   ☐ ↓ w/activity
☐ getting worse ☒ getting better ☐ no change
treatment received _stretching_

List Daily Activities Limited by Condition

Work _N/A_

Home/Family _gardening, vacuuming_

Sleep/Self-care _sleep, exercise_

Social/Recreational _play w/ grandchildren, dancing, bowling, bridge group_

List Self-Care Routines

How do you reduce stress? _watch sports, garden_
Pain? _heat, back brace, meds_

List current medications (include pain relievers and herbal remedies) _____
   hydrocodone 500 mg every 4 hrs

Have you ever received massage therapy before? _no_ Frequency? _____

What are your goals for receiving massage therapy? _get around easier, less pain_

C. Health History

List and Explain. Include dates and treatment received.
Surgeries _appendicitis 1949 removed, torn meniscus Ⓡ knee 1980 arthoscopy_

Injuries _bowling injury Ⓡ knee 1979 no treatment until surgery 1980_

Major Illnesses _scoliosis 1949_ _____
Milwaukee brace, exercise, pain meds

FIGURE 5-5A   Health Information—Health History

C. Health History
List and Explain. Include dates and treatment received.
Surgeries ___none___

Injuries ___Broken arm Ⓡ fell out of tree house in 1987, cast for 8 wks___

Major Illnesses ___none___

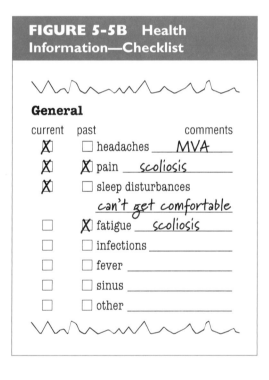

FIGURE 5-5B   Health Information—Checklist

General

current	past		comments
☒	☐	headaches	MVA
☒	☒	pain	scoliosis
☒	☐	sleep disturbances	
			can't get comfortable
☐	☒	fatigue	scoliosis
☐	☐	infections	
☐	☐	fever	
☐	☐	sinus	
☐	☐	other	

(see Figure 5-5B). You can then apply your knowledge of indications and contraindications to the development of your treatment plan. Health history can provide insight into the origin of current conditions and identify factors that may influence those conditions.

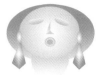

STORY TELLER
Health History Affects Current Condition

Physical trauma can result in weakness and compensational posture or movement patterns, especially when untreated. These complications may cause concomitant dysfunction or may contribute to chronic conditions. In one of our staff meetings, we discovered that the majority of patients treated for chronic repetitive stress injuries at the clinic also had a history of previous soft tissue trauma—with whiplash topping the list. Sara, for example, was in a car accident as a teenager. She bounced right back and never thought about the experience again. Twenty years later, she suffers from recurring thoracic outlet syndrome. A pattern was emerging: In the winter, she painted every wall and ceiling in her house; in the summer, she refinished the hardwood floors; and every spring after long gardening sprees, she came to the clinic complaining of numbness and tingling in her right arm and hand. It wasn't until we discussed her case as a group that we considered how her past history was influencing her present condition. The accident was so long ago that no one gave it much thought, especially Sara. Once we determined that Sara had a poorly healed cervical sprain-strain injury, her treatment plan shifted and her condition subsided. Sara's case demonstrates that careful consideration of the chronological chart can help you identify pre-existing conditions that are adversely affecting current conditions. This prompts you to adjust the treatment plan to address the old trauma.

The health history section of the health information form is helpful for identifying pre-existing conditions that are currently symptomatic. This information is critical in the event of a motor vehicle collision (MVC). In personal injury cases, patients can expect that every attempt will be made to return them to pre-injury status and that their insurance will cover the health care necessary to the full extent of their benefits. This coverage should include treatment for pre-existing conditions that were exacerbated by the collision.[1]

Contract and Consent for Care

The contract for care is an invitation for the patient to participate in treatment and share the responsibility for the result. It delineates the patient's commitment to the healing relationship. The goal is to empower the patient to become active in the healing process and to promise goodwill on behalf of the manual therapist.

The consent for care states that the patient is actively choosing manual therapy and giving permission to the practitioner to provide treatment. It may warn of possible risks and limitations of the therapy. Know the limits of your scope of practice and state them clearly here. Include a statement about your practice philosophy and how you intend to assist the patient toward greater health.

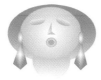
End the health information form with a dated signature confirming that the information provided is complete and accurate and that the patient is consenting to receive treatment. Require the signature of a parent or legal guardian when the patient is under age 18. This signed statement is sometimes referred to as a treatment disclaimer or waiver. The patient's signature on the form may not protect you legally if something goes awry, but it demonstrates informed decisions regarding safe care. However, the most important element of the contract and consent for care is the verbal discussion that leads to an agreement to engage in a therapeutic relationship. As Jerry A. Green, a malpractice attorney in California and president of the Medical Decision Making Institute, states, "Remember: Legal problems begin as disagreements. You prevent legal problems by making meaningful agreements."[3]

TIMING AND APPLICATION

A thorough history takes time to document. Instruct the patient to arrive 15 to 30 minutes before the initial appointment to ensure adequate time for filling out the forms. You may choose to save time by mailing out the health information form and all other applicable intake forms to the patient the week before the first session. People may breeze through the forms in your office because they are eager to get on with the session. When given their own time to think about the questions, to look things up when necessary, or to ask family members for help in reconstructing events, their information tends to be more complete. Occasionally, people forget to bring the forms to the initial session, but most remember and make it worth the trouble of mailing the forms in advance. Even when they forget the forms, filling them out a second time goes much more quickly.

Regardless of individual goals for treatment, each patient should complete a basic health information form annually. If the patient has progressive or degenerative health problems or if the patient's health changes, the form should be updated semiannually or quarterly.

Use the form as an information database and refer to it for interviewing the patient, designing the treatment plan, identifying possible cautions for care, and contacting the patient throughout the relationship. If an insurance case manager or an attorney requests the patient's file, this document may be used to substantiate the patient's injury and to determine the presence of pre-existing conditions.

Fees and Policies

CONTENT

Fees and policies include a fee schedule, payment options, and miscellaneous office policies. Publish your fees and policies and distribute them to all patients. Determine the policies that allow you to be financially sound and that provide clear boundaries. You can always be more lenient later (if special circumstances arise), but it is difficult to get tough after the fact. Ensure your safety by defining the patient behavior necessary for you to relax and enjoy your practice.

Fee Schedules

Fee schedules describe the various services you offer and the costs associated with them. Fees may be delineated by techniques and modalities, such as manual lymphatic drainage or hot/cold packs; by style or intent, such as wellness care or curative care; or by service codes, such as 97124 for massage therapy or CBEBF for Swedish massage. If you are billing for your services using CPT codes, such as 97124, or ABC service codes, such as CBEBF, break down your fees on your fee schedule according to the time specified in the service description. For example: CPT codes designate most physical medicine procedures to 15-minute units, so your fee schedule should delineate your rates in 15-minute increments (see Figure 5-6).

Define your services clearly, both for the purpose of explaining what you offer to your patients (so they may choose appropriately based on their goals for health) and for the purpose of insurance reimbursement so they can pay you appropriately based on the services you provide. If you submit claims to insurance companies, you may need to define your services according to insurance standards to ensure reimbursement. For example: The **Current Procedural Terminology (CPT)** codebook—a set of codes published by the

---

FIGURE 5-6   Fees and Policies—Fee Schedule

A. Fee Schedule

Fees for services are as follows:

- CranioSacral/Lymph Drainage (97140) $100 per hour ($25 per 15 minute unit)
- Feldenkrais (97112) $100 per hour ($25 per 15 minute unit)
- Hot and Cold Packs (97010) $15 per session ($15 per session)
- Therapeutic Massage (97124) $80 Per Hour ($20 per 15 minute unit)

American Medical Association—defines standard therapeutic procedures and modalities, assigns time frames for the purposes of insurance billing and reimbursement, and designates all health care services by categorizing like techniques, such as 97124—defined as massage, including effleurage, petrissage, and tapotement (stroking, compression, percussion). The code 97140 is defined as manual therapy techniques, such as mobilization/manipulation, manual lymphatic drainage, manual traction, including myofascial release. The code 97112 is defined as neuromuscular reeducation of movement, balance, coordination, kinesthetic sense, posture, proprioception, or all these, and for sitting and standing activities.[5] When describing your services to your patients, use specific terms rather than general categories or codes, such as deep tissue massage instead of 97124, CranioSacral therapy instead of 97140, or Feldenkrais instead of 97112 (see Appendix E for billing codes).

However, it is important to note that there is no standard terminology in the CPT codebook defining a style of massage such as wellness, treatment, therapeutic, or medical. If you submit claims using CPT codes and you choose to delineate different fees for these "styles" of massage, do so with a clear definition in mind and make sure that specific techniques and modalities do not overlap. In other words, if you differentiate between wellness care and curative care on your fee schedule, the techniques and modalities you employ should be unique to the type of service provided—Swedish massage for wellness care and Structural Integration for curative care. If you submit claims using **Advanced Billing Concepts (ABC) codes**—a set of codes designed for use in alternative medicine, nursing, and other integrative health care practices—then services for wellness visits are given separate codes. Wellness visits are defined as "clients without medical or physical complaints."[5] (Note: ABC codes are new to the health care industry and are not widely recognized by insurance companies.) Alternative Link, the publisher of ABC codes makes no representation that the use of these codes will result in coverage of described interventions or reimbursement of insurance claims.[5] With that in mind, use CPT code procedure descriptions as guidelines for defining your services and assigning your fees when providing billing services for patients until you verify that ABC codes are reimbursable.

When establishing your fees, keep in mind that it is discriminatory and fraudulent to charge different rates for the same service. In other words, you cannot have one rate for cash patients and another rate for insurance patients. You must charge the same rate for a service regardless of how the patient is paying. If an insurance auditor finds that you used myofascial release and lymph drainage on a patient who paid cash at the time of service but you charged the individual less than you are charging the insurance company for the same techniques and modalities, you may be required to refund the difference. If an auditor determines that your billing practices are fraudulent, you could be asked to reimburse the company for overcharges—retroactive to seven years.

In many states, it is legal to offer discounts to patients who pay at the time service is rendered. Discounts are allowed within reason as long as they apply to insurance patients as well as to cash-paying patients. Publish all discounts on your fee schedule, including prepaid package discounts and financial hardship discounts, as well as discounts that apply when payment is made at the time of service. Check your local laws and abide by any requirements and exceptions (see Chapter 9 for a discussion on the ethics of fee schedules).

Another method for setting your fee schedule is to charge by time rather than by modality. This method is known as **bundling** services. A flat fee includes any manual therapy applied that can be billed under one procedural code. For example, you may use Swedish massage, myofascial release, lymph drainage, trigger point therapy, acupressure, and muscle energy techniques in varying combinations, but find it difficult to break everything down into time per modality. You may choose to bill using the general massage therapy procedural code and not bother with five different procedure codes and five different rates. Bundling services is common in cash practices and can be used with a billing practice as long as you do not bundle procedures that would be reimbursed at a lower rate than the one under which you are billing. This is a fraudulent practice known as **upcoding**.

Payment Policies

The payment policies section states the payment methods available and clarifies the type of insurance reimbursement you will accept and under what circumstances. Insurance reimbursement arrangements vary from manual therapist to manual therapist, from state to state, and from country to country, depending on the scope of practice of the individual therapies and the insurance climate of the region. Inform yourself about the specific risks and benefits of insurance billing for your unique situation before setting a policy.

Here is an example of a policy statement to use when billing a patient's automobile insurance company:

The usual policy of this office is for patients to pay for services as they are rendered. In the case of billing an automotive insurance claim, the therapist may exercise the option of billing your insurance company directly for your health care treatments. Payment is ultimately your obligation, regardless of insurance or other third-party involvement.

It is the policy of this office that your payment of the therapist's fees may be deferred until your personal injury claim is settled or a judgement is obtained, *provided the following conditions are fully satisfied:*

◆ The therapist retains the option to request that you be represented by an attorney who specializes in personal injury law.

◆ A guarantee of payment for health care services contract is signed by you *and* your attorney. This permits the therapist's fees to be paid from the final settlement when obtained.

◆ The merits of your personal injury claim are established by your attorney and communicated to the therapist.

◆ All accounts not paid in full within 60 days of the date billed will be charged interest. Interest rates are calculated at 12% annually and are charged at 1% monthly. Interest is calculated on the principal amount; interest is not compounded.

◆ You will be charged for any appointments missed without 24-hour notification of cancellation (this office does not charge the insurance company for missed appointments).

◆ You acknowledge responsibility for all outstanding payments should the insurance company refuse to pay for services rendered.

◆ You make a good faith payment for services on a monthly basis until your claim is concluded.

It is acceptable to charge interest on past due accounts. Many states have laws regarding interest terms and start dates as they apply to medical services, such as 12% per year simple interest beginning 60 days after the billing date. Know what those are in your state and specify your terms clearly. It is generally mandated that the patient be made aware of interest rates in writing before the rates accrue.

100

HANDS HEAL:
COMMUNICATION,
DOCUMENTATION,
AND INSURANCE BILLING
FOR MANUAL THERAPISTS

Office Policies

Provide written statements of your office policies. Make sure your patients read them and agree to abide by them. Require a signature demonstrating that the patient has read and understood your fees and policies. It is generally easier to enforce a policy statement when it is in writing and has been signed and dated. Keep the signed form in your patients' files. You may have to remind patients of these policies at a later date.

Cancellation policies are common in practices in which one session makes up a significant percentage of the daily income. Set a standard cancellation fee or charge the full price of the session whenever the patient fails to cancel within a specified number of hours before the scheduled time. Consider abiding by your own cancellation policy. For example, offer a similar discount to those patients whose appointments you cancel without a 24-hour notice. Demonstrate that you value their time, particularly when you are asking them to value your time. Another way to show respect when you are the one canceling without 24-hour notice is to give the patient a certificate for a free "no-show" or late cancellation on their part.

Right of refusal is another common office policy. This policy can be helpful for turning away people who are impaired by alcohol or drugs, have an infectious illness, push for treatment outside your scope of practice, or behave inappropriately. It is important to set boundaries, to feel safe in your practice, and to take care of yourself. Use this policy any time you have a gut instinct to do so.

TIMING AND APPLICATION

The patient should read and sign your fees and policies form before the first session begins. Include the policy statement with the health information form and any other intake forms completed by the patient at the initial visit. Post your fees and policies clearly to reinforce what you are requiring the patients to agree to and to demonstrate your professionalism toward potential patients who walk in off the street. Revisit your fees and policies annually and update them as necessary.

Health Report
CONTENT

The health report provides a snapshot of the patient's health (see Appendix B for a blank form). In just a few minutes, the patient can chart the location of pain, stiffness, and numbness—by writing the letters P for pain, S for stiffness, and N for numbness—on the human figures and can rate his or her pain and loss of function by placing a dash on the lines of the analog scales. The drawings provide a map of the patient's symptoms that is accurate and easy to read. Below the figures are two analog scales or lines of continuum: one denoting pain, the other activity level. The mark on the line is measured and a numerical score is calculated and recorded, making references to progress quick and easy.

The health report is the form mentioned in the opening case study of Sandee in Chapter 4. The benefits of this form are great for the patient and the practitioner. Progress is recorded in the patient's own handwriting, convincing even the most frustrated patients of their health improvements. The manual therapist can use this form to support the health history interview, gathering pertinent information from tentative patients and streamlining the discussion with the chatty ones.

Human Figures

Diversity in learning styles is widely recognized in today's classrooms. Visual, auditory, and tactile learners have different ways of processing and storing information. The same is true of patients. Some enjoy filling out forms, yet others would rather tell you about themselves (and often do so in story format). Still others can draw images more easily than filling in blanks on a form or talking. Provide a variety of ways to gather information, including multiple choice forms, one-on-one communication, and pictures to draw on, such as the ones on the health report (see Figure 5-7).

Coaxing information from some patients can feel like pulling teeth. Maybe they were taught not to complain or they are just not comfortable speaking to people they do not know well. For those patients, drawing symptoms on pictures may be easier than having to talk about their pain or disability.

With other patients, trying to keep the interview under five minutes is challenging. Some would rather talk about their problems than solve them. Others chatter when they get

FIGURE 5-7 Health Report—Figures

A. Draw today's symptoms on the figures.

1. Identify CURRENT symptomatic areas in your body by marking letters on the figures below. Use the letters provided in the key to identify the symptoms you are feeling today.
2. Circle the area around each letter, representing the size and shape of each symptom location.

Key
P = pain or tenderness
S = joint or muscle stiffness
N = numbness or tingling

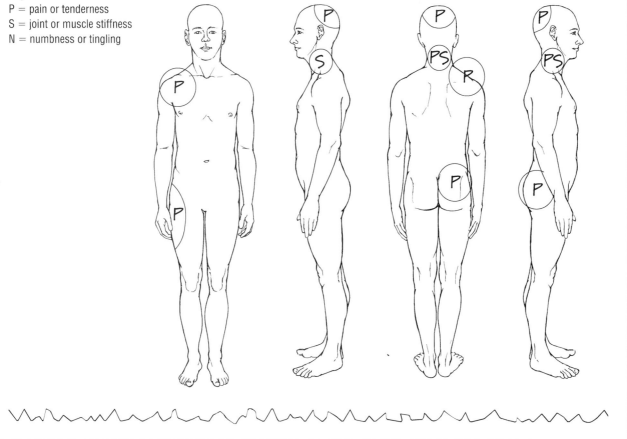

102

HANDS HEAL:
COMMUNICATION,
DOCUMENTATION,
AND INSURANCE BILLING
FOR MANUAL THERAPISTS

nervous. Gather the salient pieces of information on a form every 30 days or as needed to update you on the details of their health. Once the current information is recorded and reviewed, a few brief questions may suffice to assess their progress and prepare for the session.

Analog Scales

An **analog scale** is a method of measurement that uses a line of continuum and places one extreme on one end and the opposite extreme on the other end. For example, on this form the patient's pain or loss of function is measured. On the line of continuum, pain-free is at one end and debilitating pain is at the other end. The patient places a mark at a point between the two extremes that best represents how he or she feels at the moment (see Figure 5-8).

Analog scales are reliable and more accurate than numerical rating scales, such as 0 to 10. The literature suggests that numbers can be remembered from session to session, which decreases the validity of the responses. A malingerer may remember a previous response and manipulate the answer accordingly.[1] It is cumbersome to use these scales with every subjective complaint or objective finding. A verbal response is indicated during the session using a number scale (0 to10) or the word *values* (mild, moderate, severe). Used on the health report and filled out prior to the session, the analog scale is fast and effective, and it addresses the two primary concerns in health care outcomes: function and pain.

To use the analog scale, the patient simply places a mark on the lines to indicate his or her pain level at that moment. The line represents a continuum ranging from pain-free to unbearable pain or from full activity to no activity. The line is 10 centimeters long, making it easy to score the patient's mark on a scale of 0 to 10. The patient does not know the rating system. On a scale of pain-free to unbearable pain, for example, pain-free is given the value 0, and unbearable pain is given the value 10. The mark is placed between the two values, and the measurement is assigned a value 0 to 10. The measurement is the score. After the session, measure the mark on the line and record the score in the comments section.

TIMING AND APPLICATION

Patients with injuries or chronic conditions should complete the health report at the initial session and at each reevaluation session—about every 30 days or every 6 to 8 sessions. If the patient has no subjective complaints, such as pain, loss of function, stiff joints, or neuropathies, simply include the report in the packet of intake forms at the initial visit and the annual updates to ensure that you have all the health information you need.

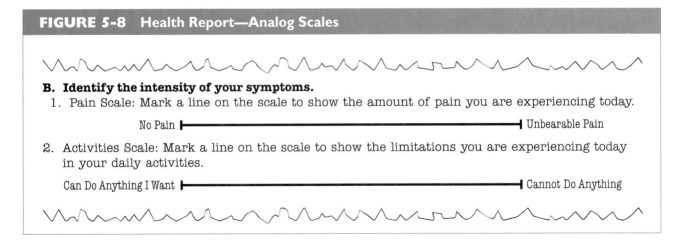

FIGURE 5-8   Health Report—Analog Scales

B. Identify the intensity of your symptoms.
1. Pain Scale: Mark a line on the scale to show the amount of pain you are experiencing today.

   No Pain |———————————————————————————————————————| Unbearable Pain

2. Activities Scale: Mark a line on the scale to show the limitations you are experiencing today in your daily activities.

   Can Do Anything I Want |———————————————————————————————| Cannot Do Anything

If motivating yourself to chart is an issue, use the form to ease into the habit of regular documentation by having the patient do most of the charting for you! Use a two-sided copy of the health report. Before the session, have the patient draw on the human figures and mark the analog scale on the front side of the form. Use the comments section to record your treatment notes. After the session, have the patient draw on the figures and mark the analog scale on the back of the form. Use the comments section on the back to record self-care exercises for the patient and any notes regarding a treatment plan for the next session. This shortcut is not recommended for insurance patients or for long-term care, but it is a good way to get started. As you proceed through this book, you will discover the limitations of using this form for all your daily charting needs, but if necessary, begin with the health report for your daily notetaking.

Pain Questionnaires

Research shows that pain questionnaires are a reliable and effective tool for measuring the extent and nature of a patient's injury and improvement with treatment (refer to Wise One Speaks: The Reliability of Pain Questionnaires in this chapter). Proof of significant injury is provided through the disability percentage. The treatment plan is justified with ongoing use of the questionnaires.

Pain questionnaires consist of questions regarding the patient's ability to sit, stand, wash, dress, walk, sleep, read, drive, travel, work, concentrate, and participate in recreation. The patient answers the questions by checking one of six options provided (Revised Oswestry and Vernon-Mior) or by circling one of five numbers (Functional Rating Index). The manual therapist collects the form and scores the answers using a disability percentage scale. Over time, the scores can be compared and progress can be concluded based on the change in scores.

Several pain questionnaires are available. Three are presented in this text: (1) the Revised Oswestry Low Back Pain and Disability Index, (2) the Vernon-Mior Neck Pain and Disability Index, and (3) the Functional Rating Index (see Appendix B for blank forms). All three indices are backed by strong research. Two are almost identical in content but focus on different areas of the body—Oswestry on the lowback and Vernon-Mior on the neck. Both can be used creatively for other areas of dysfunction—the Vernon-Mior for the upper extremities and the Oswestry for the lower extremities. The Functional Rating Index is for general use and does not ask questions specific to areas of the body. It made its debut recently in the health care industry and is quickly becoming the preferred instrument for measuring pain and function.[6] See Figure 5-9 (from Freise RJ, Menke JM. Functional rating index: A new valid and reliable instrument to measure the magnitude of clinical change in spinal conditions. Spine 2001;26:78–87).

When used throughout a treatment series, pain questionnaires can record functional progress. A progressive increase in functional abilities throughout the treatment assists in demonstrating that the treatment is reasonable and necessary. Functional progress reassures the patient, the referring HCP, and the medical-legal team that the treatment is returning the patient to pre-injury status.

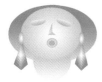

WISE ONE SPEAKS
The Reliability of Pain Questionnaires

Traditionally, objective measurements of soft tissue injury, such as palpable spasm and loss of lordotic curve on x-ray, have been thought reliable as "hard" evidence when measuring the extent of injury and the effectiveness of treatment. At the same time, subjective pain and function assessments were criticized as "soft" evidence. However, subjective pain assessments as measured through time-tested pain questionnaires have gained substantial acceptance in use and are now considered "hard evidence."[6,7,8,9]

A pain questionnaire, when used together with objective physical measurements, is considered the most reliable assessment of function and disability in the area in which there is no universal norm. One such pain questionnaire is the Oswestry Index, which was developed in 1976 in a hospital unit in Oswestry, Shropshire, England. It scores patients' disability in 10 different areas including intensity of pain; ability to lift, walk, sit, and stand; ability for self-care; and impact on social interactions, sex life, sleep, and travel.

Studies have confirmed that the Oswestry Index has good validity (scores improve as patient disability lessens) and reliability (scores are consistent when answered on different occasions by a patient remaining in the same condition).[9] After many refinements, this questionnaire is widely used in both research and clinical practice in Britain. Self-rating disability questionnaires are also in wide use in North America.

The Functional Rating Index is a relatively new pain questionnaire and is getting recognition as a reliable, valid, and responsive instrument. Also, some claim that it is superior to other instruments with regard to clinical utility.[6]

As health care providers know, all tools that assist in documenting the nature and extent of a patient's injury and the patient's improvement with treatment are vital. A well-formatted and consistently used pain questionnaire offers many benefits, including:

• Provides a reliable means to measure change in the patient's physical condition
• Assists in documenting the nature and extent of injury and need for care
• Illustrates improvements in function resulting from treatment
• Supports the reasonableness and necessity of treatment
• Satisfies the provider's duty to monitor changes in subjective and objective findings
• Aids the provider in writing reports or testifying at depositions or trial
• Aids the provider in assessing residual limitations related to activities of daily living

TIMING AND APPLICATION

Pain questionnaires are easy to use and involve a minimal time commitment. There is no need to use all three; simply choose the one most appropriate for the patient's presenting condition. You or your staff may provide the questionnaire to patients at the initial session and again at every reevaluation session—every 30 days or 6 to 8 sessions. The patient fills it out before the session begins. You collect the form, check it for completeness, score it, review it, and file it in the patient's chart.

FIGURE 5-9 Functional Rating Index

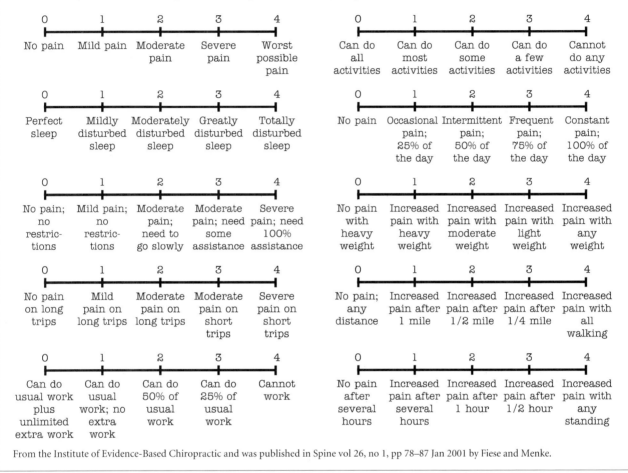

FUNCTIONAL RATING INDEX

Name _____ ID#/DOB _____ Date _____

In order to properly assess your condition, we must understand how much your _____ have affected your ability to manage everyday activities. For each item below, please circle the number which most closely describes your condition right now.

0	1	2	3	4
No pain	Mild pain	Moderate pain	Severe pain	Worst possible pain

0	1	2	3	4
Can do all activities	Can do most activities	Can do some activities	Can do a few activities	Cannot do any activities

0	1	2	3	4
Perfect sleep	Mildly disturbed sleep	Moderately disturbed sleep	Greatly disturbed sleep	Totally disturbed sleep

0	1	2	3	4
No pain	Occasional pain; 25% of the day	Intermittent pain; 50% of the day	Frequent pain; 75% of the day	Constant pain; 100% of the day

0	1	2	3	4
No pain; no restrictions	Mild pain; no restrictions	Moderate pain; need to go slowly	Moderate pain; need some assistance	Severe pain; need 100% assistance

0	1	2	3	4
No pain with heavy weight	Increased pain with heavy weight	Increased pain with moderate weight	Increased pain with light weight	Increased pain with any weight

0	1	2	3	4
No pain on long trips	Mild pain on long trips	Moderate pain on long trips	Moderate pain on short trips	Severe pain on short trips

0	1	2	3	4
No pain; any distance	Increased pain after 1 mile	Increased pain after 1/2 mile	Increased pain after 1/4 mile	Increased pain with all walking

0	1	2	3	4
Can do usual work plus unlimited extra work	Can do usual work; no extra work	Can do 50% of usual work	Can do 25% of usual work	Cannot work

0	1	2	3	4
No pain after several hours	Increased pain after several hours	Increased pain after 1 hour	Increased pain after 1/2 hour	Increased pain with any standing

From the Institute of Evidence-Based Chiropractic and was published in Spine vol 26, no 1, pp 78–87 Jan 2001 by Fiese and Menke.

To use the pain questionnaires, instruct your patient to read the instructions at the top and to fill out the form completely. If a section is left incomplete, return it to the patient for completion. Avoid discussing with the patient the reason for using the pain questionnaire. Advising patients on how the process works may influence responses on subsequent questionnaires. You may reiterate that the questions should be answered according to the patient's current condition—how they feel right now. Remember, timing can be a factor when filling out these forms. For example: If the form is completed on a Friday after a long work week, the answers may be different than if the form is completed on a Monday after a relaxing weekend. Keep this in mind when scheduling your reevaluation sessions.

Score, review, and look for areas of impaired function. If there is no loss of function indicated on the health information form, you may chose to omit the pain questionnaire from the pack of reevaluation forms for that particular patient. If the patient has no functional limitations, simply include a questionnaire in the packet of intake forms at the initial visit and at the annual updates to ensure that you have all the health information you need.

106

HANDS HEAL:
COMMUNICATION,
DOCUMENTATION,
AND INSURANCE BILLING
FOR MANUAL THERAPISTS

SCORING THE OSWESTRY AND VERNON-MIOR PAIN QUESTIONNAIRES

To score the questionnaires, a value is assigned to each answer. There are 10 sections per questionnaire and six possible answers in each section. The top answer has a pain value of 0. The bottom answer has a pain value of 5. Assign each section a score of 0 to 5, depending on the answer.

Add all 10 scores together. The highest possible score (worst pain) would be 5 for each section, or a total score of 50 (5 x 10 = 50). Multiply this number by two to reach the overall rating of disability, or (50 x 2 = 100%). This number is your disability percentage (see Figure 5-10)

The rating scale is as follows:

0 to 20%	Minimal disability
20 to 40%	Moderate disability
40 to 60%	Severe disability
60 to 80%	Crippled
80 to 100%	Bedbound or exaggerating

Injury Information Form
CONTENT

The health information form is sufficient for wellness care and most illnesses or injuries. Additional information is necessary when a patient has been involved in an on-the-job injury or a car collision. Different types of insurance cover different kinds of injuries or benefits. Workers' compensation covers on-the-job injuries and illnesses. Private and group insurance (through an employer) cover general injuries and illnesses. **Personal Injury Protection (PIP) coverage** includes injuries related to MVCs. In-depth documentation is recommended to address the specific needs of litigation and of national and state workers' compensation regulations.

As with any insurance case, documentation is vital. The primary difference between recordkeeping for cash-paying patients and for patients with insurance reimbursement is that care can be discontinued and payment can be reversed or even denied by the insurance company based on the documentation.[1] The injury information form (see Appendix B for a blank form) records specific data that may assist in substantiating patients' claims and in providing information required by insurance companies to continue coverage for your services. The mechanics of the injury, symptoms, daily activities affected by the injuries, and any possible health complications resulting from the incident must be documented. The goal is to gather information to substantiate that the injuries are significant and were incurred as a result of the incident and, thus, justify care.

Personal Identification and Contact Information

The five identifiers—name, date, date of birth, insurance identification or claim number, and date of injury—should appear at the top of each form. The address and phone numbers are not included, as this form is used with the health information form.

FIGURE 5-10 Pain Questionnaire with Disability Percentage

Helena LaLuna, CR
123 Sun Moon and Stars Drive
Capitol Hill, WA   98119
Tel   206 555 4446

Ⓡ shoulder   (revised Vernon-Mior)
NECK PAⓍN & DISABILITY INDEX

Patient Name _Zamora Hostetter_   Date _4-4-04_

Date of Injury _3-31-04_   ID#/DOB _C98-7654321_

This questionnaire has been designed to give the health care provider information as to how your neck pain has affected your ability to manage everyday life. Please answer every section and mark in each section only the **ONE** box which applies to you. We realize you may consider that two of the statements in any one section relate to you, but please just mark the box which most closely describes your problem today.

3 **Section 1 - Pain Intensity**
- ☐ I have no pain at the moment.
- ☐ The pain is very mild at the moment.
- ☐ The pain is moderate at the moment.
- ☒ The pain is fairly severe at the moment.
- ☐ The pain is very severe at the moment.
- ☐ The pain is the worst imaginable at the moment.

3 **Section 2 - Personal Care**
(washing, dressing, etc.)
- ☐ I can look after myself normally without causing pain.
- ☐ I can look after myself normally but it causes extra pain.
- ☐ It is painful to look after myself and I am slow and careful.
- ☒ I need some help but manage most of my personal care.
- ☐ I need help every day in most aspects of self care.
- ☐ I do not get dressed, I wash myself with difficulty and I stay in bed.

5 **Section 3 - Lifting**
- ☐ I can lift heavy weights without extra pain.
- ☐ I can lift heavy weights but it causes extra pain.
- ☐ Pain prevents me from lifting heavy weights off the floor, but I can manage if they are conveniently positioned, e.g. on a table.
- ☐ Pain prevents me from lifting heavy weights, but I can manage light to medium weights if they are conveniently positioned.
- ☐ I can lift very light weights.
- ☒ I cannot lift or carry anything at all.

1 **Section 4 - Reading**
- ☐ I can read as much as I want to with no pain in my neck.
- ☒ I can read as much as I want to with slight pain in my neck.
- ☐ I can read as much as I want to with moderate pain in my neck.
- ☐ I can't read as much as I want to because of moderate pain in my neck.
- ☐ I can hardly read at all because of severe pain in my neck.
- ☐ I cannot read at all.

3 **Section 5 - Headaches**
- ☐ I have no headaches at all.
- ☐ I have slight headaches which come infrequently.
- ☐ I have moderate headaches which come infrequently.
- ☒ I have moderate headaches which come frequently.
- ☐ I have severe headaches which come frequently.
- ☐ I have headaches almost all of the time.

1 **Section 6 - Concentration**
- ☐ I can concentrate fully when I want to with no difficulty.
- ☒ I can concentrate fully when I want to with slight difficulty.
- ☐ I have a fair degree of difficulty in concentrating when I want to.
- ☐ I have a lot of difficulty concentrating when I want to.
- ☐ I have a great deal of difficulty in concentrating when I want to.
- ☐ I cannot concentrate at all.

5 **Section 7 - Work**
- ☐ I can do as much work as I want to.
- ☐ I can do my usual work but no more.
- ☐ I can do most of my usual work but no more.
- ☐ I cannot do my usual work.
- ☐ I can hardly do any work at all.
- ☒ I can't do any work at all.

1 **Section 8 - Driving**
- ☐ I can drive my car without any neck pain.
- ☒ I can drive my car as long as I want with slight pain in my neck.
- ☐ I can drive my car as long as I want with moderate pain in my neck.
- ☐ I can't drive my car as long as I want because of moderate pain in my neck.
- ☐ I can hardly drive at all because of severe pain in my neck.
- ☐ I can't drive my car at all.

4 **Section 9 - Sleeping**
- ☐ I have no trouble sleeping.
- ☐ My sleep is slightly disturbed (less than 1 hour sleepless).
- ☐ My sleep is mildly disturbed (1-2 hours sleepless).
- ☐ My sleep is moderately disturbed (2-3 hours sleepless).
- ☒ My sleep is greatly disturbed (3-5 hours sleepless).
- ☐ My sleep is completely disturbed (5-7 hours sleepless).

30 x 2 = 60%

4 **Section 10 - Recreation**
- ☐ I am able to engage in all my recreational activities with no neck pain at all.
- ☐ I am able to engage in all my recreational activities with some pain in my neck.
- ☐ I am able to engage in most, but not all of my usual recreational activities because of pain in my neck.
- ☐ I am able to engage in a few of my usual recreation activities because of pain in my neck.
- ☒ I can hardly do any recreational activities because of pain in my neck.
- ☐ I can't do recreational activities at all.

Signature _Zamora Hostetter_   Date _4-4-04_

108

HANDS HEAL:
COMMUNICATION,
DOCUMENTATION,
AND INSURANCE BILLING
FOR MANUAL THERAPISTS

General Injury Information

The first page of the injury information form is filled out by people with any of the three types of injuries: on-the-job, MVCs, and other personal injuries. The second page is only for people involved in MVCs. For a personal injury case, differentiate between an MVC and other types of injury. Examples of a personal injury case other than a car collision include patients injured after falling off the roof of a house while cleaning the gutters, slipping on a commercial premise, or being impaled by debris flying from a construction site while walking nearby.

Type of Injury

On-the-job injuries and MVCs typically result in musculoskeletal dysfunction and therefore are common in manual therapy practices. Musculoskeletal complaints are the primary reason people seek manual therapy.[10] Differentiate between workers' compensation claims and personal injury cases on the injury information form.

Establish whether a record of the incident is on file somewhere other than in your patient's chart. Such records are helpful in substantiating particulars surrounding the injury. For example, a person involved in an MVC might have a police report on file or someone injured on the job may have filed an incident report. Both may apply if the person had an MVC while on the job. If a police report has been filed, request a copy.

Description of the Injury

Information provided by the patient about the onset of the injury might explain the presence and severity of symptoms and functional limitations (see Figure 5-11). On-the-job injuries and personal injuries other than car collisions vary widely, making it impossible to standardize the questions about onset. Prompt those patients to be as specific as possible when describing how the injury or injuries occurred.

The second page of this form provides a list of standard questions for recording specific information about the mechanics of MVCs. However, it is important to focus on how the patient got hurt, rather than how the collision occurred. The questions on the injury information form must be stated clearly, and you need to review the answers thoroughly with the patient to ensure that the answers are accurate and suitable.

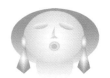

STORY TELLER
Mechanisms of Injury

Describing the mechanisms of injury helps explain the type and extent of injury. In the example presented in Figure 5-11, Zamora fell on a hard surface. This injury is more damaging than if she had fallen on grass or other bags of rice. As a result, the severity of her injuries may be substantial. Her arms, hips, back, and head hit an unforgiving tile floor, complicating the overall injury. How she made contact with the ground may explain the location of her shoulder injury. Encourage the patient to describe the details about how the injury took place, including the environment and the interplay between the body and the objects involved, in addition to the obvious symptoms or physical expressions of the injury.

(Continued)

STORY TELLER   *(Continued)*

Describe the details of the injury, but avoid documenting the events that led up to the injury. At the massage clinic, we treated a patient who had been hit by a car while riding her bicycle. She was meticulous on the injury information form in describing the collision. Something that occurred in a fraction of a second seemed to happen in slow motion from the patient's perspective. She described it as it had appeared to her, with no reference to actual time. Unfortunately, the way in which she recorded her description of the accident made it appear that she had time to prevent it. This impression complicated her personal injury case, making it difficult to receive reimbursement for her health care. Her case went to court.

The lesson in this experience was to let the police report speak to the incident and use the injury information form to describe the injury itself. Had she focused on the mechanics of the injury—how she fell and what body parts hit the pavement—rather than on how the car approached her and what went through her mind leading up to the impact, she might have been able to settle out of court quickly and without disruption in medical payments.

Symptoms

Have the patient record all symptoms since the incident. Establish a time line for the onset of the injuries. Not all symptoms surface immediately, and some patients take weeks to seek manual therapy. The time line will help chart the progression of the injuries and the healing (see Figure 5-12).

Effect of Injuries on Daily Activities

An easy way to determine whether an injury is affecting the patient's quality of life is to look at the patient's ability to function in day-to-day activities (see Figure 5-13). If the patient's ability to earn a living is impaired, the injury is significant. Such an impairment may include loss of time at work, restrictions of responsibilities (such as assignment to light duty), and loss of productivity. Documentation of changes in work-related activities is critical with many claims, particularly ones involving on-the-job injuries.

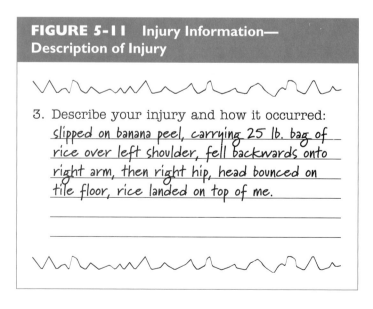

FIGURE 5-11   Injury Information— Description of Injury

3. Describe your injury and how it occurred:
slipped on banana peel, carrying 25 lb. bag of rice over left shoulder, fell backwards onto right arm, then right hip, head bounced on tile floor, rice landed on top of me.

110

HANDS HEAL:
COMMUNICATION,
DOCUMENTATION,
AND INSURANCE BILLING
FOR MANUAL THERAPISTS

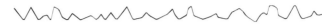

FIGURE 5-12   Injury Information— Symptom Time Line

4. Describe how you felt during and immediately after the injury: shoulder "popped"–immediate pain, head throbbing

Later that same day: backache

The next day: neck stiff, back stiff, can't use right arm at all

The next week: N/A

The next month: N/A

Describe any bruises, cuts, or abrasions as a result of the injury: bruise on right hip

FIGURE 5-13   Injury Information—Functional Limitations

7. What are your work responsibilities? cooking, prep, stocking supplies

Which work activities are affected by this injury? everything

Have your work responsibilities changed as a result of this injury?   ☒ Yes   ☐ No
Explain   unable to work

What other daily activities are affected by this injury?   everything using my right arm

Activities other than work are also important to one's quality of life. Inability to participate normally in exercise, self-care, and household responsibilities should be recorded. Anything that detracts from the patient's quality of life may be included for personal injuries and for injuries covered by major medical plans. Focus on work-related impairments for workers' compensation cases. Follow up with a pain questionnaire every 30 days or 6 to 8 sessions to note changes in the patient's ability to function at work and home.

Adjunctive Care

Have the patient list all care received for the injury (see Figure 5-14). This is helpful information for communicating with the health care team and assists in reducing the chance of duplicating treatment and in coordinating treatment plans. Record the primary HCP's diagnosis. You can then refer to the diagnosis in your charts.

Typically, insurance peer reviewers red-flag a case whenever manual therapy is the only source of treatment, unless the manual therapist has primary care status. The combination of allopathic and complementary care is more acceptable. Noting additional care may help justify the treatment and speed up claims processing.

Pre-existing Conditions

Establish the presence of pre-existing conditions right away. Avoid the unpleasant surprise of the insurance company disallowing payment for services because the symptoms treated were present before the accident.

The information recorded here and on the health information form can help establish that current symptoms, even when associated with pre-existing conditions, are related to the collision (see Figure 5-15). The information in this section will be compiled with the information in the health history section of the health information form. If the documents state that none of the symptoms were present before or that the pre-existing symptoms were exacerbated by the current injury, it is easier for the attorney or claims adjuster to conclude that the symptoms were a direct result of the collision or work injury.

FIGURE 5-14 Injury Information— Adjunctive Care

8. Did you go to the emergency room?
X Yes   ☐ No

Were you hospitalized?   ☐ Yes   X No

List the health care providers who have treated you for this injury, the type of treatment provided, and their diagnosis.

ER—separated shoulder—sling

DC—whiplash, spinal subluxations, muscle

spasms—adjust, ice

112

HANDS HEAL:
COMMUNICATION,
DOCUMENTATION,
AND INSURANCE BILLING
FOR MANUAL THERAPISTS

FIGURE 5-15 Injury Information—
Pre-existing Conditions

9. Have you ever had this type of injury
   before? ☐ Yes   ☒ No

   Explain _____

   _____

   Did you have any physical complaints
   before the injury? ☐ Yes   ☒ No

   Explain _____

   _____

   Do you have any illnesses or previous
   injuries that may have been affected by
   this injury? ☐ Yes   ☒ No

   Explain _____

   _____

Motor Vehicle Collision Information

Mechanisms of Whiplash

The second page of the injury information form highlights the mechanisms that influence the severity of a whiplash injury (see Figure 5-16). Severity of injury is critical for establishing whether extensive, ongoing treatment is required in order to return the patient to pre-injury status. Some research studies suggest that people heal from MVCs in 6 to 8 weeks, regardless of treatment. This may be true for very minor soft tissue injuries, but not for more complex sprain-strain syndromes or injuries presenting with neurological dysfunction.[1]

Symptoms

Symptoms are gathered on several intake forms. The symptoms checklist on page 2 of the injury information form are specific to head trauma sustained in whiplash injuries and may indicate neurological damage. This information influences the type of care you provide and the type of referrals you suggest, but it generally does not come up in an interview unless specifically asked. Loss of memory is not as obvious as the pounding headache or the bruises. The patient may forget to tell you about them unless prompted on the form.

Other questions about symptoms are more general than the head injury questions, but they also concern symptoms common with whiplash trauma. Breathing difficulties are often associated with seatbelt trauma. Sleeping comfort may be used later in the SOAP charts as a tool for mapping progress. Track the number of hours of restful sleep, the number of times waking (and why), and how the patient feels upon rising to show the progression of health.

External proof of impact is concrete data. Record any visible trauma. Take pictures of bruises, cuts, and abrasions.

FIGURE 5-16 Injury Information—MVC

John Olson, LMP, GCFP
345 Moon River Rd. Ste. 6
Minnehaha, MN   55987
TEL   612 555 9889

HANDS HEAL

INJURY INFORMATION page 2

B. Motor Vehicle Collision Information

1. Did the police arrive at the crash site?
   ☒ Yes   ☐ No

2. How was your vehicle hit?
   ☒ Rear end   ☐ Head on   ☐ Side swipe
   OR Did your vehicle hit another vehicle/object?
   ☐ Rear end   ☐ Head on   ☐ Side swipe
   If you were hit from behind, was your vehicle pushed forward upon impact?
   ☒ Yes   ☐ No   If yes, how much?
   about 50 feet

   Did your vehicle hit anything else after the initial impact?   ☐ Yes   ☐ No
   Explain _____
   _____
   _____
   _____

3. Were you at a stop or moving at the time of impact?   ☐ Stopped   ☒ Moving
   If you were stopped, was your foot on the brake?   ☐ Yes   ☐ No
   If you were moving, were you:
   ☐ Increasing speed
   ☒ Decreasing speed
   ☐ Traveling at a steady speed

   Was the other vehicle moving at the time of impact?   ☒ Yes   ☐ No
   If yes, was it: ☒ Increasing speed
   ☐ Decreasing speed   ☐ Traveling at a steady speed

4. Where were you seated in the vehicle?
   passenger side–front seat
   _____

5. Which way was your head facing upon impact?
   facing nephew–driver, we were talking
   _____

6. Were you aware of the approaching vehicle or did the impact catch you by surprise?
   ☐ Aware   ☒ Surprise

7. Did you lose consciousness?
   ☐ Yes   ☒ No

8. Were you wearing a seat belt?   ☐ No
   ☐ Lap belt   ☐ Shoulder harness   ☒ Both

9. Is your vehicle equipped with an airbag?
   ☐ Yes ☒ No
   Did it activate?   ☐ Yes   ☐ No

10. Is the top of your head rest:
    ☐ Above your head   ☒ Below your head
    Does your head touch the head rest?
    ☐ Yes   ☒ No
    If no, how far in front of the head rest is your head?
    a few inches

11. What were the road conditions?
    ☐ Wet   ☐ Dry   ☒ Icy   ☐ Oily

12. What type of vehicle were you in? (make, model, year)
    '82 Honda Accord
    What type of vehicle hit you? (make, model, year)
    '91 Ford F250 Truck

13. Did any part of your body come into contact with the vehicle?   ☐ Yes   ☒ No
    Explain _____
    _____
    _____

    Did any parts of the vehicle break?
    ☒ Yes   ☐ No
    Explain _fender damage_
    _____
    _____

14. Check all of the following symptoms that you have experienced since the collision:
    ☐ Loss of memory _____
    ☐ Loss of balance _____
    ☒ Visual disturbances _eye strain_
    ☐ Hearing difficulties _____
    ☒ Difficulty breathing _tight & painful_
    ☒ Sleep disturbances _pain keeps me up_

15. Anything else you want to tell me about the accident or how you feel?
    _____
    _____
    _____

Patient Signature _Darnel G. Washington_   Date _2-6-04_

113

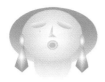

At the massage clinic, we had a patient who, after five car accidents in eight years, began taking public transportation. When she stepped off the bus one day, the bus hit her. Bruises marked by the headlights were imprinted on her chest and abdomen. Some pictures are worth a thousand words.

Space is left at the end of the form for the patient to add comments. It is impossible to cover all possibilities in a standardized form. Additional pertinent information unique to the individual may be written in this space.

TIMING AND APPLICATION

The patient completes this form before the initial session begins. The injury information form may accompany the health information form in a packet of intake forms sent to the patient the week before the first treatment. The patient fills out the forms at home and brings them to the office. The injury information form needs to be completed only once per incident.

All patients fill out a health information form. Personal injury and workers' compensation patients also fill out the injury information form, but only those involved in an MVC need to fill out the second page of the injury information form. Keep the health information and the injury information forms separate, so other patients are not burdened with unnecessary paperwork.

Injury information is useful in the interview and in the development of a treatment plan. The information recorded is vital to workers' compensation and personal injury cases and is used to substantiate the injury and justify the treatment.

Billing Information Form
CONTENT

The billing information form (see Appendix B for blank forms) states your billing policies and gathers financial information necessary to verify benefits and to authorize treatment and is used to complete the top half of the HCFA 1500—the standard billing form for insurance companies (see Figure 5-17). Information on this form includes:

- Personal identification and contact information—patient and insured—together with information found on the health information
- Insurance information—specific to workers' compensation, personal injury, and private health insurance
- Assignment of benefits
- Release of medical records
- Statement of financial responsibility

See Chapter 8 for instructions on filling out the remainder of the HCFA 1500 form.

Personal Identification and Contact Information

All pertinent contact information for the insured, the insurance company and adjuster, the attorney, and the primary care provider is included on the billing information form,

FIGURE 5-17 HCFA 1500—Patient and Insurance Information

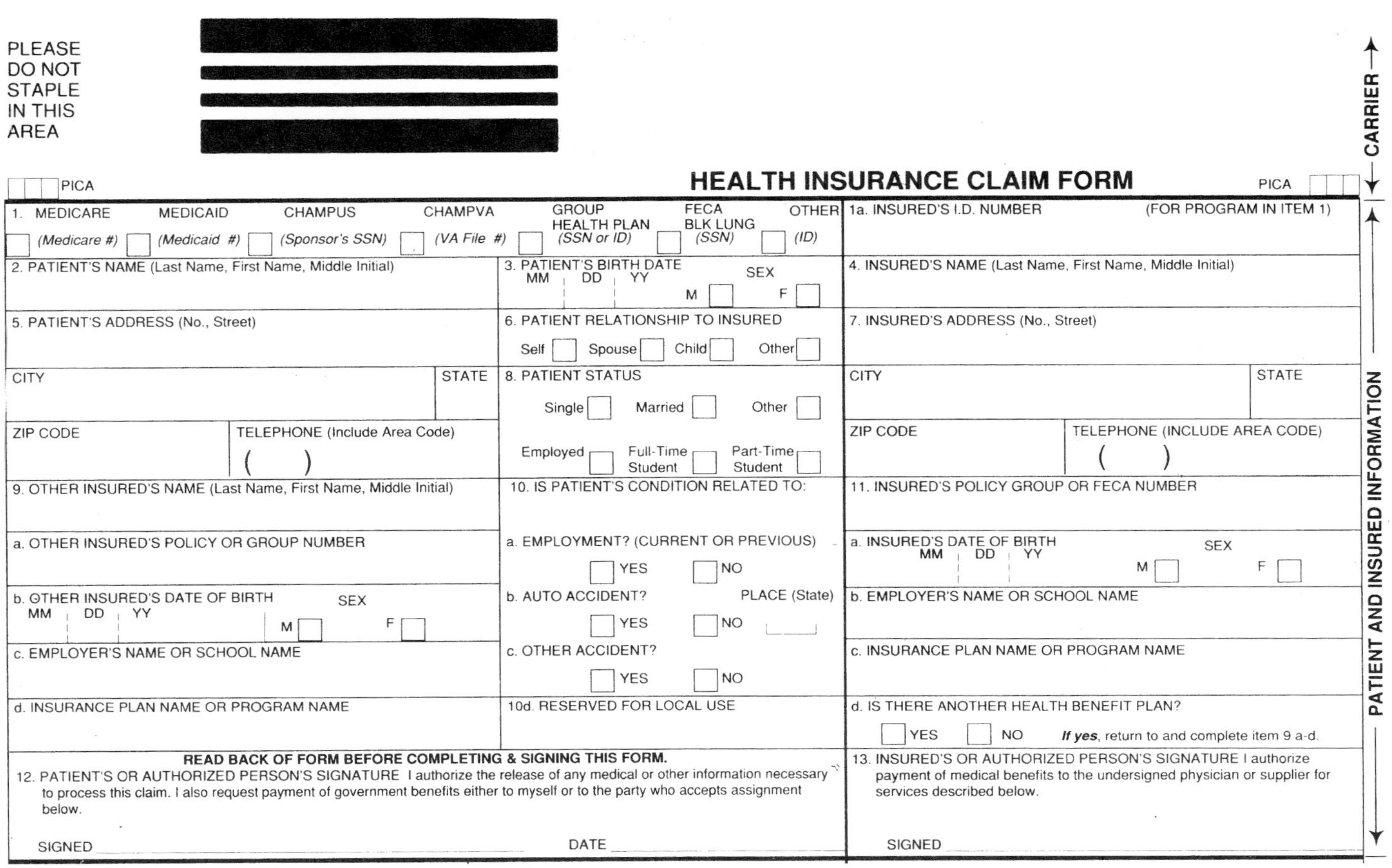

PLEASE
DO NOT
STAPLE
IN THIS
AREA

HEALTH INSURANCE CLAIM FORM

PICA

| PICA | | | | | | | |

PATIENT AND INSURED INFORMATION

CARRIER

1. MEDICARE (Medicare #)　MEDICAID (Medicaid #)　CHAMPUS (Sponsor's SSN)　CHAMPVA (VA File #)　GROUP HEALTH PLAN (SSN or ID)　FECA BLK LUNG (SSN)　OTHER (ID)

1a. INSURED'S I.D. NUMBER　(FOR PROGRAM IN ITEM 1)

2. PATIENT'S NAME (Last Name, First Name, Middle Initial)

3. PATIENT'S BIRTH DATE
MM　DD　YY
SEX
M　F

4. INSURED'S NAME (Last Name, First Name, Middle Initial)

5. PATIENT'S ADDRESS (No., Street)

6. PATIENT RELATIONSHIP TO INSURED
Self　Spouse　Child　Other

7. INSURED'S ADDRESS (No., Street)

CITY　STATE

8. PATIENT STATUS
Single　Married　Other
Employed　Full-Time Student　Part-Time Student

CITY　STATE

ZIP CODE　TELEPHONE (Include Area Code)
(　)

ZIP CODE　TELEPHONE (INCLUDE AREA CODE)
(　)

9. OTHER INSURED'S NAME (Last Name, First Name, Middle Initial)

10. IS PATIENT'S CONDITION RELATED TO:

11. INSURED'S POLICY GROUP OR FECA NUMBER

a. OTHER INSURED'S POLICY OR GROUP NUMBER

a. EMPLOYMENT? (CURRENT OR PREVIOUS)
YES　NO

a. INSURED'S DATE OF BIRTH
MM　DD　YY
SEX
M　F

b. OTHER INSURED'S DATE OF BIRTH
MM　DD　YY
SEX
M　F

b. AUTO ACCIDENT?
YES　NO
PLACE (State)

b. EMPLOYER'S NAME OR SCHOOL NAME

c. EMPLOYER'S NAME OR SCHOOL NAME

c. OTHER ACCIDENT?
YES　NO

c. INSURANCE PLAN NAME OR PROGRAM NAME

d. INSURANCE PLAN NAME OR PROGRAM NAME

10d. RESERVED FOR LOCAL USE

d. IS THERE ANOTHER HEALTH BENEFIT PLAN?
YES　NO　*If yes,* return to and complete item 9 a-d.

READ BACK OF FORM BEFORE COMPLETING & SIGNING THIS FORM.
12. PATIENT'S OR AUTHORIZED PERSON'S SIGNATURE I authorize the release of any medical or other information necessary to process this claim. I also request payment of government benefits either to myself or to the party who accepts assignment below.

SIGNED　DATE

13. INSURED'S OR AUTHORIZED PERSON'S SIGNATURE I authorize payment of medical benefits to the undersigned physician or supplier for services described below.

SIGNED

115

116

HANDS HEAL:
COMMUNICATION,
DOCUMENTATION,
AND INSURANCE BILLING
FOR MANUAL THERAPISTS

unless it has been recorded on the health information form. The HCP listed on the health information form may not be the primary provider for the current injury. For example: The patient's general practitioner may be listed on the health information form, but the patient's chiropractor is the referring HCP for the motor vehicle case. If the patient was injured in a motor vehicle collision, an attorney may have been retained. The attorney may monitor the bills and collect and send bills from all the health care providers to the insurance company, or simply wish to stay apprised of the billing status. Know where to send the bills and to whom. Having a direct contact expedites the payment process.

Billing Information

The billing information form records data about the patient's benefits, depending on the types of insurance coverage (see Figure 5-18). Here are three examples with the same patient but different insurance scenarios:

> Example 1: The patient is Sarah Lobos. She has private health insurance through her work. She is the patient and the insured.
>
> Example 2: Sarah is the patient. Her partner, Jackie Shenge, has insurance for both of them through her city job. Section A of the billing information is for Sarah's information, and sections B and C are for Jackie's information.
>
> Example 3: Sarah was injured in a motor vehicle accident while driving her insured car. She is the patient and the insured, and her car insurance information would be recorded as the primary insurance information. If her car insurance does not cover medical expenses or her injuries require coverage beyond her car insurance plan, the secondary coverage is Jackie's health insurance (see Chapter 8 for in-depth information on insurance coverage).

Assignment of Benefits and Release of Medical Records

The upper portion of the HCFA 1500 billing form is for patient identification and insurance information, as well as for two signatures of the patient: one to authorize the insurance company to pay the provider directly (assignment of benefits) and the other to authorize the provider to release medical records to the insurance company for the purpose of processing claims (release of medical records). It is acceptable to obtain the patient's signature and keep it on file rather than have the patient sign every billing form you send out. The signed billing information form (see Figure 5-19) serves this purpose.

An attorney retained for litigation in a personal injury insurance case may ask the patient to sign an exclusive medical release form that restricts the release of health care information to the attorney only (refer to Figure 3-3 for an example). This means that the signature on all medical release forms, including the one on our form, is null and void. The intent here is to prevent the insurance company of the at-fault party from obtaining information without the knowledge and consent of the attorney. Verify the date of the patient's signature and compare it with the one on the attorney's form before sending out information.

Financial Responsibility

It is appropriate and legal to remind patients that they are financially responsible for your services, even though the insurance company is expected to pay for the treatments. Ultimately, the patient is responsible for the balance due if the insurance reimbursement is

FIGURE 5-18 Billing Information—Insurance Information

Patient Information

Is patient's condition related to:

☒ auto collision—In what state? __MN__
☐ other accident _____
☐ employment ☐ illness

Patient status: ☒ male ☐ female
☐ single ☒ married/partnered ☐ other

Patient relationship to insured
☐ self ☐ spouse/partner ☐ child ☒ other

Insured's Information (if other than patient)

Name __James Washington__
Address __32 W. Holden Court__
City _____Minnehaha_____ State __MN__ Zip __55987__
Phone: __612-555-7654__
Date of birth __5-31-60__
Sex: ☒ Male ☐ Female
Employer's Name or School Name _____
__Maad Printing and Design__

Insurance Information

Insurance plan name or program name: __Farmington States__
Member ID#: __989-76-6789__ Group #: _____
Customer service phone #: __612-555-7887__ Date and time you called: __2-6-04__
Name of customer service representative: __Clifford Glens__
Insurance claim address: __P.O. Box 3778 O-Claire__ State: __MN__ Zip: __55987__
Does the plan include a Physical Medicine and Rehabilitation benefit? ☒ Yes ☐ No
Who may provide the services? ☒ Massage Therapist ☐ Physical Therapist ☐ Other
Is pre-authorization required? ☐ Yes ☒ No Who can authorize the services? _____
Is a prescription required? ☒ Yes ☐ No Is a referral required? ☐ Yes ☒ No
Who may refer? ☒ MD ☒ DC ☒ ND ☐ PT ☐ Other _____
How often does the referral need to be updated to ensure continuous coverage? __N/A__
Is there a Preferred Provider list for Manual Therapists? ☐ Yes ☒ No
Is _____ on the list? ☐ Yes ☐ No

denied or reversed, or if partial payment is considered payment in full. If you have contracted with the insurance company at a discounted rate, then you cannot, by the terms of your contract, seek payment from the patient for the remaining amount. Otherwise, the patient is responsible for the balance (refer to Figure 5-19).

TIMING AND APPLICATION

This form should be completed and insurance coverage verified before treatment is provided without immediate payment, or as otherwise stated in your payment policies (see Chapter 8 for in-depth coverage of insurance verification). Unless the insurance coverage changes, the form only needs to be completed once per incident.

Every patient who wants the insurance company to pay the manual therapist directly for health care treatment fills out the billing information form.

Amending the Forms

You may want to make slight changes, additions, or corrections to the information recorded on any of the forms in the patient's file without asking the patient to complete

FIGURE 5-19 Billing Information—Patient Authorization

Assignment of Benefits

My signature below authorizes and directs payment of medical benefits for services billed to my health care provider: _____

Release of Medical Records

My signature below authorizes the release of my medical records including intake forms, chart notes, reports, and billing statements to my attorneys, health care providers, and insurance case managers, for the purpose of processing my claims. (I will inform my practitioner immediately upon signing any exclusive Release of Medical Records with my attorney.)

Financial Responsibility

It is my responsibility to pay for all services provided. In the event that my insurance company denies payment or makes a partial payment, I agree to be and remain responsible for the balance. It is also my understanding and agreement that if you have contracted with my insurance company at a discount rate and the agreed-upon fee has been satisfied, the balance owed on those specific visits will be waived.

Signature _____ Date _____

an entirely new form. The patient's perspective may change or she may wish to include new perceptions. Changes can be made by either the patient or the practitioner, regardless of who filled out the form originally. There are two options for updating the existing form:

1. Write the new information on the original form. If you are replacing existing information, draw a single line through the outdated information, making sure that the previous information is still legible. Date and initial all changes and additions. Never use correction fluid or an eraser to delete information (see Figure 5-20).
2. Attach an amendment to the document. Write the new information on a separate sheet of paper and staple it to the original. Date and initial the attachment.

All medical documents may be amended or updated as needed. Patients have a right to access their files and to make sure the information recorded is accurate. Make a habit

FIGURE 5-20   Amending Forms

10-10-04 HLL

Habits   resumed smoking

current   past   comments

☒   ☒ tobacco ~~quit 1998~~

☒   ☐ alcohol *mild use*

☐   ☐ drugs _____

☐   ☐ coffee, soda _____

of recording information in the presence of the patient. Avoid giving misinformation or interpreting information incorrectly. Reiterate the information provided to you and verbally confirm your interpretation of the patient's history and current status.

SUMMARY

A variety of intake forms are used to document the therapeutic relationship. All of these forms are completed before the first treatment, and some are completed before every session or periodically to evaluate progress.

Every patient fills out a health information form and reads and signs a fee schedule and office policy form. Patients who have health concerns and are seeking treatment for injuries or illnesses are to fill out a health report and pain questionnaire periodically to document subjective data and to assist the manual therapist in evaluating progress. Patients seeking insurance reimbursement complete a billing information form, both initially and when the insurance coverage changes. The injury information form is completed by patients injured on the job or in a motor vehicle collision—filled out once per incident.

REFERENCES

1. Adler RH. Whiplash, Spinal Trauma, and the Personal Injury Case. Seattle: Adler ◆ Giersch PS, 2005.
2. Werner R. A Massage Therapist's Guide to Pathology. Baltimore: Lippincott Williams & Wilkins, 2002.
3. Green JA. Holistic Practice Forum, HP–100, Green, Mill Valley, 1990.
4. Current Procedural Terminology (CPT). Chicago: AMA, 2004.
5. Practitioner's Guide to Billable Interventions Using ABC Codes, 7th Ed. Albuquerque: Alternative Link, 2005.
6. Freise RJ, Menke JM. Functional rating index: A new valid and reliable instrument to measure the magnitude of clinical change in spinal conditions. Spine 2001;26:78–87.
7. Deyo RA, Diehl AK. Measuring physical and psycho-social function in patients with low back pain. Spine 1983;8:635–642.
8. McDowell I, Newell C. Measuring Health: A Guide to Rating Scales and Questionnaires. New York and Oxford: Oxford University Press, 1997.
9. Fairbank J, Davies J, Coupar J, O'Brien JP. The Oswestry Low Back Pain Disability Questionnaire. Physiotherapy 1980;66:271–273.
10. Cherkin D, Deyo RA, Eisenberg D, et al. National Alternative Medicine Ambulatory Care Study, preliminary findings, 1999.

*D*ocumentation: SOAP Charting

CHAPTER OUTLINE

A medical director of an insurance carrier in Idaho was questioned by a group of manual therapists: "Why isn't massage therapy a covered benefit in any of your plans?" He replied, "If every manual therapist can show me six months of SOAP charts on every patient, we will consider it."

Introduction

SOAP (Subjective, Objective, Assessment, Plan) **charting** is a standard format for documenting treatment sessions in the health care field. It is used routinely by physicians, physical therapists, chiropractors, nurses, manual therapists, and other medical and allied health professionals.[1] The rapid and widespread adoption of the SOAP format is a tribute to its simple structure and inherent flexibility. Any health concern, method of evaluation, and treatment style can be recorded in the SOAP format. The SOAP structure meets the needs of a variety of health care professionals in many settings.

The SOAP chart documents the patient's health information and goals, the practitioner's findings and treatment, and the patient's self-care routine; and it records the patient's response to the solutions and progress toward the goals. The information is organized into four categories:

◆ **S**ubjective—data provided by the patient (symptoms and functional limitations)
◆ **O**bjective—data from the practitioner's perspective (movement tests, palpation findings, visual observations, as well as treatment and the patient's immediate response to the treatment)
◆ **A**ssessment—functional goals and outcomes based in activities of daily living
◆ **P**lan—treatment recommendations and self-care education

This structure prompts comprehensive information gathering and makes data storage and retrieval easy.

Adaptations of the SOAP format have been created for massage therapists, for example SOTAP[2] and CARE.[3] This chapter provides basic information for manual therapists on how to use the traditional SOAP format with a focus on **functional outcomes reporting**. Some clinics, hospitals, and schools may require a standard of documentation that varies slightly from that presented here; however, the skills acquired through this book can be adapted easily to suit any system of documentation. When massage therapists master the basics most common to all health care providers, the transition will be easy when an employer requires another format or the therapist chooses something more appropriate for his or her needs. For example, SOAP charting can be adapted into the CARE format, as noted below:

◆ **C**ondition of the patient—measurable data regarding the patient's medical condition, such as pain or tension (split between the Subjective and Objective sections)
◆ **A**ction taken—types of massage provided, location, and duration of treatment (part of the Objective section)
◆ **R**esponse of patient—measurable physiological changes and verbal and non-verbal feedback (part of Assessment; however, proponents of CARE charting do not advocate using the functional outcomes style of reporting. This is conceivable if your patients are relatively healthy and without functional limitiations)
◆ **E**valuation—recommendations for future treatment, such as massage, patient homework, and suggestions to other caregivers (Plan)

The advantages of using the SOAP format include:

◆ Consistency across professions
◆ Common language and communication style
◆ Demonstration of professionalism
◆ Proof of progress and **functional outcomes**
◆ Brevity and comprehensiveness
◆ Fast retrieval of information

Another recent trend in documentation is functional outcomes reporting. This style of charting—writing notes that address the patient's ability to function in everyday activities and setting goals and designing treatments to improve function—is quickly being adopted by physical therapists and massage therapists alike. Functional outcomes reporting fits into the SOAP format and shifts the focus of documentation to the patient's quality of life. The practitioner records the patient's functional limitations and works with the patient to develop goals for returning to personally meaningful activities, and together, the practitioner and patient implement solutions to reach those goals. Because this style of recording information is patient-focused, relying less on the diagnostic capabilities of the practitioner, it is a natural addition to the charting regimen for manual therapists and is therefore emphasized in this book.

Guidelines for Charting

First and foremost, charting should contribute to the therapeutic relationship, not detract from it. Don't let charting become a distraction. Follow the patient's lead in the interview.[4] You do not need to follow the SOAP format in order. The beauty of the SOAP structure is that you can organize your information in a linear fashion without having to think or speak in a linear manner. As information is presented, place it in the appropriate section.

Be attentive and maintain good listening skills, as discussed in Chapter 1. If the patient is emotional and needs your undivided attention, record the information later. It is more important to be attentive to the patient in a moment of need than to write on the chart. Reflect your understanding of the patient's experience after she is composed and record the data appropriate to her health concern once she verifies the information.

Be brief. Jot down just enough to jog your memory later, such as words, dates, or short phrases.[5] It can be difficult to discern important information about the patient's health as you are listening to her story. Things often make more sense later, after you have heard the whole story. Take brief notes and fill in the blanks after you summarize the pertinent information to the patient and get confirmation of your interpretation. Make sure you accurately represent the patient's concerns.

Measure everything. Gather as much detail as possible to document the injury or health concern and write it down. It is difficult to prove progress when there is nothing to mark progress against. For example, pain may still be present but diminished, occurring less frequently, with a shorter duration and fewer exacerbations than at the previous session. Be thorough. If information is worth writing down, it is worth measuring.

Avoid vague statements. It is not enough to write "feeling better," "condition is improved," or "pain increases with sitting." Be specific. Rate the intensity of pain, describe the activities that are limited, and state how long the patient is able to perform the activity before the symptoms increase or the activity must cease. Use measurable data to explain the symptoms and compare the symptoms to those from the previous session to demonstrate progress. For example: Mild pain, intermittent, increasing to moderate pain

124

HANDS HEAL:
COMMUNICATION,
DOCUMENTATION,
AND INSURANCE BILLING
FOR MANUAL THERAPISTS

with sitting for one hour or more expresses a decrease in pain when compared with last week's SOAP note: moderate pain, constant, unable to sit for 30 minutes or more. The information should be able to stand alone. "Feeling better" is not only vague, but it can be taken out of context and can signal to an insurance company to discontinue care because the patient no longer requires treatment.[5] If the patient is feeling better, the insurance company could determine that she no longer requires treatment.

Use consistent terminology to measure your findings and patient symptoms, such as mild, moderate, or severe. It is difficult to note progress when comparing "hurts pretty bad" to "kinda sore" or "sorta achey." If you are unclear about the best term to use that fits the patient's symptoms, use the following guidelines:

◆ Normal (0 out of 10) should be noted when a symptom is resolved.
◆ Mild (1, 2, or 3 out of 10) describes the severity of a symptom, but that the symptom does not interfer with the patient's ability to function.
◆ Moderate (4, 5, or 6 out of 10) describes the severity of a symptom, and as a result of that symptom, the patient is forced to modify daily activities.
◆ Severe (7, 8, or 9 out of 10) describes the severity of a symptom, and as a result of that symptom, the patient is unable to perform some activities of daily living.
◆ Disabled or bedridden (10 out of 10) is reserved for patients who are unable to function normally in any area of life as a result of the symptoms.

Chart only information applicable to the patient's condition and goals for health. Often, a story surrounds pertinent details. Pay attention to the details of the story, but be selective when choosing the information to document. Record only data that substantiate the concern or contribute to the solution. For example: Lin experiences an increase in allergies at work when Sally, a coworker from marketing, wears heavy perfume. It is not important to mention information about work or the coworker. The important thing to note is that Lin's allergy symptoms increase when she is exposed to perfume.

Be objective. State everything in a factual manner. Leave your opinions off the chart. For example, omit: "I believe the patient doesn't want to get better and is avoiding going back to work." Instead, quote the patient directly in the Subjective section. He may comment on the situation in ways that adequately represent his state of mind, opinions, or emotions. Chart specific, measurable information and let his lack of progress, as an example, demonstrate that the treatment is not producing results. The information should pertain to the patient, not to you.[5] If the relationship isn't productive, step up the communication and reconsider your approach (review discussion of this topic in Chapter 1).

As you ask the patient specific questions to confirm an assessment or rule out a particular condition, record the positive and negative findings. Negative findings include "All active cervical ranges of motion (ROM) normal . . . ." The positive finding includes ". . .except left lateral flexion—moderately limited with mild pain at tissue stretch." If the negative findings are not recorded, it will be difficult to remember 30 days later, at the reevaluation session, which ROM tests were done at the initial assessment.

Consider another example in which "no" answers are as important as "yes" answers: Jose has shoulder pain. The pain increases when he raises his arm to the side, but there is no pain with any other shoulder movement. If you are identifying a rotator cuff injury or determining bursitis versus tendonitis, knowing that there is no pain with a particular action could affect your treatment plan as much as knowing that there is pain with an action. Record all answers that contribute to the case. Even if your scope of practice does not permit you to state on your SOAP note whether the patient has bursitis or tendonitis, the information is critical to your treatment plan—bursitis and tendonitis are treated very differently.

State only that there is pain with all ranges of motion, not that the patient has bursitis unless you have diagnostic scope and can treat accordingly.

Use common medical terms and become fluent with standard abbreviations (see Appendix D). Many standardized medical abbreviations and symbols used by all types of health care providers are applicable to manual therapy. The medical terms referred to here are descriptive, not diagnostic. Use terms familiar to the health care community to describe your findings, such as hypertonic (HT), spastic (SP), fibrotic (fib), ischemic (IS); rather than tight, lumpy, ropey, or mushy. Use the shorthand available for these terms to make charting quick and easy.

▼

BONE GAME
Translation

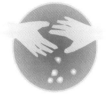

Headache pain, pounding, left frontal, moderate minus, 2 to 3 days, monthly, with menses for 10 plus yr

Abbreviation: HA Ⓟ, pounding, Ⓛ frontal, M–, 2 to 3 day/mth, c̄ menses 10+ yr

The trigger point was moderately painful with digital pressure at the trigger point site and mildly painful at the referral site.

Abbreviation: TP M Ⓟ c̄ dig. pres. @ TP site & L Ⓟ @ ref. site

Cervical flexion passive range of motion was limited moderate minus with mild pain at end range.

Abbreviation: C-flex P-ROM↓M– c̄ L Ⓟ @ end range

Right shoulder active abduction moderate segmented movement occurred with mild compensational shoulder elevation at end range.

Abbreviation: Ⓡsh-abd A-ROM M seg c̄ L comp. sh-elev @ end range.

Moderate trigger point site pain changed to mild pain, mild referred pain changed to no pain.

Abbreviation: TP site M Ⓟ Δ L Ⓟ, L ref. Ⓟ Δ P̷

Moderate segmented movement in right shoulder active abduction changed to smooth movement without compensational shoulder elevation.

Abbreviation: M seg. mvm't Ⓡsh-abd A-ROM WNL s̄ comp. sh-elev

Patient supine, anterior-lateral view, deep inhalation, mild plus mobility restriction upper right.

Abbreviation: pt supine, ant-lat view, deep inhal., mob L+ restr. upper Ⓡ

Left biceps insertion moderate pain with mild digital pressure, mild plus referred pain into left elbow.

Abbreviation: Ⓛ biceps insert. M Ⓟ c̄ L dig. pres., L+ ref. Ⓟ → Ⓛ elbow

1-hour full-body Swedish massage; 30-minute foot reflexology; or 90-minute Hellerwork—inspiration.

Abbreviation: 1 hr FB Sw Ⓜ; 30 min foot reflex.; 90 min HW—inspir.

Muscle energy with cervical flexion, direct pressure on scalene trigger point, myofascial release on diaphragm.

Abbreviation: MET c̄ C-flex, DP scal. TP, MFR diaph.

Craniosacral therapy with attention to the thoracic cage, muscle energy for cervical flexion and extension, and lymph drainage for upper quadrants.

Abbreviation: CST T cage, MET C-flex & ext, LDT UQ ⒝ⓛ

126

HANDS HEAL:
COMMUNICATION,
DOCUMENTATION,
AND INSURANCE BILLING
FOR MANUAL THERAPISTS

Add personalized abbreviations to the list of standard ones to meet the needs of your practice. Do not use abbreviations that are not on your list, even if they are abbreviated words that you believe are common, such as quads for quadriceps muscles or hams for hamstring muscles. Others who read the patient file must be able to interpret everything on the chart with accuracy. Payment of your bill may depend on a claims representative understanding your notes. If you use a series of tests or treatment techniques that do not have standard abbreviations, create your own shorthand and produce a legend to attach to the standardized list. For example, many of Sari's patients have been in motor vehicle collisions (MVC). She finds it helpful to abbreviate information regarding the crash and whiplash-related injuries, but the abbreviations list she uses does not have the medical terms she requires for her practice. Therefore, she includes her own shorthand legend with the standard list she sends out when her charts are requested (see Figure 6-1).

Never use correction fluid or an eraser to eliminate information. Cross out mistakes with a single line. Initial and date the error. Do not leave blank spaces where data could be altered (see Amending the Forms section in Chapter 5).

Sign your legal name or initials to the end of every chart entry. Never use nicknames—SOAP charts are legal documents. Stay current with legal name changes, which are common with marriage or divorce. Include your health care credentials with your signature. The supervising practitioner signs the chart in addition to student, aide, or apprentice in learning environments or clinic settings.[8]

Write legibly. Insurance carriers can refuse payment if they are unable to ascertain whether the treatment was reasonable and necessary or whether the symptoms warranted the type of treatment.[9] Chart notes are the primary source for verifying this information.

FIGURE 6-1 Addendum to Standard Abbreviations, Showing Motor Vehicle Collision Treatment and Billing Information

Motor Vehicle Collision Treatment and Billing Abbreviations

accel	acceleration
CADS	cervical acceleration deceleration syndrome
CPT	Current Procedural Terminology
G-Force	acceleration force
HCFA-1500	Health Care Financing Administration current billing form
HCP	health care provider
ICD	International Classification for Disease
ICE	independent chiropractic examination
IME	independent medical examination
MVC	motor vehicle collision
PCP	primary care provider
PIP	personal injury protection
PR	peer review
pre-IS	pre-injury status
pre-XC	pre-existing conditions
+SB	wearing seat belt
SBD	not wearing seat belt
WAD	whiplash associated disorder

If the notes are illegible, payment can legitimately be denied. Charting is intended to facilitate communication. Make it easy for others to read the information you are trying to share. It is acceptable for your signature to be illegible. Just make sure you have your name, address, and phone number stamped clearly on each page in the patient's file so others can determine who the practitioner is and how to reach you.

▼

STORY TELLER
Who to Pay?

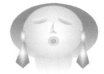

An insurance adjuster called needing more information on a patient before she could authorize payment. She couldn't read the patient's name written on the SOAP chart, and there was no identifying information about the patient, such as insurance identification number or date of birth. I asked her to fax me the charts because I couldn't place who the patient might be. As the charts came over the fax, I was taken aback. The handwriting was not mine. The initials signing the chart entries were not mine, and the patient was not mine! The charts were not only missing patient information, there was no contact information for the massage therapist. The only legible name on the chart was mine—next to the little copyright symbol (©) in the lower right hand corner of the form. I tried to explain to her that I created the form, but I did not write the chart note. I don't know if the correct massage therapist was ever paid for her services.

Components of the SOAP Format

SOAP notes were created as part of a documentation system called the **problem-oriented medical record (POMR)**, introduced by Dr. Lawrence Weed in the 1960s. Historically, the POMR listed patient problems in the front of the chart, and the practitioner wrote a separate SOAP note to address each problem.[1] Currently, it is acceptable to write one SOAP note for each session, addressing all of the "problems" on the same SOAP note. The SOAP format was developed to help structure the practitioner's efforts to solve the patient's health issues. The practitioner records the patient's health concerns, the practitioner's findings, sets goals with the patient, and develops a treatment plan based on the findings and goals. Practical and easy to use, the SOAP note has become the charting standard in the health care industry.

SUBJECTIVE

Subjective information provided by the patient includes a health history and current health information. Data collected on the intake forms is considered subjective information and is used to provide comprehensive documentation of the patient's health at the onset of treatment. Use the Subjective section of the SOAP chart as an ongoing record of details about the patient's current health status: current concerns, physical symptoms, emotional complications, changes in functional ability, and impact on the patient's daily routine.

On a SOAP chart, subjective information is divided into three parts:

◆ A prioritized list of health concerns or goals for the session
◆ Symptoms relating to the current health concerns
◆ Activities that aggravate or relieve the symptoms

128

HANDS HEAL:
COMMUNICATION,
DOCUMENTATION,
AND INSURANCE BILLING
FOR MANUAL THERAPISTS

Health Concerns

Place the patient's health concerns at the top of the SOAP chart. Remain mindful of the reasons why the patient is seeking care. The patient's health concerns may be defined as injuries, medical conditions, symptoms, or as goals for maintaining health or preventing disease. For example, Darnel is seeking care for injuries sustained in a motor vehicle collision, Tham wants to be able to work without pain or numbness, and Lin is eager to prevent complications of diabetes and learn relaxation skills. Include pertinent information that directly affects the care you provide for the current date of service.

Some of the information may not come directly from the patient. A prescription may provide the diagnosis or contributing information may come from test results you did not perform. Darnel's x-rays, for example, show degenerative scoliosis; Tham has a diagnosed repetitive stress disorder; and Lin has a family history of heart disease that potentially could complicate her diabetes. This information is critical to the direction of subjective information gathering and the formation of the treatment plan, but may or may not have originated with the patient. Typically, this information is found on the health information form, but if diagnoses come trickling in after the fact, write it in the Subjective section under Health Concerns. References to spinal stenosis or carpel tunnel syndrome will not be misconstrued as operating outside your scope of practice. It is appropriate to list diagnostic terms in this section of the SOAP chart, because the information comes from the patient or the HCP.

Prioritize multiple concerns. For example, Darnel has limited neck range of motion, back pain, and headaches. In Chapter 1, we discussed his strong desire to reduce the back pain so he could interact with his granddaughter Madi. His headaches are more distressing than his limited neck mobility. Therefore, we would prioritize his health concerns or needs in the following order: Treat injuries and symptoms associated with the motor vehicle collision including secondary scoliosis recurrence.

1. Reduce low back pain.
2. Reduce headache pain.
3. Increase neck mobility.

It is imperative to ask patients to prioritize their health concerns, rather than to assume one symptom is more critical than another. For example, Jack has a list of four concerns he asks to be addressed in his manual: sharp pain in the right hip, low back stiffness, achey right knee, and swelling in the left thumb. Assuming that the lower body complex is the most pressing concern for Jack, his manual therapist gets busy working on the low back, hip and knee. She does a thorough job, but runs out of time before addressing the swollen thumb. By the time Jack is up and off the table, the low back, hip and knee feel fantastic. The manual therapist feels confident the session was a success, having accomplished three of Jack's four concerns. He, however, leaves disappointed. He knows he doesn't have a chance at winning the arm wrestling contest at the pub this weekend with a swollen thumb. Avoid any misunderstandings by asking patients to prioritize their goals for the session. In addition, review your treatment plan with them before you begin the manual.

Symptoms

Obtain a complete list of symptoms from the patient in the initial interview. Much of this information is recorded on the intake forms. Synthesize and condense the information into the **initial SOAP notes**. Inquire about specific areas that have bearing on your treatment applications and are within your scope of practice. Commonly, manual therapists inquire about signs and symptoms in these categories:

◆ General—fatigue, pain, signs of stress, allergies, fever, posture, and general function
◆ Lymphatic—swollen nodes, edema
◆ Musculo-skeletal—tension, weakness, muscle or joint pain, stiffness, swelling
◆ Peripheral vascular—cramps, varicose veins, cold hands or feet, color or pallor
◆ Neurological—numbness, tingling, local weakness, memory, tremors, fainting, blackouts, seizures, paralysis
◆ Psychosocial—lifestyle, home situation, a typical day, important experiences, religious beliefs that may pertain to treatment or illness, perceptions of health, attitude, and outlook for future[4]

Other systems that come into play may not be adequately represented in the intake forms. For further information regarding the systems of the body and examination techniques, consult Bates' *Guide to Physical Examination and History Taking* (8th edition)[4] or Magee's *Orthopaedic Physical Assessment* (2nd edition).[6]

Once you have identified symptoms—pain, stiffness, weakness, and the like—ask the patient to describe the symptom's specific location, intensity, duration, frequency, and the setting in which it occurred and recurs. Record that information. For example: headache pain, pounding, left frontal, moderate minus, 2 to 3 days, monthly, with menses for 10 plus years.

Description

Once the patient has identified the symptoms, ask him or her to describe them further. For example: If the symptom is pain, it may be described as sharp, shooting, dull, or aching. A patient once described her numbness as "cold and wet." Record any information that qualifies the symptom and is helpful in assessing and treating it or in marking progress.

Location

Ask the patient to identify the precise location of the symptom. In addition to locating the symptom, this information can be helpful in identifying the source of the dysfunction and in substantiating progress. As explained in Travell and Simons, the location of the trigger point pain can lead to proper treatment application. For example: If Moira's headache pain is located in the forehead over her right eye, the trigger point is likely to be found in the right sternocleidomastoid.[7] Progress can be demonstrated when the area of pain diminishes in size. In the story of Sandee in Chapter 4, her back pain originally covered her entire low back area. Eventually, the location of her pain was reduced to a small area around her sacrum. Be specific about the location to assist with symptom identification, assessment of the condition, and treatment application.

Intensity

Measure all symptoms by quantifying their expression. Ask patients to rate the intensity of their symptoms on a numerical scale of 0 to 10, a value scale of mild or light (L), moderate (M), and severe (S), or a descriptive scale of normal (N), good (G), fair (F), and poor (P). The value scale can stand alone as a three-point scale, or can be extended into a nine-point scale with the addition of pluses and minuses (L–, L, L+, M–, M, M+, S–, S, S+).

Choose the rating scale that works best for you. Be consistent. If you choose a nine-point value scale, use that scale for all patients at every session.

130

HANDS HEAL:
COMMUNICATION,
DOCUMENTATION,
AND INSURANCE BILLING
FOR MANUAL THERAPISTS

Frequency and Duration

Note how often the symptom occurs. Use general terms like seldom, intermittent, frequent or constant; or specific descriptions like twice a day, three times a week, or hourly to note the frequency.

Record how long the symptom lasts when it occurs. Use time to denote the duration: seconds, minutes, days, weeks, months, or years.

Onset

The onset describes the setting in which the injury or condition occurred or the external factors affecting the injury and the date of the occurrence. Include the biomechanics of the body positions and movements involved in the injury. For example, Moira lifted a box of books from the floor to a shelf above her head. She turned to the left to pick up the box and turned to her right to set the box up on the shelf.

In the case of a fall, it is important to note the body parts that came into contact with the type of surface and the order in which this occurred. Zamora, for example, was carrying a 25-pound bag of rice when she slipped on a banana peel at work. She fell backward with her arm outstretched to break her fall, landed on a tile floor on her right hand and right hip, and ended up on her back, with her head hitting the floor and bouncing a few times. The heavy bag of rice landed on top of her. This information helps determine the treatment plan by identifying the points of impact and the angles of entry.

In the case of a repetitive movement injury, the onset includes the repeated action and a description of any other contributing data. For example: Clint hammers repeatedly at shoulder height with right hand, 20-ounce hammer, 8 hours per day, 5 days per week, 5 years at job, carrying heavy nail pouch on left hip.

Include the date of the onset. Be specific to a day, month, and year, rather than a casual reference to "since last Friday," or "when I was sixteen." The latter requires you to make a calculation every time you refer back to the initial SOAP note. Keep it simple.

In situations involving repetitive movement injuries, the date of the onset may be difficult to determine. As in the scenario above, help Clint determine the approximate year the symptoms began occurring. To Clint, it may feel like the pain has been going on forever, but if you prod his memory a bit by suggesting 10 years or 20 years, he's likely to chuckle and remind you that he's only 23 years old and has been working construction for five years. Record a month or a time of year as well as the year of onset, if possible. Noting "Summer of '42" or "January '93" is more helpful than a simple "for many years."

Having a clear record of the mechanisms of injury will help justify treating a broader area. For example, with Moira's lift and twist injury, the diagnosis may be a low back sprain-strain. Treatment to her neck and shoulders may seem luxurious and unnecessary to a referring HCP or an insurance representative unless you can clearly explain the biomechanical links and compensating symptoms involved.

Activities of Daily Living–Aggravating and Relieving

Emphasize function, such as how well the patient is able to perform daily activities, when charting subjective information. Record the patient's current and prior level of function, how the symptoms affect his ability to function, and how his ability to function affects his life at home and work.

The documentation process—inquiry, discussion, and charting—increases patients' awareness of their role in exacerbating or reducing the symptoms. Record events of everyday life that aggravate or relieve symptoms to document significant injury, note progress, and educate patients to use activities that relieve rather than aggravate their symptoms.

The information regarding patients' activities of daily living will assist you in proving functional progress and providing effective self-care education. Functional limitations that have the most effect on their quality of life will be used to determine long-term and short-term goals. Use relieving activities when planning their homework and self-care regime. Goals and outcomes are documented in the Assessment section; homework is described in the Plan section.

Activities That Aggravate Symptoms

When documenting activities that aggravate the patient's symptoms, be specific about home and work responsibilities, including hobbies and play activities. Generally speaking, activities involve basic functions: sitting, standing, walking, lifting, sleeping, and the like. Use the Pain Questionnaires to identify the basic functions with which patients experience difficulty. In this section of the SOAP chart, however, explain how each function personally relates to the individual's daily activities. Include the relevance of the specific activity to the patient's life, how long the patient can perform the activity before the symptoms begin or worsen, and compare with the patient's previous ability. For example: Pain increases from mild to moderate with sitting or standing more than 30 minutes. Sits at computer 7 to 8 hours per day for work, stands in kitchen 1 to 2 hours per day doing household chores, and reads for recreation. Unable to drive comfortably for more than 10 minutes—35-mile commute to work, picks children up from day care, next week a road trip with the family through the Canyon Lands is scheduled—planned for 6 months.

Include activities the patient can no longer perform because of the symptoms. For example: Unable to lift objects heavier than 25 pounds—job requires lifting objects up to 60 pounds, exercise routine included weight lifting, small children at home require lifting for care. Address endurance by describing an activity and stating the amount tolerated before signs of fatigue are exhibited. For example: Must stop reading after 20 minutes and housework after 10 minutes because of pain and fatigue.

When daily activities change noticeably but symptoms remain constant, a look at aggravating activities may reveal progress that might otherwise go undetected. Often, when patients are recovering from injuries that have limited them, the better they feel, the more they attempt to do. They are eager to return to work, get out of the house, and feel useful again. The weeds in the garden are nagging them, the stack of laundry is piling up, and the kids want to get the flat tire fixed on the bike. When the activity level increases, there may be little to no improvement in symptoms—symptoms may even worsen. Rather than assuming there is no progress, document the changes in activities. This will explain the lack of progress with the symptoms and show improvement in the patient's health based on activity level.

▼

STORY TELLER
Pain Threshold Affects Patient Perceptions of Progress

I was a bit lazy charting sessions with a fellow massage therapist who had been in a car collision. Angela's knee was injured in the crash and required surgery. At first, I was diligently recording her functional limitations and helping her set functional goals. For example, she was ambitious about attending the opening of a basket exhibition, and we worked together to set reasonable goals regarding her ability to walk around the gallery. With frequent stops to sit and rest, she was able to see each basket in the exhibit!

(Continued)

132

HANDS HEAL:
COMMUNICATION,
DOCUMENTATION,
AND INSURANCE BILLING
FOR MANUAL THERAPISTS

STORY TELLER *(Continued)*

Six weeks later, Angela seemed very down about her condition. She complained that she felt little progress and was experiencing pain every day while walking and standing. Realizing that weeks had gone by since I questioned her regarding her daily activities, I asked her how much walking she was doing. "I'm walking to and from work every day, and it always hurts!" I knew she lived a mile from her office atop a hill. Angela had returned to walking the two miles round trip just four weeks after her stop-and-go limp around a gallery. I was impressed! As her therapist, I was able to maintain perspective of Angela's progress, but Angela couldn't see beyond the fact that today she was in pain. Somehow, I needed to help Angela remain cognizant of her progress.

I told Angela my painful story of being introduced to 100 MDs at the CAM symposium and what I had learned from the Chronic Low Back Pain study[8] (refer to the Story Teller in Chapter 1). After discussing how one's threshold of pain can affect one's perception of progress, she agreed that we had not focused adequately on her functional successes; namely, the dramatic shift in her ability to walk. We made a commitment to set goals every month and regularly evaluate her functional progress until all her goals for health were met.

Activities That Relieve Symptoms

List activities that alleviate symptoms. Include modifying necessary activities, self-care, exercises, or remedies that relieve the symptoms. Changing positions, taking frequent breaks, stretching exercises, self-massage, topical analgesics, and hot or cold packs are also considered activities that alleviate symptoms.

Investigate closely the steps the patient has taken to care for herself. Uncover as many ways as possible that the patient participates in her health care. Document specific activities that you want to reinforce or that have been particularly effective. For example: Catherine Ann applies ice to low back as needed for pain, sits on a tennis ball to relieve trigger point pain, and squeezes tennis ball throughout day to exercise hands. You may choose not to record all the information uncovered, but use it to compliment the patient, build her self-esteem, and encourage her to continue to participate in her health care.

OBJECTIVE

This section of the SOAP chart stores information from the practitioner's perspective:

◆ Measurable data—movement tests, palpatory findings, visual observations
◆ Treatment applications—techniques, location, duration
◆ Patient's response to the massage

State information clearly and concisely. Stick to details within your scope of practice. Do not chart treatment techniques for which you cannot explain the physiological effects clearly and consistently. Avoid data that cannot be measured or reproduced.

Measurable Findings

Massage therapists primarily gather the following objective, measurable data: visual observations, such as posture and breath; palpatory findings, such as spasms and trigger points; movement and strength tests, such as gait analysis and active, passive, and resistive ROM tests. Document all tests uniformly and consistently.

Follow these simple guidelines when gathering and charting your objective findings:

◆ Document a full range of data.
◆ Measure every finding.
◆ Measure before and after treatment application.
◆ Perform the post-assessment in the same way as the pre-assessment.
◆ Use consistent terminology and symbols.

The data you record should represent the full scope of your practice. Do not limit yourself by narrowly focusing on one aspect of your expertise. This can cause problems when others in your profession exercise the full extent of the professional scope.

STORY TELLER
The Laundry List of Hypertonicities

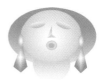

I attended a meeting with reviewers and medical directors from a few insurance companies. I was there to defend the scope of practice of massage therapists as a result of a narrowing interpretation of our assessment and treatment abilities. The medical director of one of the health plans claimed she was getting hypertonicities from reading about all the hypertonicities on therapists' SOAP charts. She wanted to know why the providers in her network insisted on listing every tight muscle in the body and nothing else, and whether indeed the therapists were capable of noting inflammation, spasms, trigger points, joint dysfunction, and such. Tight muscles alone do not provide a convincing argument for medical necessity. Balance your objective charting by noting a variety of findings.

Measure all information. Quantify and qualify data based on deviations from normal. Normal is determined by:

◆ Comparing bilaterally when possible
◆ Defining normal for a general population of similar constitution
◆ Asking the patient to define normal for himself or herself

Quantify data by rating the intensity of its expression. For example: trigger point moderately painful with light digital pressure at the trigger point site and mildly painful at the referral site; or, cervical flexion passive range of motion was limited 4/10 with 2/10 pain at end range.

Qualify data by describing its expression. For example: right shoulder active abduction moderate segmented movement with mild compensatory shoulder elevation at end range; or, moderate plus sharp shooting pain with movement from prone to supine position while turning on treatment table.

Assess the condition before and after treatment. It is difficult to document progress or determine the effectiveness of a treatment modality without being able to do a before-and-after comparison. For example: moderate trigger point site pain changed to mild pain, mild

134

HANDS HEAL:
COMMUNICATION,
DOCUMENTATION,
AND INSURANCE BILLING
FOR MANUAL THERAPISTS

referred pain changed to no pain; or, moderate segmented movement in right shoulder active abduction changed to smooth movement without compensatory shoulder elevation.

Perform tests identically for pre-treatment and post-treatment. Data must be comparable. For example, postural analysis in a standing position (weight bearing) provides different information from postural analysis in a supine or seated position (non-weight bearing). Therefore, the patient should be in the same position for both tests. Also, reproduce the test in the original environment. For example: If the patient was sitting in a chair for the pre-treatment range of motion assessment, he should be sitting in the same chair, not on the treatment table, for the post-treatment assessment.

Be consistent from session to session. It is difficult to compare data over time when the range of motion testing was done standing initially, seated last session, and supine this session. Also, take into consideration the timing of the tests. If the initial test was done on a Friday afternoon after a long week at work, and the test was reassessed on a Monday morning after a relaxing weekend, the data will not be comparable.

Pick qualifying and quantifying terms and use them consistently. Smooth, segmented, and spastic may describe the quality of the range of motion. Sharp and dull can be used to qualify pain. Numerical scales (0 to 10) or value scales (L, M, S) can quantify data. Select terms that adequately represent your assessment test results. Create abbreviations for the terms when necessary and add them to your legend. Most importantly, use the same terms consistently from session to session and patient to patient.

Visual Observations

Visual findings stem from observing movement patterns such as posture, muscle atrophy, skin abnormalities, swelling, and signs of trauma (such as bruises, abrasions, and scars). Much of the visual data can be recorded on the SOAP chart by drawing symbols on the human figures. For example: Posture is easily noted on the figures by drawing skewed lines to depict elevations and arrows in the direction of rotations. Use standard symbols to represent visual findings, or you may add your own to the key. Functional movement patterns, such as gait or respiration, and comments about general appearance are more easily noted in the space provided for written information (see Figure 6-2).

Follow these guidelines for documenting posture and movement patterns:

◆ Note the position of the patient—seated, standing, prone, supine
◆ Record the angle of the observation—anterior, lateral, posterior
◆ Describe the activity being observed—breathing, walking, lifting, standing
◆ Follow the guidelines for gathering and charting objective findings (listed previously)

For example: patient supine, anterior-lateral view, deep inhalation, mild plus mobility restriction upper right quadrant.

Posture can be quantified by rating the amount of deviation from normal. Simply mark a number or letter denoting the intensity of the deviation near the line or arrow as it is drawn on the figures.

Chart irregularities: forward head posture, leg length variations, spinal curvatures, and the like. Note elevations, rotations, inversions, and eversions. Common sites for observing posture are at the ears, shoulders, superior and inferior angles of the scapulae, anterior and posterior superior iliac spine, knees, and the medial and lateral malleoli.

Breath can be measured by qualifying the pattern and rate of breath, describing sounds associated with breathing, and quantifying the mobility of the ribs with inhalation. Note irregularities such as a rattling noise or shallow, rapid, weak, uneven, or inconsistent patterns in breathing. Observe the rise and fall of the ribs and chart the restrictions.

FIGURE 6-2 **Objective Section: Visual and Palpable Observations**

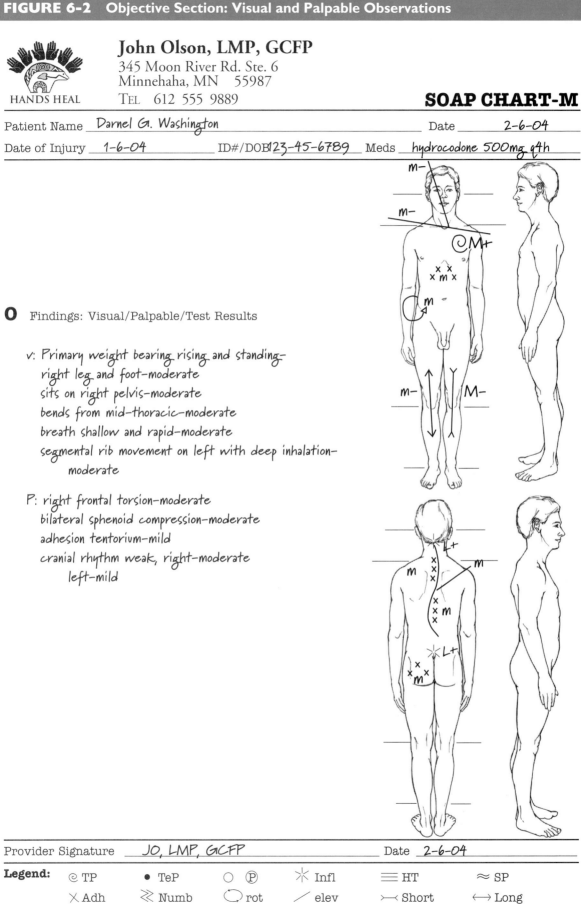

John Olson, LMP, GCFP
345 Moon River Rd. Ste. 6
Minnehaha, MN   55987
TEL   612 555 9889

HANDS HEAL

SOAP CHART-M

Patient Name __Darnel G. Washington__   Date ____2-6-04____

Date of Injury __1-6-04__   ID#/DOB__123-45-6789__ Meds __hydrocodone 500mg q4h__

O   Findings: Visual/Palpable/Test Results

v: Primary weight bearing rising and standing-
    right leg and foot-moderate
    sits on right pelvis-moderate
    bends from mid-thoracic-moderate
    breath shallow and rapid-moderate
    segmental rib movement on left with deep inhalation-
        moderate

P: right frontal torsion-moderate
    bilateral sphenoid compression-moderate
    adhesion tentorium-mild
    cranial rhythm weak, right-moderate
        left-mild

Provider Signature ___JO, LMP, GCFP___   Date __2-6-04__

Legend: ☾ TP   ● TeP   ○ Ⓟ   ✳ Infl   ≡ HT   ≈ SP

  ✕ Adh   ≋ Numb   ◯ rot   ╱ elev   ⟩─ Short   ⟷ Long

136

HANDS HEAL:
COMMUNICATION,
DOCUMENTATION,
AND INSURANCE BILLING
FOR MANUAL THERAPISTS

Functional movement patterns can be qualified and quantified by noting the amount of movement, how well the movement is performed, and how long the patient can sustain the movement before experiencing fatigue. Note sensations caused by movement and rate their expression.

Palpation Findings

Palpation is an objective test used to locate and assess inconsistencies in various rhythms, pulses, and systems of the body such as soft tissue, joints, viscera, and lymph. Massage therapists tend to be highly trained and adept at sensing subtle discrepancies and changes under their fingers. As a result, detailed palpatory information is a valuable resource for all caregivers involved in the patient's health care team, and the information can be shared through SOAP charts and progress reports.

Document palpation findings by noting and describing abnormalities and conditions. Terminology varies among professions and specialties. Compile a comprehensive list of evaluative terms for your practice and use the terms consistently. Your list may include:

◆ Muscle tone—including tension, hypertonic, hypotonic, spastic, rigid, splinting, contracture, spasm, lines of tension, holding patterns
◆ Pain—including trigger points, tender points, meridian points, Jones points, absence of sensation, spasm-pain-spasm cycle. (Note: Pain is usually considered subjective information. Pain becomes objective when it is elicited by the practitioner through touch, testing, and the like.)
◆ Scar tissue—adhesions, fibrosis, fibrotic tissue, granulation tissue
◆ Inflammation—including swelling, edema, active hyperemia, ischemia, congestion, stagnation, heat, pitted edema

Avoid diagnostic terms—such as grade 2 sprain or strain and lymphedema—to describe findings if you do not have diagnostic scope or if the referring HCP or the patient did not provide you with diagnostic information.

Measure the palpation data by rating the intensity of the finding, such as with severe spasm, or quantifying the size, such as with right ankle edema 20 centimeters in circumference.

Much of the data collected through palpation is documented easily on human figures using symbols found in the legend. Write the quantifying or qualifying terms next to the figure. Whenever necessary, tie the letter or number to the symbol with a connecting line. Anything too complicated or cumbersome to draw on the figures can be written out in the space provided (refer to Figure 6-2). The figures are intended to increase the speed and ease of documentation and to aid in fast recall. This intent is defeated if the figures are overburdened with symbols. When the data are abundant, draw the primary information on the figures and list the secondary data in the space provided under Objective.

Follow these guidelines when documenting palpation findings:

◆ Identify the specific location.
◆ Rate or describe the type of touch that triggers the finding (for example: light, medium, or deep).
◆ Include any referred sensation, if applicable.
◆ Identify connections or relationships, if any.
◆ Follow the guidelines for gathering and charting objective findings (listed earlier in this chapter).

For example: left biceps insertion moderate pain with light digital pressure, mild plus referred pain into left elbow.

The most common standardized testing for massage therapists is range of motion (ROM) testing (see Appendix B for blank forms). It is used in many professions and is familiar to lay people as a means of assessing health. A popular television commercial shows a person bending over and touching his toes, at first with limitation and pain, then—after taking the product—with greater range and ease. The message: Greater movement with less discomfort equals better health. As a result, many patients expect ROM testing from any practitioner assessing and treating joint pain.

ROM testing is a valuable assessment tool for determining the stage of inflammation, the level of severity of sprains and strains, joint trauma, and muscle weakness. Gather and record ROM test results to substantiate dysfunction, validate progress, and identify conditions. Assessing ROM before treatment substantiates the limitations for the patient. Retesting ROM after intervention demonstrates the effectiveness of the treatment plan and proves progress resulting from the session. Periodic testing at pre-treatment and post-treatment times shows continued progress and gives the patient, the referring caregivers, and the insurance reviewers evidence that the treatment is working.

Document the test:

◆ Identify the position of the patient—standing, seated, prone, supine, sidelying
◆ Identify the type of test—active, active assisted, passive, resistive
◆ Name the joint—including right shoulder, left hip, cervical spine
◆ Name the action—including flexion, extension, left rotation, right lateral flexion

Chart the results of the test (see Figure 6-3):

◆ Rate the amount of movement as a deviation from normal—hypermobile, hypomobile, within normal limits (for example: moderate decrease in seated active cervical flexion . . .)
◆ Rate the presence of pain with movement or stretch (for example: . . . with moderate pain)
◆ Rate the quality of the movement—including smooth, segmented, spastic, rigid (for example: . . . with mild segmented movement)

ROM test results are commonly expressed in degrees or percentages of normal. If you are not using measuring devices such as goniometers, use the numerical scale of 0 to 10 or the value scale of mild, moderate, and severe to rate ROM test results. You will be able to show deviations from normal with enough detail to note progress as changes develop. (For information on how to perform ROM tests or use goniometric measurements, see Kendall et al.[9] or Norkin and White.[10])

Treatment

Document the length of the session, the massage techniques and modalities used, and the location of the treatments that were applied. Record the treatment in two ways. First, provide a big picture of the session—the length of the session, techniques, and general body parts treated. For example: 1-hour full-body Swedish massage; 30-minute foot reflexology; or 90-minute Hellerwork—inspiration. Second, fill in the details– particular techniques used to treat specific findings. For example: muscle energy technique with cervical flexion, direct pressure on scalene trigger point, or myofascial release on diaphragm. You do not need to write down everything you do; just give the highlights. Chart enough information to recall the important events of the session at a later date.

FIGURE 6-3 Range of Motion (ROM) Charts

John Olson, LMP, GCFP
345 Moon River Rd. Ste. 6
Minnehaha, MN   55987
HANDS HEAL   TEL 612 555 9889

RANGE OF MOTION

Patient Name _Darnel G. Washington_ _____ Date _2-6-04_ _____

Date of Injury _1-6-04_ _____ ID#/DOB _123-45-6789_ _____

PRE-TEST 1 Initials _JO_   Date _2-6-04_ _____

Position of patient: prone, sidelying, sitting, (standing,) supine, other: _____

Type of test: (active,) active assisted, passive, resistive, other: _____

Joint: C-spine, T-spine, (L-spine,) hip, knee, ankle, shoulder, elbow, wrist, other: _____

Action	Quantify ↓ or ↑		Rate Pain		Rate Quality	
	ⓇR	ⓁL	ⓇR	ⓁL	ⓇR	ⓁL
flex	M⁻ →	↓	L⁺		L⁻	seg
ext	M⁺ →	↓	M⁻		M⁻	seg
SB	L↓	M↓	L	M	N	Mseg

POST-TEST 1 Initials _JO_   Date _2-6-04_ _____

Position of patient: prone, sidelying, sitting, (standing,) supine, other: _____

Type of test: (active,) active assisted, passive, resistive, other: _____

Joint: C-spine, T-spine, (L-spine,) hip, knee, ankle, shoulder, elbow, wrist, other: _____

Action	Quantify ↓ or ↑		Rate Pain		Rate Quality	
	ⓇR	ⓁL	ⓇR	ⓁL	ⓇR	ⓁL
flex	L →	↓	θ⁺		N →	
ext	M →	↓	M↑		L →	seg
SB	∆̸	∆̸	∆̸	L	N	L seg

Patient's Response to Treatment

Every subjective and objective finding should be reassessed during the session. This may happen as you go—immediately after a specific technique is applied to address a particular symptom—or at the end of the session.

Quantify and qualify the changes. Include positive and negative responses to treatment. Record the updated information on the chart above or alongside the original entry. Use the delta symbol (Δ) to distinguish the pre-treatment data from the post-treatment entry (see Figure 6-4). This is an efficient way to document the patient's response and avoid rewriting in several places on the chart.

Note symptoms and measurable data that did not change. This may help you determine areas of focus for the next session. Identify whether the treatment was ineffective or that time did not permit addressing the issue. In either case, you will want to address the problem in the treatment plan; make the issue a priority for the next session or select another technique to use. "No change" is easily abbreviated with a line drawn through the delta symbol. (∆̸)

ASSESSMENT

Traditionally, the Assessment section of the SOAP chart records the practitioner's interpretation of the subjective and objective findings. Conclusions are drawn, the condition is named (diagnosis), and the prognosis—probable course of the disease—is determined and recorded on the SOAP chart. However, practitioners without diagnostic scope are not permitted to assess the patient's condition in these terms.

In functional outcomes reporting, assessment is the place to summarize the patient's functional ability—to set goals that, when accomplished, demonstrate functional

FIGURE 6-4 **Objective: Response to Treatment**

HANDS HEAL

John Olson, LMP, GCFP
345 Moon River Rd. Ste. 6
Minnehaha, MN   55987
Tel   612 555 9889

SOAP CHART-M

Patient Name _Darnel G. Washington_   Date _2-6-04_

Date of Injury _1-6-04_   ID#/DOB _123-45-6789_ Meds _hydrocodone 500mg q4h_

S Symptoms: Location/Intensity/Frequency/Duration/Onset

   Neck, mid, low back pain moderate
   constant since car accident Δ L
   headache Pain moderate intermittant
   daily since car accident Δ Ⓟ

O Findings: Visual/Palpable/Test Results

   V: Primary weight bearing rising and standing-
        right leg and foot-moderate Δ̸
        sits on right pelvis-moderate Δ̸
        bends from mid-thoracic-moderate Δ L
        breath shallow and rapid-moderate Δ L
        segmental rib movement on left with deep inhalation-
             moderate Δ smooth

   P: right frontal torsion-moderate Δ L
        bilateral sphenoid compression-moderate Δ M⁻
        adhesion tentorium-mild Δ̸
        cranial rhythm weak, right-moderate Δ L
             left-mild Δ Normal

Provider Signature   _JO, LMP, GCFP_   Date _2-6-04_

Legend:

☾ TP	● TeP	○ Ⓟ	✳ Infl	☰ HT	≈ SP
✕ Adh	≋ Numb	◯ rot	╱ elev	⊱ Short	↔ Long

140

HANDS HEAL:
COMMUNICATION,
DOCUMENTATION,
AND INSURANCE BILLING
FOR MANUAL THERAPISTS

progress. Every practitioner using the functional approach to SOAP charting will record functional goals and outcomes in the Assessment section. If the patient does not have any functional limitations, but does have a medical condition that warrants SOAP charting, leave this section blank. Before you fall back on this option, however, question the patient regarding his or her sleep patterns. Most people living with pain have disruptions in their sleep, even when they are still able to perform all other activities of daily living without modification. If they are waking during the night because of pain or are waking in the morning feeling fatigued, set measurable goals regarding sleep and note measurable progress as they achieve their goals.

Record the following under Assessment:

◆ Long-term and short-term functional goals based in activities of daily living
◆ Functional outcomes

▼

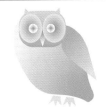

WISE ONE SPEAKS
Follow the Patient's Lead

"You should never have expectations for other people. . . . setting goals for others can be aggressive—really wanting a success story for ourselves. When we do this to others, we are asking them to live up to our ideals. Instead, just be kind." This quote from Trungpa Rinpoche reminds us to follow the patient's lead in setting goals. Remember that the patient is in charge in the therapeutic relationship. SOAP notes were designed to help formulate a high-quality treatment plan and promote the practitioner's problem-solving skills. This same format can be equally effective in promoting the patient's problem-solving skills by adding the functional outcomes approach to our information gathering and charting. Focus on the therapeutic relationship and prioritize the patient's goals above our own in every step of SOAP charting.

The functional outcomes style of documentation is increasingly popular and benefits the patient, the practitioner, and all who read the chart because it directly addresses the basic needs of the patient, monitors effective treatment, and makes the results easily understood—not just to the experts.

Reprinted by permission from Chödrön P. Stant where you are: a guide to compassionate living. Boston: Shambhala, 1994.

Functional Outcomes Begin as Goals

Functional outcomes are written in the form of functional goals, set by the patient with practitioner guidance. Goals are determined through the activities with which the patient is having difficulty and with which the patient is motivated to resume. As they are accomplished, the goals are identified as functional outcomes.

Develop goals that address the needs of the patient and lead to an effective treatment plan—one that will resolve the patient's concerns. With the patient, follow these steps:

◆ Summarize and prioritize verbally the patient's functional limitations, referring to what is already written in the Subjective section of the SOAP chart.
◆ Relate these functional limitations to all meaningful and pertinent activities of daily living (ADLs) and review these with the patient.

◆ Select one activity that is adversely affected by the patient's condition—one to which the patient is most motivated to return.

◆ Create and record long-term and short-term SMART goals (LTG, STG) based on that ADL.

Setting SMART Goals

To ensure that the goals will lead to productive treatment plans and produce functional outcomes that serve the patient's needs, follow the **SMART goals** criteria.[11] The acronym SMART stands for the following:

Specific—to a daily activity

Measurable—quantified and qualified to note incremental progress

Attainable—able to be accomplished given the patient's condition

Relevant—critical to the patient's daily life

Time-bound—defined to be successful in a specific amount of time

With the patient, build functional goals that meet the SMART criteria.

SMART—Specific and Relevant Activity

Select activities that are specific and functional. This can include vacuuming, mowing the lawn, washing hair, lifting boxes onto a conveyor belt, loading and unloading furniture to a truck, rowing a boat, and the like. The more specific the activity, the better. "Work," "exercise," "child care," and "housework" are not specific enough to base a functional goal on. If house cleaning is the work, explore the activity that increases the symptoms—is it standing at the sink, pushing a vacuum cleaner, pulling sheets off a bed, lifting laundry, scrubbing floors? If computer programming is the work, is it sitting still, staring at the screen, moving the mouse? If the exercise is playing tennis, is it the forehand stroke, backhand, serve, lateral moves? What part of child care is problematic—lifting the child, leaning over to play with her, picking up the toys?

Reducing pain is a common goal of the patient, but is not functional—based on an activity. Pain is a qualifier, measuring the success of a goal. If a patient states "pain free" as his goal, guide him to a specific activity by exploring activities that cause the pain.

Select the activity that is most relevant to the patient's life. Address work, home, family, exercise, and play activities. The goal should be based on an activity that is critical to the patient's ability to earn a living or care for himself, his family, or his household. If the injury occurred on the job and industrial insurance is paying for the treatment, select a work-related activity.

SMART—Measurable and Time-Bound

Once the specific and relevant activity is selected, specify how the success of the goal will be gauged.

1. Quantify the outcome by measuring the activity—number of units, amount of weight, repetitions, duration, or frequency
2. Qualify the outcome by projecting how the patient will feel upon completion—amount of pain, fatigue, or functional limitations
3. Schedule a time limit for completion—commonly 30 to 60 days for LTG or about 1 to 2 weeks for STG. Be specific: 45 days, not 30 to 60 days

142

HANDS HEAL:
COMMUNICATION,
DOCUMENTATION,
AND INSURANCE BILLING
FOR MANUAL THERAPISTS

For example: Lift 25-pound boxes from a three-foot-high, moving conveyor belt and stack them onto hand trucks for 30 minutes keeping pace with the conveyor with no more than mild pain within six weeks.

1. Quantify the outcome—Lift 25-pound boxes from a three-foot-high, moving conveyor belt and stack them onto hand trucks for 30 minutes keeping pace with the conveyor
2. Qualify the outcome—with no more than mild pain
3. Time-bound—within six weeks

Climb up and down four standard steps at a moderate pace three times a day with moderate pain and mild fatigue within one week.

1. Quantify the outcome—Climb up and down four standard steps at a moderate pace three times a day
2. Qualify the outcome—with moderate pain and mild fatigue
3. Time-bound—within one week

Sleep restfully for three hours without waking once each night with mild fatigue upon waking within two weeks.

1. Quantify the outcome—Sleep restfully for three hours without waking once each night
2. Qualify the outcome—with mild fatigue upon waking
3. Time-bound—within two weeks

Two standard time frames can be used: long-term and short-term. LTGs are developed first. Identify the desired end result of the treatment. If it is not possible to reach the goal in 30 to 60 days, write one or two intermediary LTGs, each one attainable within 30 to 60 days.

STGs are established to support the LTG and are often written as incremental stages of the LTG. Think of them as baby steps toward the end result. If the end result is to lift boxes up to 50-pounds from the floor to a truck up to 100 times a day for five days a week, write STGs that are fractions of the original goal. For example:

STG #1: Lift 10 pounds from a three-foot-high shelf 10 times a day within 12 days

STG #2: Lift 20 pounds from a two-foot-high shelf 10 times, two times a day within 20 days

STG #3: Lift 30 pounds from a one-foot-high shelf 20 times, three times a day within 12 days

Write STGs that provide encouragement and motivation for the patient, even if the STG does not appear to be directly related to the original goal. For example: LTG—pain free and fully functional while swimming the breast stroke for1,500 meters within 30 days. If the breast stroke is painful because of a neck injury but the patient is eager to experience success in the water, set a goal that provides a feeling of success in the water. STG—one-week goal of 30 minutes of water aerobics with moderate pain. The aerobic exercises may not require the patient to extend her neck—the function that causes her pain—and being in the water may be very comforting for her. The result is an immediate feeling of accomplishment that may not be realized with long-term goals.

The time limit for LTGs is often dictated by the prescription length. One or two STGs should be written for each LTG. Determine the measurements for the time frames by assessing the possibilities for each patient, given his or her condition and constitution.

Be reasonable when writing goals. A goal that is too vast—pain free and fully functional while swimming the breast stroke for 1,500 meters within 30 days—can be frustrating to reach when the patient is currently unable to swim at all. If we are to eliminate the patient's feelings of powerlessness and inspire her to work hard to achieve her goals, we must develop goals that are not only meaningful but continually are within her reach. Evaluate the severity of the injury, the patient's constitution, and functional status, then determine whether the goal as stated is attainable for the patient in the allotted time.

It is helpful to pre-determine how the patient's body will respond to treatment. Don't worry if you misjudge this; you can adjust the goal at the following session by renegotiating the time limit or the outcome measurements. Instead of swimming 1,500 meters with no pain, adjust the outcome to:

The patient will be able to swim 500 meters with moderate pain within 30 days.

PLAN

The Plan section charts the future treatment protocol and records self-care exercises. Set treatment goals and list probable treatment options for obtaining the goals. Outline the frequency of the sessions and duration of each and settle on an approximate reevaluation date. Chart specific instructions for homework suggestions. Document your referrals and recommendations for outside interventions and tests.

Treatment Plan

The initial note projects the plans for the first series of treatments. First, given the information shared in the extensive initial interview and full-body assessment, determine and prioritize your goals for the series:

1. Reduce inflammation in the neck
2. Reduce pain in the neck and shoulders
3. Increase ROM of the neck

Next, the practitioner and the patient select massage techniques and modalities to employ that will accomplish your goals and the patient's functional goals. Base your decision about treatment techniques on what has worked for the patient in the past and what has worked for others who have had similar conditions and constitution. List the techniques projected and the general locations for applying the massage. For example:

1. Lymphatic drainage and ice packs on the neck to reduce the inflammation
2. Swedish massage and trigger point therapy on the neck and shoulders to reduce pain
3. Muscle energy technique to the levator scapulae and sternocleidomastoid to increase ROM

Record the frequency of the subsequent sessions—3 times a week, weekly, or monthly; duration of sessions—30 minutes, 1 hour, 90 minutes; and the reevaluation date. The plan should cover the length of the prescription or the time allotted for the LTG. If you are treating the patient twice a week, a 30-day reevaluation date is appropriate. If the treatment frequency is once a week, 45 days between reevaluations may feel adequate. For example: 45-minute sessions, twice a week for three weeks; reevaluation during week of 6-15-04.

Update the plan every 30 days or more, depending on the treatment frequency. Modify the plan more frequently whenever the patient's condition changes or the plan is no longer appropriate based on the patient's response to the previous treatments. Let the

144

HANDS HEAL:
COMMUNICATION,
DOCUMENTATION,
AND INSURANCE BILLING
FOR MANUAL THERAPISTS

treatment plan guide you, but do not let it dictate the sessions. Be flexible and respond to individual needs as they arise. Remain mindful of the goals at the same time.

Self-Care

Record **self-care** exercises and homework assignments that support the goals. Self-care is a broad term that includes modifying activities to decrease pain and effort and increase safety, stretching and strengthening exercises, and home remedies such as ice packs, Epson salt baths, poltices, ointments, and self-massage techniques. Compliment the patient on everything he currently does to improve his condition and reinforce his efforts by charting the self-care exercises that are most productive.

Be specific and provide detailed instructions when assigning homework. Support the patient's self-care routine by recording the homework assignment and the specific instructions or attaching a copy of the instruction sheet to the chart. This is difficult to do if we cannot remember the assignment. For example: Stand up and stretch for two minutes for every hour of work at the computer. Hold all stretches for 30 seconds. Stretches include

1. bending over slowly and touching toes, return to standing
2. bending over to each side, return to standing
3. pulling arms behind back using filing cabinet; before sitting down, walk to the water fountain and drink

Keep homework simple. Make sure it fits into the patient's lifestyle. If the patient is very busy, homework should not be too time-consuming. New exercises should not be too complex, so assign activities the patient will find familiar and comfortable. Ideally, homework should be the patient's idea or a modification of something the patient suggests.

Remember, do not provide homework to people who are not ready for it. Some patients do not yet believe that change is possible. Assign awareness exercises for patients who are unaware of their role in the healing process and don't seem to recognize change when it occurs. Invite them to notice the way they feel when they are performing an activity that exacerbates their condition. For example: For every hour spent at the computer, stop and take a break. Notice how your neck, back, arms, and hands feel. Notice whether anything you do makes that feeling better or worse.

Initial Notes, Subsequent Notes, Progress Notes, and Discharge Notes

Four types of notes are recorded on the two SOAP formats: the extended version and the sort version. The extended version is a full-page SOAP chart with multiple prompting categories. The short version is a half-page form with only the SOAP sections noted (see Appendix B for blank forms).

◆ Initial notes (extended version)
◆ Subsequent notes (short version)
◆ Progress notes (extended version)
◆ Discharge notes (extended version)

The initial notes are comprehensive and include extensive information regarding the patient's health and current situation. Much of the information recorded on an initial SOAP chart does not need to be repeated on subsequent notes.

- List and prioritize all the patient's health concerns
- Evaluate the full body, including the way the patient is responding to his or her current health situation from head to toe
- Include all symptoms that relate to the patient's health concerns, the impact of the condition on the patient's life, and all objective findings, including compensational holding patterns and concomitant dysfunctions
- Discuss and create functional goals—after the initial assessment and treatment—that can be used as a measurement of the success of the relationship in language to which the patient can relate
- Determine the treatment plan that will best address the needs of the patient and move toward accomplishing the goals

Use the extended version of the SOAP form (see Figure 6-5).

Subsequent SOAP notes are brief and primarily record the treatment provided. The focus is on the patient's immediate presenting concerns with consideration to the proposed treatment plan. The notes are less comprehensive in regards to assessment and are more specific to the data directly related to the treatment provided. For example: On Darnel's initial SOAP chart, all cervical actions and ranges of motion were tested and recorded. On a subsequent note in which the focus of treatment was to decrease neck stiffness, only the cervical active range of motion for lateral flexion was tested, charted, treated, and retested. The intent is to spend more time accomplishing goals than assessing the condition and determining the plan. The treatment plan is projected initially and reviewed during reevaluation sessions. Subsequent sessions carry out the treatment plan. The chart should reflect that and not repeat the goals or treatment plans unless changes are necessary. Often, the Assessment and Plan sections of the SOAP chart are left blank on subsequent notes. The Assessment section should only reflect functional outcomes or changes to the goals. The Plan section in a subsequent note need only chart additional homework assignments or self-care education, unless the treatment plan needs to be altered. A shorter version of the initial SOAP form is adequate for recording information between the initial visit and the reevaluation sessions (see Figure 6-6).

Progress SOAP notes are used to chart reevaluation sessions. Reevaluation sessions are nearly as extensive as initial visits. Time is spent assessing progress, setting new goals, and creating new treatment plans. Schedule reevaluation sessions at every 6 to 8 visits and document them thoroughly. The notes for these sessions should be comprehensive and include a full-body evaluation.

Address everything mentioned in the initial note. There is no need to introduce new assessment tests unless new symptoms arise. It is critical, however, to revisit all previous assessments, even if the corresponding symptoms are no longer an issue. The intent is to put to rest some data and to measure the progress of the remaining data. For example: Initially, Darnel had moderate, constant, low back pain; moderate, frequent headaches; and mild, constant neck stiffness. Thirty days later, in the first progress note, Darnel reported moderate, constant, low back pain; mild, intermittent headaches; but no neck stiffness (It is important to record the fact that there is no neck stiffness). Without a record of that information, one could question whether the neck stiffness was resolved or whether or not the practitioner simply forgot to note its existence. Once a symptom or objective finding is noted as a non-issue, it does not need to be revisited in any future progress note unless the symptom or finding returns.

FIGURE 6-5 Initial SOAP Chart

HANDS HEAL

John Olson, LMP, GCFP
345 Moon River Rd. Ste. 6
Minnehaha, MN 55987
TEL 612 555 9889

SOAP CHART-M

Patient Name Darnel G. Washington Date 2-6-04

Date of Injury 1-6-04 ID#/DOB 123-45-6789 Meds hydrocodone 500mg q4h

S Focus for Today ↓ Pain in head, neck, back

Symptoms: Location/Intensity/Frequency/Duration/Onset
Neck, midback, low back pain moderate
constant since car accident Δ L
headache Pain moderate intermittant
daily since car accident Δ Ⓟ

Activities of Daily Living: Aggravating/Relieving
A: 1. lifting granddaughter—necessary for care: in & out of car seat, high chair, bed etc.— Ⓟ M+ pain every time
2. gardening—vegetable and flower garden, bonding time with wife—unable to garden over 5 min.
3. unable to sit & play bridge over 30 min.
R: rest, heat

O Findings: Visual/Palpable/Test Results
V: Primary weight bearing rising and standing-
right leg and foot Δ̸
sits on right pelvis Δ L ↓ balance
bends from mid thoracic Δ̸
breath moderately shallow and rapid Δ L & even
mild to moderate segmental movement—left ribs
with deep inhalation Δ smooth
P: moderate right frontal torsion Δ L
moderate plus bilateral sphenoid compression Δ M⁻
mild plus adhesion tentorium Δ̸
cranial rhythm moderately weak right Δ L
mild left Δ Normal

Modalities: Applications/Locations
97140 Lymph Drainage—trunk
60 min. Craniosacral-head
Feldenkrais—eyes and feet

Response to Treatment (see Δ)

A Goals: Long-term/Short-term
LTG: Lift granddaughter at least 10 times per day from the floor and carry her for 10 minutes with mild pain and fatigue 5 days per week in 60 days
STG: Lift light weight toys from floor 10 times per day 3 days per week in 2 weeks with mild pain

Functional Outcomes

P Future Treatment/Frequency
2 times per week for 3 weeks, 60 min. sessions, continue with lymph drainage, craniosacral and Feldenkrais, focus on ribs, diaphragms, increase mobility and decrease adhesions

Homework/Self-care
continue using heat on mid back but avoid it on neck and low back—switch to ice. Deep breathing exercises

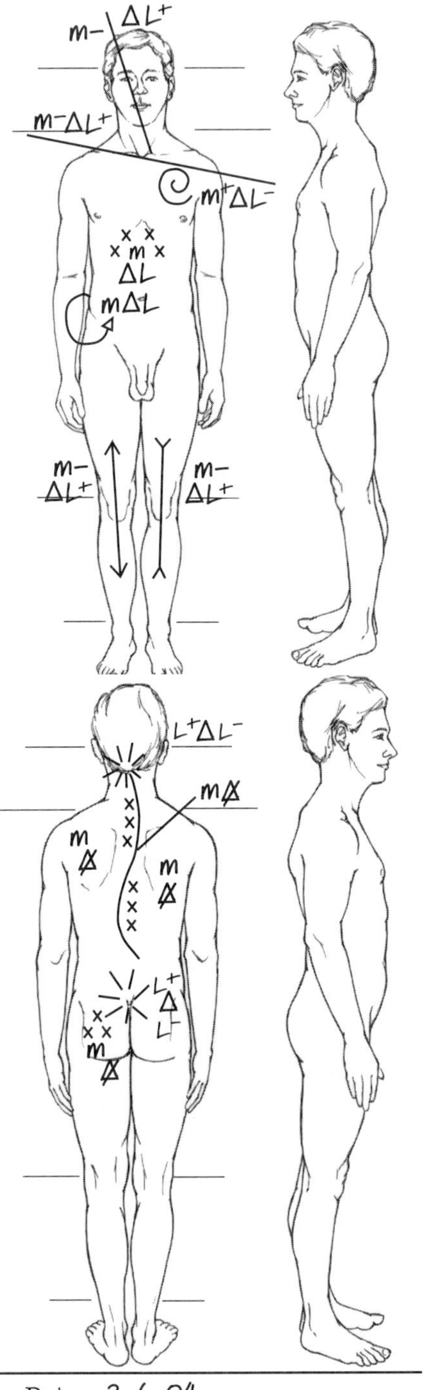

Provider Signature JO, LMP, GCFP Date 2-6-04

Legend: TP • TeP ○ Ⓟ Infl HT ≈ SP
× Adh Numb rot elev Short ⟷ Long

FIGURE 6-6 Subsequent SOAP Chart

John Olson, LMP, GCFP
345 Moon River Rd. Ste. 6
Minnehaha, MN   55987
TEL   612 555 9889

HANDS HEAL

SOAP CHART-M

Patient Name Darnel G. Washington   Date 2-8-04

Date of Injury 1-6-04   ID#/DOB 123-45-6789 Meds hydrocodone 500mg q4th

S Focus-decrease pain in head and neck

O 97140   60 min
Lymph Drainage neck, head

A F.O.-lifting lightweight toys from shelves with
moderate pain

P having good success with ice and breathing exercises
con't as instructed

Provider Signature ___ JO LMP GCFP ___   Date ___ 2-8-04 ___

S Focus-decrease pain in head & neck

O 97140 60 min
Lymph Drainage neck, head, chest, arms,
all passive cervical ranges of motion limited-mild
minus-with mild pain at end ranges Δ N
with L⁻ pain
A con't

P con't

Provider Signature ___ JO LMP GCFP ___   Date ___ 2-11-04 ___

Legend: ℮ TP   • TeP   ○ ℗   ☀ Infl   ≡ HT   ≈ SP
              ✕ Adh   ≋ Numb   ⟲ rot   ╱ elev   ⊢ Short   ⟷ Long

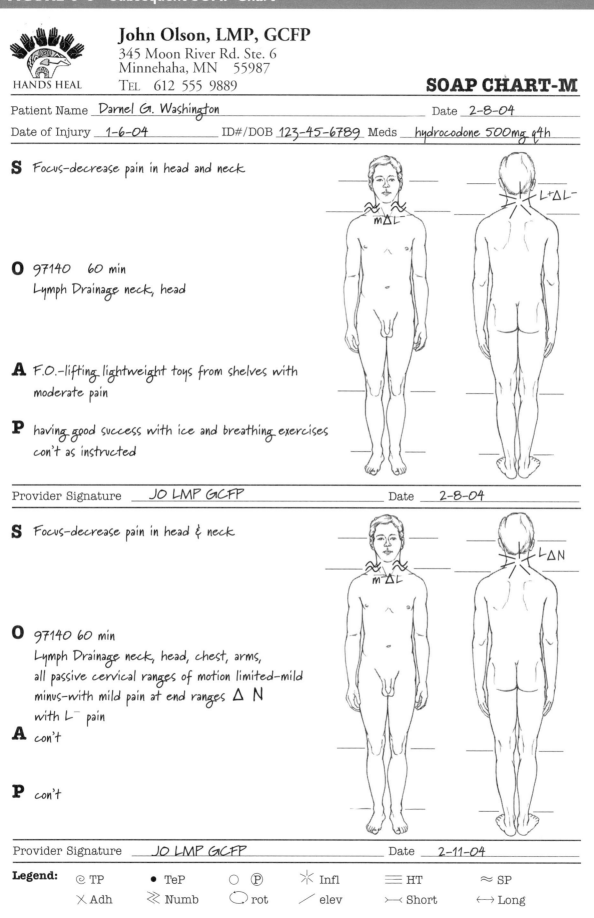

148

HANDS HEAL:
COMMUNICATION,
DOCUMENTATION,
AND INSURANCE BILLING
FOR MANUAL THERAPISTS

The intent of the progress note is to present a complete, current picture of the patient's health. A comparison of the initial note and a progress note (or two consecutive progress notes) will provide summary information for **progress reports**, which are typed on letterhead stationary and sent as a courtesy to referring the HCP. Progress notes are recorded on the extended version of a SOAP form and are similar to the initial SOAP chart (see Figure 6-7).

▼

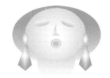

STORY TELLER
Assessment Is Treatment

A manual therapist in the Bay Area conducted a case study of all her patients to investigate the impact of information gathering on the patients' health. In every session over a one-year span, she began with range of motion testing. After recording the results, she continued to gather data, inquire about how patients felt and how their lives were impacted by the symptoms, and record postural and palpation findings. After 10 minutes of information gathering, she repeated the range of motion test. Surprisingly, the simple act of observing and recording patients' concerns resulted in a 50% improvement, on average, in range of motion. As the therapist, it is important to believe that the treatment time is well spent. This statistic may also convince patients— who are reluctant to take time away from the hands-on portion of the session—of the importance of information gathering and charting.

Upon completion of the therapeutic relationship or when the transition is made from treatment massage to wellness care, **discharge SOAP notes** are recorded. These include a final summary of the patient's progress, health status, and any subsequent course of action. Use the same SOAP form you used for the progress notes and adapt the Plan section to cover discharge data. Write the reasons for discharge, such as sessions reached limits of referral, patient met goals for care, or patient reached plateau in progress, in place of the treatment plan. Ongoing care may be required to maintain the progress established. Document any further action to be taken by the patient. Record the self-care regimen you recommend, suggestions for additional care, and any referrals to other caregivers or back to the referring HCP (see Figure 6-7).

Discharge notes include:

◆ Current health status
◆ Summary of treatment
◆ Summary of progress
◆ Reason for ending care
◆ Recommendations for ongoing care
◆ Referrals

Timing

SOAP charting may feel time-consuming at this point. You may be just beginning to chart or you may not have charted this extensively before. Charting may feel burdensome until

FIGURE 6-7 Progress SOAP Chart with Discharge Plan

John Olson, LMP, GCFP
345 Moon River Rd. Ste. 6
Minnehaha, MN   55987
TEL   612 555 9889

HANDS HEAL

SOAP CHART-M

Patient Name _Darnel G. Washington_ Date _1-20-05_

Date of Injury _1-6-04_ ID#/DOB _123-45-6789_ Meds _θ_

S Focus for Today   decrease stiffback

Symptoms: Location/Intensity/Frequency/Duration/Onset

Stiff mid back mild constant for 4 days since bridge marathon
last weekend Δ within normal limits

Activities of Daily Living: Aggravating/Relieving

A: carrying granddaughter more than 10 minutes sitting or
    gardening for more than 2 hours ↑ Ⓟ to moderate
R: exercises, stretching, rest

O Findings: Visual/Palpable/Test Results

moderate weakness with sitting Δ L
moving from mid thoracic instead of hips
rib mobility moderately decreased Δ L
breathing restricted-mild Δ N

Modalities: Applications/Locations
97140   Feldenkrais-ribs and thoracic spine
60 min.   Craniosacral-spinal traction and unwinding
Response to Treatment (see Δ)

A Goals: Long-term/Short-term

all goals have been reached within the limits of current
health condition

Functional Outcomes
has not regained prior functional status since car accident
1-6-01
(note activities of daily living listed above)

P Future Treatment/Frequency
continue awareness through movement classes once per month,
more often as needed, released from care and referred back to
Dr. Redtree.

Homework/Self-care
Remember to breathe and roll ribs when sitting for long periods-
take breaks and do exercises before stiffness sets in

Provider Signature _JO LMP GCFP_ Date _1-20-05_

Legend: ℮ TP   • TeP   ○ Ⓟ   ⚹ Infl   ≡ HT   ≈ SP
✕ Adh   ≋ Numb   ⟳ rot   ╱ elev   ⤙ Short   ↔ Long

150

HANDS HEAL:
COMMUNICATION,
DOCUMENTATION,
AND INSURANCE BILLING
FOR MANUAL THERAPISTS

it becomes habitual and you memorize the standard abbreviations. In time, you can expect to spend considerably less time charting outside each appointment time. Most charting occurs during the session with your patients. Charting in your patients' presence effectively includes them in the healing process. Do this to ensure accuracy and completeness and present an air of professionalism.

Write down subjective and objective information as you gather it from the patient. If you are performing hands-on tests or evaluating data at pre-treatment, during the massage, or in post-treatment take breaks to record information. Recording information as you go will prevent you from forgetting data and will give the patient time to rest and integrate your treatment.

After the session is over, review the goals and write new ones. Evaluate the progress and share feedback. Sharing the results of the session aloud immediately after the treatment assists the patient in integrating the results, verbalizing his or her needs for the session, and formulating ideas for future solutions. Discuss homework options and write down all assignments. Record the results of the session and status of the goals, write new goals, and work out the treatment plan together before the session ends.

The only thing left to do after the patient leaves is to review the subjective and objective data and fill in any details that will assist you in remembering information later. Otherwise, all charting is a part of the session and done with the patient present.

Remember, chart extensively every 30 days. Prepare your patients for these comprehensive evaluation sessions by telling them at the initial session what they can expect from the series, including how you work, the importance of gathering information, and how the feedback from the evaluations shapes your treatment plan (and ultimately the results). Impress upon them the importance of the information on your ability to be effective and efficient with your massage, and they will look forward to the information they receive from the assessments you provide.

SUMMARY

SOAP charting is a standard format routinely used by medical, chiropractic, and allied health professionals for documenting health care sessions. SOAP is an acronym that stands for:

- Subjective—data provided by the patient (symptoms and functional limitations)
- Objective—data from the practitioner's perspective (movement tests, palpation findings, visual observations, and treatment and the patient's immediate response to the treatment)
- Assessment—functional goals and outcomes based in activities of daily living
- Plan—treatment recommendations and self-care education

  Documentation guidelines include:

- Be attentive and practice good listening skills.
- Be clear and concise.
- Measure everything.
- Be specific—avoid vague statements such as improved, better, or less pain.
- Use consistent terminology.
- Chart information pertinent to patient's health.
- Be objective.
- Record positive and negative findings.
- Use common medical terms and standard abbreviations.
- Never use correction fluid or eraser to eliminate information.
- Sign or initial each entry with your legal name and credentials.

- Co-sign for students, aides, and apprentices.
- Write legibly.
- Print (or stamp) your name, address, and phone number on each page in the file.

Use a functional outcomes style of reporting information. Set long-term and short-term goals that will clearly demonstrate functional outcomes. Follow SMART criteria for functional goal setting. The SMART acronym stands for:

- Specific—to an activity of daily living.
- Measurable—quantify and qualify results to measure progress.
- Attainable—success is probable given the patient's condition, constitution, and attitude.
- Relevant—activity is critical to patient's ability to earn a living or care for self, family, or household.
- Time-bound—success within a specified time—long-term goals (typically 30 to 60 days) and short-term goals (generally about 1 to 2 weeks).

Describe the symptoms in detail in the Subjective section of the SOAP chart:

- Describe the symptom.
- Note the location.
- Rate the intensity.
- State the duration and frequency.
- Give a detailed description of the onset on the initial SOAP note.

Record functional limitations:

- Identify daily activities the patient can no longer do or cannot do without increasing symptoms.
- State the patient's previous ability to perform the activities listed.
- State, in measurable terms, the patient's current situation regarding the activities.
- Record activities that relieve the patient's condition.

Follow these guidelines for documenting objective data:

- Document the full range of data.
- Measure every finding.
- Base measurements on deviations from normal by (1) making bilateral comparison when possible, (2) defining normal for a general population of similar constitution, (3) asking patients to define normal for themselves.
- Measure the data before and after treatment.
- Perform the pre-evaluations and post-evaluations identically.
- Chart posture and movement by (1) noting the position of the patient, (2) noting the angle of the observation, (3) describing the activity.
- Chart palpation by (1) identifying the specific location, (2) rating or describing the touch that triggers the finding, (3) including referred sensations, (4) identifying connections or relationships between findings.
- Chart the ROM test by (1) identifying the position of the patient, (2) identifying the type of test, (3) naming the joint, (4) naming the action.
- Chart the results of the ROM test by (1) rating the amount of movement, (2) rating the pain associated with the movement, (3) rating the quality of the movement.

There are four types of SOAP notes (see Figure 6-8):

- Initial—comprehensive, prioritized list of concerns or desired results of the sessions, full-body evaluation, projected goals and treatment plan.
- Subsequent—focus on treatment, address current concerns and short-term goals and site-specific evaluation.

FIGURE 6-8 Types of SOAP Charts: Comparisons of Content

	Initial (First visit)	Subsequent	Progress (every 30 Days)	Subsequent	Discharge (last treatment)
S	All Health Concerns ALL Symptoms ALL Activities of Daily Living	Tx Focus Sx: significant changes only ADLs: significant changes only	Remaining Health Concerns ALL Sx ALL ADLs	Tx Focus Sx: significant changes only ADLs: significant changes only	Remaining Health Concerns ALL Sx ALL ADLs
O	ALL findings: Visual, palp., mvmt Tx, Δ	findings: significant changes only Tx, Δ	ALL findings Tx, Δ	findings: significant changes only Tx, Δ	ALL findings Tx, Δ
A	Long-term goals (LTG) Short-term goals (STG)	Functional Outcomes (FOs)	New LTG STG (s)	FOs	any remaining LTG summarize FOs
P	tx plan Homework Selfcare Ex (HW/SC)	HW/SC	New tx plan HW/SC	HW/SC	referral back to HCP long-term HW/SC

The ⟶ means that all data on the previous chart must be addressed in the current chart.

- ◆ Progress—comprehensive review of concerns, full-body evaluation, evaluate progress and reestablish goals and treatment plan.
- ◆ Discharge—full-body evaluation, summarize health status, summarize progress and functional outcomes, state reason for discharge, make recommendations for ongoing care.

Chart throughout the session in the presence of the patient to prevent charts from piling up on your desk. Memorize abbreviations and, in time, you will become fast and efficient at SOAP charting.

REFERENCES

1. Kettenbach G. Writing SOAP Notes. 2nd Ed. Philadelphia: F.A. Davis, 1995.

2. Dolan DW. Insurance Reimbursement and Specialty Physician Referrals. Jacksonville: American Health Press, 1999.

3. Rose, MK. The Art of the Chart: Documenting Manual Therapy with CARE Notes. massage and Bodywork Quarterly April/May, 2003.

4. Bates B. Guide to Physical Examination and History Taking. 8th Ed. Philadelphia: Lippincott Williams & Wilkins, 1998.

5. Adler RH, Giersch P. Whiplash, Spinal Trauma and the Chiropractic Personal Injury Case. Seattle: Adler ◆ Giersch, 2004.

6. Magee DJ. Orthopaedic Physical Assessment, 2nd Ed. Philadelphia: WB Saunders, 1992.

7. Travell J, Simons D, Simons L. Myofascial Pain and Dysfunction: The Trigger Point Manual. Baltimore: Williams & Wilkins, 1998.

8. Chenkin DC, Eisenberg D, Sherman KJ et al. Randomized trial comparing traditional Chinese medical acupuncture, therapeutic massage, and self-care education for chronic low back pain. Arch Intern med 2001;161:1081.

9. Kendell FP, McCreary EK, Provance PG. Muscles: Testing and Function. 4th ed. Baltimore: Williams & Wilkins, 1993.

10. Norkin CC, White D. Measurement of Joint Motion: A Guide to Goniometry. Philadelphia: F.A. Davis, 1995.

11. Weaver R. The Touch Factor Foundation Manual. Montana: Weaver, 1997.

CHAPTER **7**

Wellness Charting for Manual Therapies: Energy Work and Relaxation Therapies; Event, On-Site, and Spa Venues

CHAPTER OUTLINE

*J*ose received massage therapy weekly at the Healing Arts Clinic. He never mentioned to his massage therapists, Annie and Jamie, that he had been in a car collision. It wasn't a secret; he just didn't remember either of them asking. Jose was sure his car insurance would not cover massage because his doctor wouldn't prescribe it. Jose knew he needed something to loosen up his tense muscles and decided to pay cash for his weekly massages.

Jose responded well to his therapy. Annie combined Swedish techniques with deep tissue massage and gymnastics to increase mobility, loosen tight muscles, and help Jose relax. Jamie, who specialized in sports massage, used circulatory and drainage techniques. Jose found he had more energy and felt more relaxed. He believed massage was helping him recover from his car collision.

A year into his weekly massage routine, after prompting from his attorney, Jose asked the receptionist at the Healing Arts Clinic for copies of his massage records. His attorney wanted to include the massage records and bills in the settlement package for his personal injury lawsuit. The attorney intended to use the records to substantiate Jose's injuries and to strengthen his lawsuit with the bills and documented proof of out-of-pocket expenses Jose had incurred as a direct result of the collision. Jose hadn't specified any health complications and wasn't referred by a doctor. With no insurance company paying for the sessions, Annie had chosen not to document any of the sessions. Jamie did not chart her sessions either. The receptionist didn't have any records on Jose except cash receipts. Without documentation, Jose's lawyer was unable to establish a connection between the massage sessions and the injuries from the car collision. Therefore, Jose was unable to get reimbursed for the thousands of dollars he spent on massage, even though the therapy was instrumental in his recovery.

One afternoon, Jamie and Annie were sipping herbal tea at the Sunny Café downstairs and commiserating over their misfortune in losing their steady patient, Jose. Jamie told a similar story: A woman named Claire had been a patient for many years, coming monthly for relaxation massage. Then, three months ago, she was injured at work. Claire's insurance company refused to pay for her massage therapy. The insurance adjuster claimed that because Claire had been seeing a massage therapist before the injury, she must have had pre-existing conditions that required her to continue receiving massage treatments. Therefore, the massage therapy was not necessary for treating the recent injury.

Claire asked Jamie for her records so that she could prove to the insurance company that she had been in excellent health until the injury. But Jamie had no records of the massage sessions. Even though Claire had been healthy and received massage for relaxation only, there was no documentation to prove that to the insurance company. Claire was stuck with the bills.

Jamie and Annie shook their heads in dismay. Initially, they had been under the impression that only insurance-paying patients required documentation. Gone were the days when relaxation therapy was an excuse not to do paperwork. They made a pact with each other to better serve their patients and themselves by charting all sessions. It no longer mattered whether the session was for relaxation or injury treatment, or whether payment came from an insurance company or from the patient; they were going to keep records on every patient and document every session.

Introduction

SOAP (Subjective, Objective, Assessment, Plan) **charting** assists practitioners in solving patients' medical problems. Yet, not everyone seeks manual therapy to treat an injury or care for an illness. People in good health often receive manual therapies for any number of reasons, such as to relax and reduce stress, to experience healthy touch, or to detoxify and tone the skin.

If SOAP charting is used to help assess, treat, and cure medical problems and the patient has no pre-existing conditions or current complaints, is the practitioner obligated to keep a medical record?

Yes. Manual therapy is considered a health care modality and practitioners are licensed, certified, or regulated in varying capacities throughout the United States and other countries. If you are practicing massage, bodywork, or movement therapies in a state or province that does not regulate manual therapists as health care practitioners, simply ask your patients whether or not they feel your sessions assist them in keeping with their goals for health. Research suggests that they will say yes almost every time. In a consumer survey conducted in August 2003, 90% of the respondents agreed that massage could be beneficial to one's health; 97% of the 18- to 34-year-olds surveyed agreed with this statement.[1]

Unequivocally, manual therapy makes our bodies feel better and improves our outlook on life. As a result, we may need to adopt the standards of the health care profession until the laws catch up with our professional values.

In keeping with health care standards, manual therapists must record information about their patients' health and the services provided. Obviously, treatment for healthy or injury-free patients may not require extensive documentation on a SOAP note, as would charting patient symptoms and pathophysiological findings. Documenting manual therapy sessions for healthy patients is brief in comparison, and the format can be tailored to specific environments, such as spas, airport concessions, and sporting events.

▼

157

CHAPTER 7
Wellness Charting for Manual Therapies: Energy Work and Relaxation Therapies; Event, On-Site, and Spa Venues

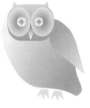

WISE ONE SPEAKS
Cost Benefits of Wellness Programs

A study described in *Wellness Management,* a newsletter of the National Wellness Association, reported the following benefits at more than 30 companies that had studied the effects of wellness programs over a 15-year period:

- **Average days of sick leave reduced by 22%**
- **Number of hospital admissions reduced by 62%**
- **Number of physician visits reduced by 16%**
- **Per capita health costs reduced by 28%**
- **Injury incidence reduced by 25%**
- **Per capita workers compensation cost reduced by 47%**

Reprinted with permission from Working in a wellness setting: New opportunities to expand your practice. Washington Massage Journal Nov/Dec 2003:6.

Wellness Format for Documenting Healthy Patients

A simple system for documenting healthy patient sessions is the Wellness chart. A Wellness chart contains a brief intake questionnaire for gathering health history information (Hx) and for recording the treatment provided (Tx). Additional information, such as personal preferences, variations from the routine, or patient progress, can be recorded under comments (C). The figures are optional and are useful for charting the therapist's findings,

158

HANDS HEAL:
COMMUNICATION,
DOCUMENTATION,
AND INSURANCE BILLING
FOR MANUAL THERAPISTS

such as muscle tension and postural deviations for patients receiving ongoing care. Three styles of Wellness charts are provided in this book: (1) Standard charts for relaxation, spa therapies, and energy work, (2) Seated charts for on-site sessions, and (3) Sports charts for sporting events (see Appendix B for blank forms).

There are only two requirements for charting wellness sessions. First, an adequate health history to ensure the patient's safety (see Chapter 5). Second, a detailed record of the therapy provided. Wellness charts must provide a historical record of wellness and health challenges over time and should recount the role of the manual therapist in the patient's progress toward health. The three components of treatment are:

◆ Type of manual therapy—techniques and modalities used
◆ Location—area where manual therapy was applied
◆ Duration—length of session

Treatment options can be provided, allowing the practitioner to simply check off or circle answers. Narrative charting is often too time-consuming for fast-paced environments with high turnover. One way to speed up charting is to provide predetermined options for treatment routines on customized Wellness charts. For example: pre-event or post-event might be the only categories you need for a sporting event; seaweed wrap, mud pack, or herbal moisturizer for a salon; stress buster, smooth and soothe, or energizer for an airport concession. Time can be noted in 15-minute increments. Location of treatment can be simplified with a checklist (see Figure 7-1) for full body (FB), upper extremities (UE), lower extremities (LE), upper trunk (UT), and lower trunk (LT). Customize your chart to fit your practice.

As discussed in Chapter 5, health information forms are completed annually. Modify the Wellness chart for repeat patients by eliminating the health history and multiplying the section that records the treatment (Tx) and comments (C). Four manual sessions can be recorded on each page (see Figures 7-2A and 7-2B). Make a point of recording pertinent

---

FIGURE 7-1 Customized Spa Wellness Chart—Treatment

3. Are you allergic to any of the following? (Please circle all that apply.) Almond Oil, Aloe Vera, Cucumber, Honey, Lavender, Milk, Mud, Olive Oil, Sandalwood, Seaweed.

4. I have provided all my known medical information. I give my consent to receive treatment.
   Signature _____ Date _____

Tx: ☐ body scrub ☐ herbal wrap ☐ Swedish massage ☐ mud pack

☐ FB ☐ UE ☐ LE ☐ UT ☐ LT ☐ facial ☐ foot reflexology

C: _____

☐ 15 ☐ 30 ☐ 45 ☐ 60 minute session   initials _____ date _____

FIGURE 7-2A Seated Wellness Chart—Second Page

Provider Name _____

WELLNESS CHART—SEATED

Name _____ ID#/DOB _____ Meds _____

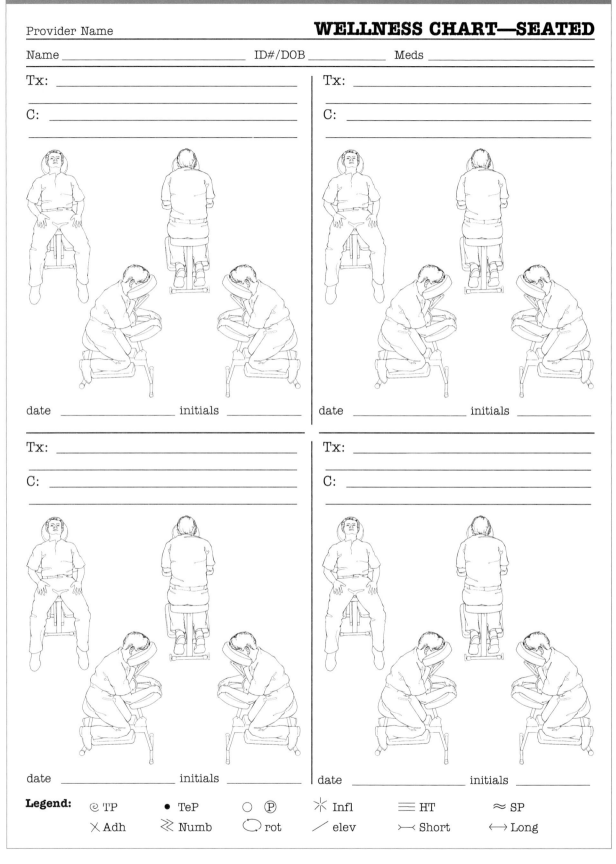

Tx: _____

C: _____
_____

date _____ initials _____

Tx: _____

C: _____
_____

date _____ initials _____

Tx: _____

C: _____
_____

date _____ initials _____

Tx: _____

C: _____
_____

date _____ initials _____

Legend: ℮ TP   ● TeP   ○ Ⓟ   ✳ Infl   ≡ HT   ≈ SP

✕ Adh   ≫ Numb   ⟲ rot   ╱ elev   ⊢ Short   ↔ Long

FIGURE 7-2B Standard Wellness Chart—Second Page

Provider Name _____ **WELLNESS CHART**

Name _____ ID#/DOB _____ Meds _____

Tx: _____

C: _____
_____

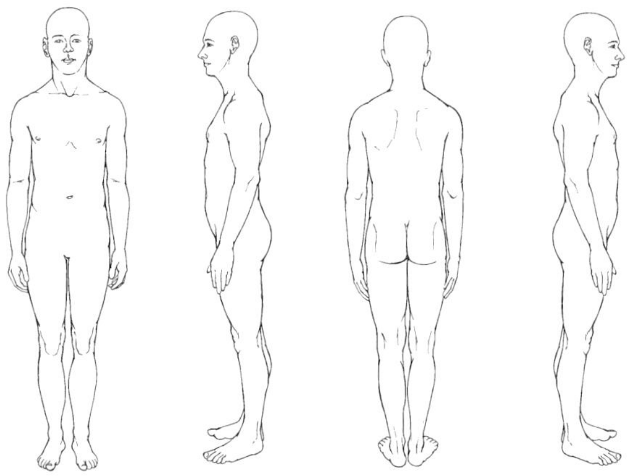

date _____ initials _____

Tx: _____

C: _____
_____

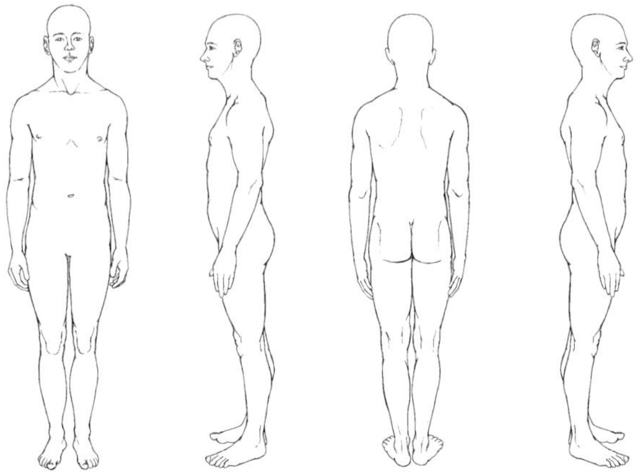

date _____ initials _____

Tx: _____

C: _____
_____

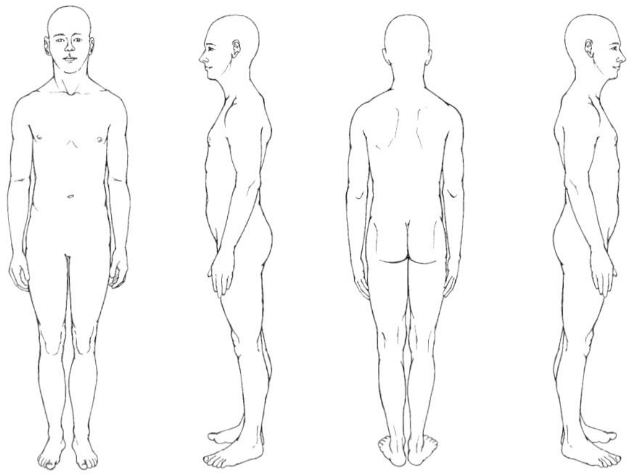

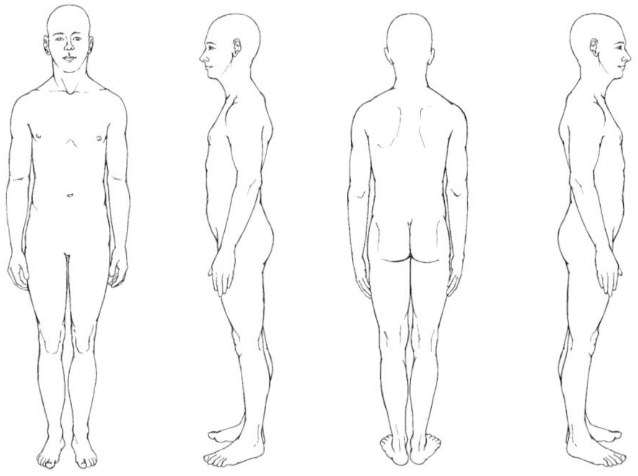

date _____ initials _____

Tx: _____

C: _____
_____

date _____ initials _____

Legend:

ℰ TP	• TeP	○ Ⓟ	✳ Infl	≡ HT	≈ SP
✕ Adh	≋ Numb	↻ rot	╱ elev	⤐ Short	↔ Long

patient data on the human figures for repeat patients. This is a quick and easy way to create a complete and accurate picture of your patient's health over time and, for ongoing manual therapy sessions, to highlight problem areas and demonstrate steady progress or reoccuring problems at a glance.

161

CHAPTER 7
Wellness Charting for Manual Therapies: Energy Work and Relaxation Therapies; Event, On-Site, and Spa Venues

SOAP Charting versus Wellness Charting

With each new patient, determine whether a SOAP note is necessary or whether a Wellness chart can be used. The question is not whether to document but rather which documentation format to use—SOAP, CARE, Wellness, Narrative, or another. It is *always* necessary to chart manual therapy sessions. Here are the factors to consider when selecting one style of documentation over another:

◆ Patient health
◆ Patient expectations
◆ Goals of treatment
◆ Treatment results
◆ Reimbursement for services

GUIDELINES FOR SELECTING THE SOAP FORMAT

SOAP charting is your best option any time extensive documentation is necessary. If any one of the following statements apply, use the standard SOAP format to document the treatment (see Chapter 6 for in-depth information on SOAP charting).

◆ The patient has health problems or symptoms and is seeking treatment to relieve them.
◆ A doctor referred the patient for treatment.
◆ Insurance is involved in reimbursement.
◆ The treatment provided varies from individual to individual and is based upon patient symptoms, conditions, and practitioner findings.
◆ The treatment results are significant, specific, and measurable.

A SOAP note is appropriate when the patient has health concerns that the manual therapist is expected to address during treatment. SOAP charts record patient symptoms, functional limitations, and objective data such as inflammation, muscle spams, trigger points, and the like. If the patient is healthy, there are no symptoms to record, no data to collect, and no condition to treat. However, patients have expectations that sometimes may be similar or different than our own regarding treatment. For example, the therapist may believe she is providing manual therapy for relaxation, but the patient may have selected the treatment specifically to heal a whiplash injury, as was the case for Jose. Remember to clarify patient goals and place them above your own or educate patients on the limitations of the treatment and discuss alternative options. The key is to reach a mutual agreement regarding goals for health.

Always use a SOAP chart with patients who have been referred by an HCP. Referring providers generally have a particular outcome in mind, making a thorough assessment warranted. You can always switch to a Wellness chart once a patient reaches his or her goals for health or when you discover that the patient's health concerns are minimal and manual therapy is primarily indicated for stress reduction.

162

HANDS HEAL:
COMMUNICATION,
DOCUMENTATION,
AND INSURANCE BILLING
FOR MANUAL THERAPISTS

If the patient is seeking insurance reimbursement, provide support by gathering information that will assist in receiving payment for your services. Insurance plans typically state that treatment must be **medically necessary**. A SOAP note will provide the documentation required to prove medical necessity. If you cannot find supportive data—proof of a medical condition that manual therapy can treat effectively and efficiently—chart the manual therapy sessions on a Wellness chart rather than stretching the truth simply to fill a SOAP chart. A common mistake when using a SOAP chart to record Wellness care is to note tight muscles as moderately or severely hypertonic, even though the patient's activity level is not affected by the tight muscle. It would be more realistic to note the tight muscles as mildly hypertonic: The tight muscle does not interfere with the patient's ability to perform daily activities. Claire, in the opening story, was hoping for documentation affirming that her regular manual therapy was addressing minor tight muscles and stiff joints, not the injury treatment the insurance company inferred.

All manual therapy treatments should be modified to meet the needs of the patient. The difference between a treatment that warrants a SOAP chart and one appropriate for a Wellness chart lies in the overall intent. Sessions where treatments vary constantly based on individual symptoms and findings and are applied in a curative manner deserve a SOAP chart. For example, if cross-fiber friction is applied directly over scar tissue with the intent to decrease adhesions and increase mobility, the treatment has curative intent and should be recorded on a SOAP chart. Manual therapy routines that vary slightly and occur in every session—as when modifications are made to ensure client safety and comfort, such as adjusting positions or providing a pillow—do not require a SOAP chart.

Treatment results that go beyond general therapeutic benefits, such as decreasing pain, increasing postural balance, or increasing mobility, should be substantiated on a SOAP chart. Document progress by measuring significant changes in subjective and objective findings. If, for example, you and your patient initially determined that treatment was strictly for general health purposes—increasing muscle relaxation, circulation, and energy—and you have been using the Wellness charting method, switch to the SOAP format once you and the patient determine that the goals of the therapy have changed.

Organize the charts in the patient's file chronologically by date regardless of format. There is no need to keep SOAP notes separate from Wellness notes. It is acceptable to mix charting formats within a single file. Patients often fluxuate between wellness care and therapeutic treatment as their needs change and they reach their goals for health.

GUIDELINES FOR SELECTING THE WELLNESS FORMAT

Use Wellness charting when the patient is healthy, treatment is routine, and sessions do not involve ongoing, curative health care. Follow these guidelines for determining whether a session warrants this style of documentation:

◆ The patient is healthy and has no specific health issues.
◆ If the patient has health issues, the specific health conditions, symptoms, and findings are not addressed in the session, other than for patient safety and comfort.
◆ Treatment is provided for general therapeutic benefits—such as improved circulation, relaxation, and energy—without the intent or expectation of altering existing health conditions or symptoms such as localized pain, numbness, compensatory postural patterns, or limited mobility.

163

CHAPTER 7
Wellness Charting for Manual
Therapies: Energy Work and
Relaxation Therapies; Event,
On-Site, and Spa Venues

◆ The treatment is routine. The practitioner does not deviate from that routine, other than to ensure patient safety and comfort, regardless of symptoms and pathophysiological findings.

◆ The patient is not using the session as ongoing, curative health care treatment for a specific condition.

RELAXATION THERAPIES: SOAP OR WELLNESS?

The style or the intent of the treatment can determine the documentation format. Drainage techniques applied as a full-body routine with general circulatory benefits may warrant Wellness charting; on the other hand, a drainage session designed to treat inflammation resulting from a swollen ankle warrants SOAP charting. Manual modalities, such as Trager, Swedish massage, and CranioSacral Therapy, can be applied with either curative or palliative intent. Follow the guidelines outlined above to determine whether to use SOAP charting or Wellness charting. Use the standard Wellness chart for documenting most relaxation therapies (see Figure 7-3).

In many cases, the guidelines for determining charting format are easy to apply.

However, situations exist in which the lines blur. For example, it is nearly impossible for many manual therapists to follow a relaxation routine and not address what they feel underneath their hands. If you find yourself treating specific findings and straying from a routine, note the variations from the routine and the objective findings in the comments section of the Wellness chart. If the patient returns for additional treatment and, together, you make the decision toward a more detailed treatment plan, switch to a SOAP format.

Relaxation is a general health benefit with widespread effects. Simple effleurage strokes can have profound analgesic benefits. Basic gymnastics can produce dramatic changes in mobility and function. Symptoms have been shown to resolve and illnesses to go into remission from healing touch.[2] The intent in providing an abbreviated format for charting is not to belittle the magnitude of hands-on healing, but rather to provide an avenue for simplifying the paperwork when appropriate. Use the Wellness format when the treatment is intended to be palliative, not curative. If the results are more profound than anticipated, describe them in the comments section.

ENERGY WORK: SOAP OR WELLNESS?

Energy work, as with any other manual therapy, can be charted on either a SOAP note or a Wellness chart, depending on the condition of the patient and the intent of the treatment. The difficulty in using a SOAP format to record energy work is one of language more than of style. Objective findings are not as tangible to the untrained hand or eye, but are equally valid. The initial challenge is in coming up with a vocabulary to define what you feel and see and to use it consistently in a way that makes sense to others who may be untrained in energetic modalities. The list of abbreviations provided in this book contains standard symbols and abbreviations for energetic findings and treatment techniques (see Appendix D). Create an addendum for additional terms to fit your practice or list additional terms directly on the Wellness chart (see Figure 7-4).

Guidelines for documenting energy work: Follow the guidelines for selecting the style of documentation. If Wellness charting is appropriate, chart the treatment routine and note the patient's response to treatment in the comment section or near the data noted on the human figures (see Figure 7-4). If SOAP charting is necessary, follow the guidelines

FIGURE 7-3 Standard Wellness Chart—Relaxation

Naomi Wachtel
567 Sunnydale Dr.
Flat Irons, CO   80302
TEL   303 555 8866

WELLNESS CHART

Name _Lin Pak_   ID#/DOB _5-31-63_   Date _7-27-04_

Phone _(303) 555-0033x253_   Address _IBM 3rd Floor_

1. What are your goals for health, and how may I assist you in achieving your goals? _Limit_
   long-term complications of diabetes through relaxation and stress reduction

2. List typical daily activities—work, exercise, home. _I sit a lot at work and watch movies_
   at home

3. Are you currently experiencing any of the following? If yes, please explain.

   pain, tenderness   ☒ No ☐ Yes: _____   stiffness ☒ No ☐ Yes: _____
   numbness or tingling   ☒ No ☐ Yes: _____   swelling   ☒ No ☐ Yes: _____
   allergies   ☒ No ☐ Yes: _____

4. List all illnesses, injuries, and health concerns you have now or have had in the past 3 years.
   (Examples: arthritis, diabetes, car crash, pregnancy) _diabetes, borderline high blood_
   pressure

5. List medications and pain relievers taken this week. _insulin_

6. I have provided all my known medical information. I acknowledge that massage therapy is
   not a substitute for medical diagnosis and treatment. I give my consent to receive treatment.

   Signature _Lin Pak_   Date _7-27-04_

   Tx: _Full Body Swedish Massage, Lymph Drainage trunk and upper extremities_
        45-minute session

   C: _Homework-relaxation exercises, check blood pressure before and after_
       massages at home

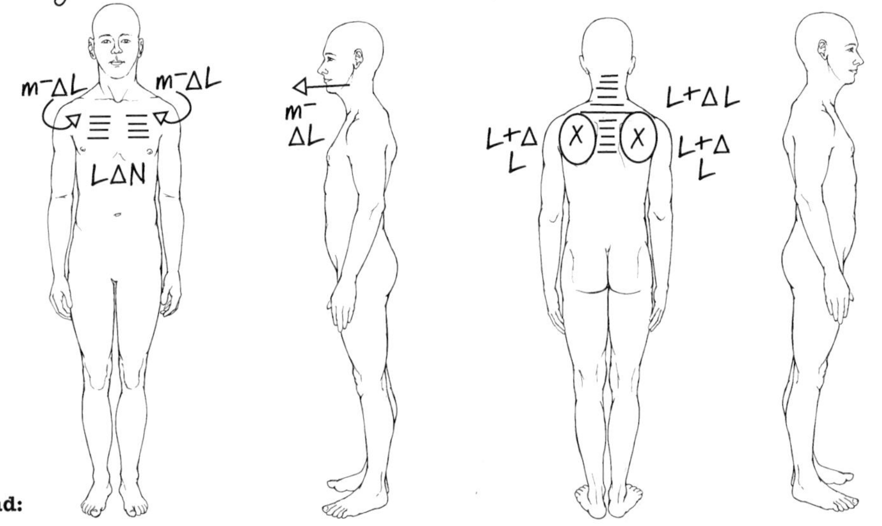

Legend:

ⓒ TP   • TeP   ○ ⓟ   ✳ Infl   ≡ HT   ≈ SP   initials _NW, LMT_

✕ Adh   ≋ Numb   ⟲ rot   ╱ elev   ⊷ Short   ⟷ Long

164

FIGURE 7-4 Standard Wellness Chart—Energy Work

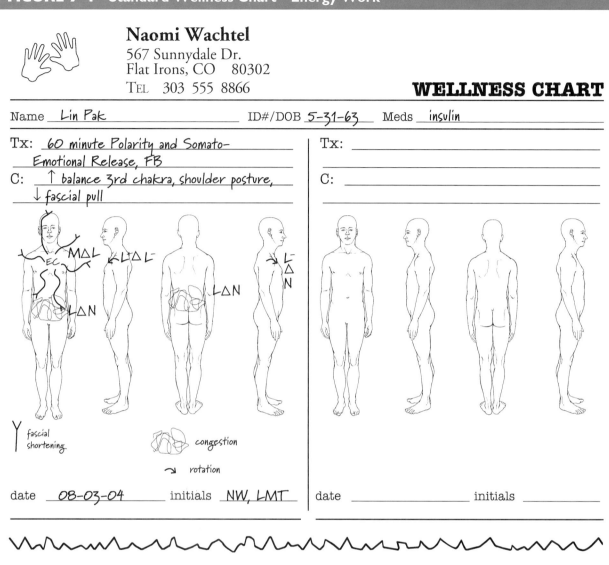

Naomi Wachtel
567 Sunnydale Dr.
Flat Irons, CO   80302
Tᴇʟ   303 555 8866

WELLNESS CHART

Name _Lin Pak_____   ID#/DOB _5-31-63___ Meds _insulin_____

Tx: _60 minute Polarity and Somato-_____   Tx: _____
___Emotional Release, FB_____
C: _↑ balance 3rd chakra, shoulder posture,___   C: _____
___↓ fascial pull_____

Y fascial
shortening

congestion

↷ rotation

date _08-03-04_____ initials _NW, LMT___   date _____ initials _____

presented in Chapter 6. Here is a modified summary of the information in the previous chapter regarding the charting of energy work:

◆ S—Note subjective information, as defined in Chapter 6 (p. 127).

◆ O—Note objective findings specific to your energetic training. Emphasize physiological findings. Use common terminology whenever possible.

◆ O—State treatment location, duration, and modalities used. Highlight specifics.

◆ O—State measurable changes in the subjective and objective data resulting from the session. Gauge the changes in intensity and quality of expression. Tell how the changes affect the patient's quality of life.

◆ A—If the patient's ability to function in everyday activities is impaired, set goals based on improving function, as defined in Chapter 6 (p. 138).

◆ P—Create a treatment plan and provide self-care instructions, as described in Chapter 6 (p. 143).

166

HANDS HEAL:
COMMUNICATION,
DOCUMENTATION,
AND INSURANCE BILLING
FOR MANUAL THERAPISTS

Energy work is often considered among insurance companies to be experimental or investigational because treatment results have not been adequately substantiated using standard scientific processes. This is also the case with other manual modalities. Lymphatic drainage is one of the few manual modalities to date with substantial international scientific evidence of effectiveness.[3] As a result, demonstrating measurable progress based in function, symptoms, and physiological findings is important for *all* manual modalities. When charting energy work—Reiki, Polarity, or therapeutic touch—or emotional bodywork, such as SomatoEmotional Release, Rosen Method, or Soma, emphasize the physical expressions of the energetic or emotional dysfunction. Highlight the results of treatment over the modalities used. Use terminology that is easily understood across professions.

Venues Befitting Wellness Charting

Wellness charting is appropriate for many venues. Two common ones are sporting events, in which participants receive pre- or post-event therapy, and spas, in which patients select from a menu of treatments designed for relaxation, detoxification, and beautification. The purpose of these sessions is specific to the venue, not to the individual, and the treatment routines do not vary much. Patients are not likely to depend on these for ongoing health care because the treatments are not tailored to meet individual needs, but rather to address general therapeutic goals.

Each venue has specific documentation needs. The following will be addressed individually:

◆ Events—sporting events and health fairs
◆ On-site venues—business offices, malls, airports, grocery stores
◆ Spas and salons

EVENT THERAPY

A common sight near the finish line at foot races or under a tent at street fairs is a large group of manual therapists with tables or chairs providing relief for participants. Manual therapy offered at venues such as these—sporting events, health fairs, and community events—require Wellness charting. The pace is fast, the turnover is frequent, the sessions are brief, and the need to document is minimal. The charts will not become permanent records of the patients' health, nor will the information be used for ongoing care. But the charts do assist the practitioner in determining whether treatment is appropriate, and they provide records that can become crucial if a patient claims later to have been injured in the course of treatment.

Treatment provided at events meets the guidelines for Wellness charting. The patients are healthy enough to be competing or walking long distances. Therapists are there to provide basic services and routine treatment. People are generally not seeking curative health care at these venues, and practitioners often do not have the time or information necessary to treat specific health conditions. Although therapists may use the event as an opportunity to market their practices, the treatment provided is likely to be the only treatment the patient will receive from these therapists. If the patient does seek out the therapist's professional services in the future, a formal intake will ensue and a decision will be made at that time regarding whether to use SOAP notes or Wellness notes for ongoing care.

Because the pace is fast and distractions are many at an event, read the intake questions out loud to the patient. Make eye contact to ensure that the patient is paying attention and understands the questions being asked. If a patient answers yes to any of the questions, the practitioner must be prepared to ask additional questions that are not on the intake form to establish the appropriateness of treatment. For example, if a patient says he has swollen feet, rule out infections and heart conditions that could be exacerbated by treatment. If a patient was injured recently, determine the treatment methods that are most appropriate and decide whether treatment to certain areas of the body should be avoided.[4] If a patient has just finished a race and is exhibiting signs of shock, first aid should be administered immediately by trained medical staff. The intake information is brief but critical in event venues, as discussed in Chapter 5. Tailor your event Wellness chart to the specific venue and the treatment routines you provide.

The nature of manual therapy at sports events is that there are no repeat visits. The event occurs once, or annually, and the tables or chairs are packed up and gone by the next day. As a result, several patient sessions can be recorded on one form—individual patient files need not be created. The intake questions are at the top of the form and are read to each individual. Space is provided below to record the athlete's name, the positive responses to intake questions, and the treatment provided, including modalities, location, and duration (see Figure 7-5).

ON-SITE MASSAGE

On-site chair massage is increasingly popular in work environments as an employee benefit. Many businesses recognize the detrimental effects of stress on job performance and long-term health[5] and offer on-site chair massage in an effort to keep productivity high and reduce sick leave.

On-site chair massage differs from event therapies in one important way—the site is often permanent. On-site companies or individual practitioners contract with businesses for regular visits, which often are weekly. When chair massage—accessible, non-threatening, and affordable—is a regular fixture in the work environment, patients who might not otherwise seek the services of a manual therapist may become repeat customers. A permanent site with repeat customers, many of whom have symptoms of repetitive stress conditions, presents some charting challenges, given the time constraints of on-site chair massage environments.

On-site chair massage, similar to event therapy, is fast-paced, has high turnover, and involves brief treatments. There is no time for extensive interviews, intake forms, or breaks between sessions for charting. However, the need for documentation is great. Charting must be quick and easy, and it must serve the needs of the patient.

In an interview, David Palmer, often called the father of on-site chair massage, said, "I don't see on-site massage . . . too closely associated with healthcare services because it's not a treatment . . . It's not designed to fix anything. It's merely designed to make people feel better and to produce what I think is the greatest value of manual, which is to simply enhance circulation."[6] In such situations, a brief Wellness chart is adequate. However, some people in the workplace have carpal tunnel syndrome, chronic headaches, or fibromyalgia. Many of those people use the on-site chair massage provided in their offices to treat their symptoms and to keep them functioning productively in the workplace. A record of their symptoms, physiological findings, and progress could benefit practitioners and patients alike. Demonstrating tangible results to business owners and to patients will increase customer satisfaction, demand, and availability.

167

CHAPTER 7
Wellness Charting for Manual
Therapies: Energy Work and
Relaxation Therapies; Event,
On-Site, and Spa Venues

FIGURE 7-5 Sports Chart

WELLNESS CHART—SPORTS

Provider Name __Naomi Wachtel, LMT__   Date __8-4-04__

Event __Mountain Aid 10K__   Location __Finish Line Tent__

Ask each athlete the following: (Note individual responses below—concerns only.)

1. Are you currently experiencing any of the following?
   - pain, tenderness, stiffness
   - swelling
   - numbness, tingling
   - dizziness
   - cold, clammy skin
   - shaking

2. How soon do you compete? / When did you finish competing?

3. Have you warmed up? / Cooled down?

4. Have you consumed water since the event?

Athlete's Name __Janelle Helm__   Athlete's initials: __JH__

Hx: (note concerns) __No water-gave her 12 oz B&A tx__

Tx: (check all that apply) _____ Pre-event __15 min__ Post-event _____ Refer-first aid/med

C: _____ Initials: __NW, LMT__

Athlete's Name __Michelle Johnson__   Athlete's initials: __MJ__

Hx: (note concerns) __Ø__

Tx: (check all that apply) _____ Pre-event __15 min__ Post-event _____ Refer-first aid/med

C: __Focus on feet & legs__ Initials: __NW, LMT__

Athlete's Name __Florence Thompson__   Athlete's initials: __FT__

Hx: (note concerns) __Ø__

Tx: (check all that apply) _____ Pre-event __10 min__ Post-event _____ Refer-first aid/med

C: __Focus on shoulders, UBack__ Initials: __NW, LMT__

Athlete's Name __Sam Bailey__   Athlete's initials: __SB__

Hx: (note concerns) __Spasm-Abd during tx__

Tx: (check all that apply) _____ Pre-event __5 min__ Post-event _____ Refer-first aid/med

C: _____ Initials: __NW, LMT__

Athlete's Name _____   Athlete's initials: _____

Hx: (note concerns) _____

Tx: (check all that apply) _____ Pre-event _____ Post-event _____ Refer-first aid/med

C: _____ Initials: _____

Athlete's Name _____   Athlete's initials: _____

Hx: (note concerns) _____

Tx: (check all that apply) _____ Pre-event _____ Post-event _____ Refer-first aid/med

C: _____ Initials: _____

The Seated Wellness chart (Figure 7-6) provides an alternative to the Sports Wellness chart. The primary addition to the chart includes illustrations of a person in a treatment chair. The practitioner draws symbols on the human figures, which allows quick charting of symptoms and objective findings and creates an easy reference for demonstrating progress and planning future treatments. The Seated Wellness chart contains an intake form, records measurable subjective and objective data, notes treatment routines, and provides space for additional comments from the practitioner.

Several treatments for the same patient may be recorded on the second page of the Seated Wellness chart to prevent repetitive health information gathering (see Figure 7-2A). Other on-site venues—airports, convention centers, shopping malls, and grocery stores—are not prone to repeat clientele. The clientele is transient, the desire to receive treatment is spontaneous, and sessions are routine. Do not attempt to record repeat visits on a single form for this type of patient. File charts by date, rather than by patient name, and have each patient fill out a new intake with each visit. Use the first page of the Seated Wellness chart for these venues or design a customized Wellness chart that meets your individual needs.

SPA AND SALON SESSIONS

Spas are traditionally located in resorts, which cater to a transient population. Increasingly, however, spas are found in downtown areas, in urban neighborhoods, and inside salons. Salons are incorporating manual therapy and hydrotherapy services with traditional pedicures, manicures, and facials. With increasing availability, people are becoming regulars of manual therapies in spas.

Spas and salons are ideal environments for Wellness charting. The need for extensive charting is low, and the turnover is fast. Treatment is routine and consistent and varies little with individual needs. Patients select treatment routines from a menu, based on the general health benefits advertised. The primary role of manual therapy in a spa environment involves pampering, facilitating relaxation, cleansing, detoxifying, and toning the skin. Patients rarely consider the treatment to be a remedy for an illness or injury, but rather may consider it a means of injury prevention and health maintenance.

Use of the Wellness chart in spas and salons is simple and practical. Practitioners use the chart to identify health conditions that contraindicate extreme temperatures or increases in circulation. Skin allergies and sensitivities are also major concerns when gathering health history. Treatment options are checked off, and comments primarily reflect the personal preferences of the patients. Use the standard Wellness chart (as shown in Figure 7-2B) or design a spa Wellness chart (see Figure 7-1) to meet your individual needs.

Space is provided for multiple sessions on one chart, because patients may return. In a curative health care environment, patient visits typically are weekly or biweekly. In a spa environment, monthly or quarterly visits more often are the norm.

SUMMARY

Document all massage therapy sessions. Two options for charting discussed in this chapter are:

◆ SOAP charting
◆ Wellness charting

169

CHAPTER 7
Wellness Charting for Manual Therapies: Energy Work and Relaxation Therapies; Event, On-Site, and Spa Venues

FIGURE 7-6   Seated Wellness Chart—First Page

Sarah Benjamin
123 Sun Moon and Stars Drive
Capitol Hill, WA   98119
TEL   206 555 4446

WELLNESS CHART—SEATED

Name ___Tham Maad___   ID#/DOB ___12-19-80___   Date ___12-12-04___

Phone ___ext 134___   Address ___Microtech N. campus 2nd floor___

1. What are your goals for health, and how may I assist you in achieving your goals? _____
   ___work without numbness, relax___

2. List typical daily activities—work, exercise, home. ___computer, reading, skateboarding___

3. Are you currently experiencing any of the following? If yes, please explain.

   pain, tenderness   ☒ No ☐ Yes: _____   stiffness ☐ No ☒ Yes: ___R SH___
   numbness or tingling   ☐ No ☒ Yes: ___R hand___   swelling   ☒ No ☐ Yes: _____
   allergies   ☒ No ☐ Yes: _____

4. List all illnesses, injuries, and health concerns you have now or have had in the past 3 years.
   (Examples: arthritis, diabetes, car crash, pregnancy) ___MVC Aug. 1993___

5. List medications and pain relievers taken this week. ___none___

6. I have provided all my known medical information. I acknowledge that massage therapy is
   not a substitute for medical diagnosis and treatment. I give my consent to receive treatment.

   Signature ___Tham Maad___   Date ___12-12-04___

   Tx: ___30 min. SW ⓜ - Focus on Ⓡ SH, arm, hand, BL neck, chest, back, light pressure___

   C: ___tingling in Ⓡ hand radiates from Ⓡ elbow, intermittant, worse in AM and late afternoon___

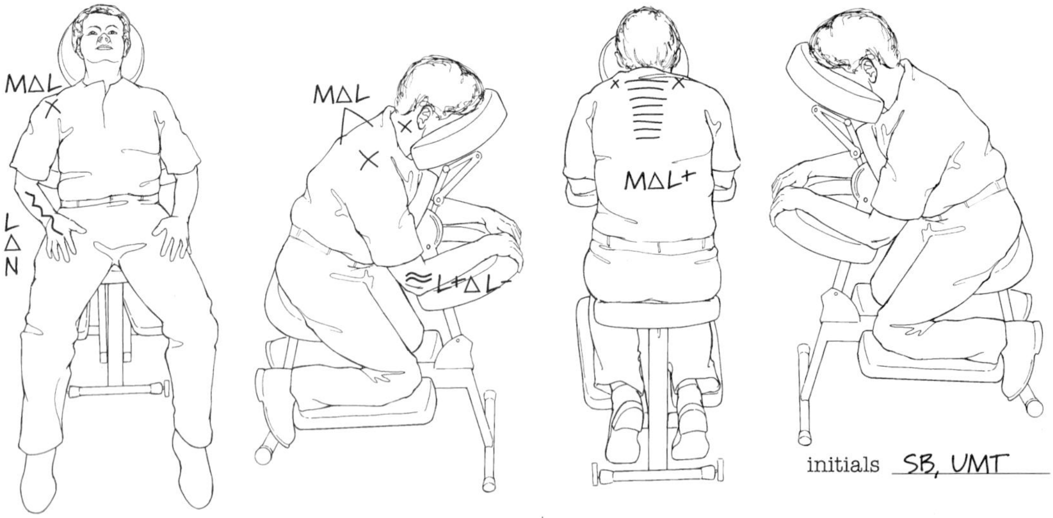

initials ___SB, UMT___

Legend:

℮ TP	● TeP	○ Ⓟ	✳ Infl	≡ HT	≈ SP
✕ Adh	≷ Numb	↻ rot	╱ elev	⊶ Short	⟷ Long

Use the Wellness format for relaxation treatments and energy work—depending on the health of the client and the intent of the treatment—and in the following venues:

171

CHAPTER 7
Wellness Charting for Manual
Therapies: Energy Work and
Relaxation Therapies; Event,
On-Site, and Spa Venues

◆ Events—sporting events and health fairs
◆ On-site locations—offices, malls, and airports
◆ Spas and salons

To ensure the effectiveness of the Wellness chart, vary the intake questions and treatment options according to the venue and the practitioner's treatment style. Use the Wellness format for charting sessions that meet the following guidelines:

◆ The patient is healthy and has no specific health issues.
◆ If the patient has health issues, the specific health conditions, symptoms, and findings are not addressed in the session.
◆ Treatment is provided for general therapeutic benefits without the intent or expectation of altering health problems or symptoms.
◆ The treatment is routine.
◆ The patient is not using the session as ongoing, curative health care treatment for a specific condition.

REFERENCES

1. Opinion Research Corporation International. Hands On: The Newsletter of the American Massage Therapy Association, November/December 2003, p. 6.
2. Carlson R, Shield B. Healers on Healing. Los Angeles. CA. Tarcher Inc. 1989.
3. Chikly B. Silent Waves: Theory and Practice of Lymphatic Drainage Therapy. Scottsdale, AZ: I.H.H. Publishing, 2002.
4. Werner R. A Massage Therapist's Guide to Pathology. Baltimore, MD: Williams & Wilkins, 2002.
5. Hafen BQ, Karren KJ, Frandsen KJ, Smith NL. Mind Body Health: The Effects of Attitudes, Emotions, and Relationships. Boston: Allyn & Bacon, 1996.
6. Mower M. The on-site massage movement: Interviews with David Palmer, Russ Borner, Raymond Blaylock. Massage Magazine March/April 1994, pp. 52–58.

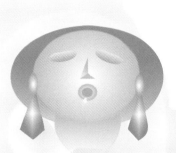

SECTION **III**

*B*illing and Ethics

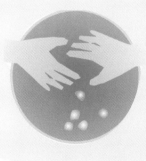

CHAPTER 8

Insurance Billing

CHAPTER OUTLINE

*S*everal years ago, I attended a panel discussion at a massage therapy convention on the integration of massage into insurance plans. The panel of physicians offered advice on participating in health care teams and billing insurance companies. The massage therapist mediating the panel opened her introduction with this joke: "I have some good news and some bad news. The good news is that we can now bill insurance for our services. The bad news is that we can now bill insurance for our services."

So far, the good news appears to outweigh the bad. Inclusion in insurance plans carries many benefits. As consumers, we have fought for the right to choose our health care providers and our preferred treatment modalities. The widespread inclusion of complementary and alternative medicine (CAM) into a variety of insurance plans proves that consumers can affect the health care industry. As health care providers, we have the opportunity to improve the lives and health of more people by participating in insurance programs.

Not only does this inclusion acknowledge our impact on patients' health, but it also permits us to promote change from inside the insurance and health care arenas. Manual therapists are hands-on, relationship-based practitioners who educate patients to ask questions and participate in their own care. All aspects of health care delivery shift as these newly empowered patients demand the same respect from other practitioners.

We also change the insurance industry by participating in insurance administration. A group of CAM providers was recently hired as consultants by an insurance company to assist with integrating acupuncture, massage, and naturopathy into the company's health plans. The goal was to educate staff and medical personnel on when and why to refer for complementary services. A massage therapist spoke at length to the medical director about the company's policies for treating lymphedema. She explained that lymphedema is a chronic condition that requires long-term treatment and self-care education and should not be treated as an acute condition with a two-week limit on care. By the next monthly meeting, the company had rewritten its entire policy on lymphedema treatment to reflect her suggestions.

Manual therapy is an industry that relies on word-of-mouth referrals. Opening our practices to health care referrals and insurance networks invites patients who may never have sought our services before, including those who are not yet aware of the benefits of manual therapy, those who cannot afford to pay out of pocket for our services, and those who would not normally seek out CAM care unless recommended by a doctor they trust. Each of these populations is large and can have an immediate impact on a manual therapist's practice.

Patients with acute conditions respond quickly to treatments. Health care referrals can offer an unparalleled learning environment. Patient files become a source for identifying effective and efficient treatments for a variety of conditions.

Accepting health care referrals and providing billing services can expand your patient load and your income. For example, I began offering insurance billing services in 1985. Before that, I had a modest practice in the evenings and on weekends. Immediately, I needed to hire three therapists just to service all the referrals. In a year and a half, my clinic had 15 manual therapists working full-time to meet the demand for services.

The panel mediator was right, however. There is bad news. Insurance billing can be complicated, costly, and time-consuming, and payment is not fully guaranteed. Billing requires frequent communication with insurance carriers and referring health care providers. The paperwork associated with insurance billing takes time, in addition to the time therapists spend treating patients. We must be willing to maintain clear paper pathways, remain flexible and pleasant in response to the demands of each carrier's protocols and procedures, and be persistent enough to see your way through to the end—payment in full.

Unfortunately, you must also be willing to discount your fees and sign restrictive contracts in order to participate in many health insurance plans. On the other hand, research shows that people are willing to pay out of pocket for our services,[1] but given the possibility of financial support from their insurance carriers, they will seek out manual therapists who participate in their plans. If we do not open our practices to insurance, we risk losing patients who go in search of a manual therapist willing to provide insurance billing services.

Colodia Owens, author of *Managed Care Organizations: Practical Implications for Medical Practices and Other Providers*, asks, "Is health care a right, a privilege, or a rationed commodity?"[2] I believe that health care is a right, and with a little tenacity and organizational skill, I can provide health care to my patients under their insurance plans. My participation in the insurance industry is a choice, and it makes me feel glad every time I look into a patient's grateful eyes—the police officer with a broken neck, the poet with lymphedema from a double mastectomy, and the professor with a closed-head injury. Together, we nod knowingly. This is care they don't get anywhere else.

Introduction

Insurance regulations and procedures vary from plan-to-plan, from state-to-state, and even among health care professions. Just when you think you have it all figured out, billing procedures change or a new CPT code (Current Procedural Terminology) is introduced and a familiar one deleted. Luckily, there are ways you can prepare for the fluctuating demands of insurance billing. This chapter provides guidelines for staying on top of the shifting information and decreasing the risks associated with accepting insurance reimbursement as payment for services.

Before you begin, ponder these questions to determine whether insurance billing services are appropriate for your practice:

1. Are peers in your area billing insurance companies? Are enough of them successful at it? Are they getting paid? Are their practices full as a result? If few of your peers are successful, you must be very creative and determined to break new ground for your profession. If many of your peers are billing insurance, you might find it difficult to compete if you choose not to participate.
2. Do you turn away people because you are unable to accommodate them? Would you like more patients? Have you ever lost a patient because you were unwilling to bill an insurance company? Have people changed their minds about scheduling with you when they found out that you do not accept insurance patients?
3. Can you afford to wait 30 to 90 days to get paid, which is the typical turnaround time for insurance reimbursement? Do you have adequate cash flow to meet your monthly expenses as you establish a consistent flow of insurance payments?
4. At what point will you feel motivated to offer insurance billing services? Many networks credentialing providers fill up quickly and close their doors to new providers within a year of offering manual therapy coverage in the plans. Will the insurance networks be closed when you are finally ready to join? Or will you retire before insurance billing is standard for your profession in your area?

If you choose not to provide billing services for your patients, are legally able to request payment up front for your services, and can provide a receipt with instructions on

178

HANDS HEAL:
COMMUNICATION,
DOCUMENTATION,
AND INSURANCE BILLING
FOR MANUAL THERAPISTS

how patients can seek insurance reimbursement on their own, you must educate yourself thoroughly to avoid burdening your patients with unnecessary risk.

Use the guidelines provided in this chapter together with information you gather that is specific to your state or region and to your **scope of practice**. Collecting this information requires some effort on your behalf, including making phone calls to peers and governing bodies, such as the Department of Health or Department of Education, insurance representatives, and attorneys. You will also need to read current research materials specific to your location and practice, including professional journals, insurance provider newsletters, and billing texts. Also, attend local workshops and seminars. Because of regional and professional differences in insurance billing and because licensing laws continue to change in many areas, it is critical to stay abreast of trends in insurance reimbursement that can affect your practice.

Playing the role of "ostrich in the sand" is not a viable option if an insurance review determines that you have received payment for services not within your scope of practice or that the fees charged were in excess of your usual fees. You can be forced to reimburse money that was paid to you and, in many instances, violations can be retroactive for several years. Follow the strategies suggested for managing insurance reimbursement and fill in the blanks with information specific to local laws and professional regulations. Carefully read Chapter 9: Ethics and ensure that your **fee schedules** are legal and ethical. Become well-informed and prepared to meet the demands of insurance billing.

Research the following before providing billing services:

◆ If you are a licensed health care provider, what services are within your legal scope of practice? Can you bill directly for your services? Do you need a prescription from a referring HCP, or do you have diagnostic scope? Which type of HCP has primary care status and can refer patients for manual therapy treatments?

◆ If you are not a licensed health care provider, do regulations exist that permit you to provide health care services under the license or supervision of an HCP with primary care status? Can you bill directly or must the supervising HCP bill for you? Do you need direct supervision or will a prescribed treatment plan and a referral suffice?

◆ Which types of insurance (for example, health insurance, worker's compensation, or personal injury protection coverage) will reimburse for manual therapy services in your state?

Once you determine that you are eligible to receive reimbursement for manual therapy services from insurance companies, confirm the billing and reimbursement procedures for each patient. For example, Blue Cross, a private health insurance company, has many plans available for consumers to purchase, and each plan has it own requirements for billing and reimbursement. Answer the following questions before providing billing services to a new patient:

◆ Is the patient's condition—such as muscle or joint pain, fibromyalgia, or cancer—covered under his or her insurance plan? Provide the insurance representative with the corresponding diagnostic code using **ICD-9** (International Classification of Diseases, Ninth Revision) **codes**. (See Appendix E for a condensed list of ICD-9 codes. For a complete listing, go online to http://www.icd9coding.com.)

◆ Are physical medicine and rehabilitation covered benefits for the patient's condition (the category of service that massage and manual therapy fall under in the CPT code manual)?

◆ Who can provide the massage or manual therapy treatment (i.e., a physical therapist, massage therapist, or occupational therapist)?

◆ Which therapeutic procedures or modalities are reimbursable when the professional therapist (i.e., licensed massage therapist) provides the service (i.e., massage, manual therapy techniques, therapeutic exercise, neuromuscular reeducation, or hot/cold packs)? Provide the CPT codes that correspond with the services being offered.

◆ What are the restrictions of each CPT code? These include services that cannot be provided on the same date of service, time limits on the duration of the treatment session, or the maximum reimbursement rate for the service.

In this chapter, forms are provided for identifying and recording information on your patients according to each individual plan. The accompanying guidelines assist you with communication and organizational skills to make the insurance billing process flow smoothly and to decrease the risks involved.

To get started, familiarize yourself with the following terms and resources:

◆ Physical Medicine and Rehabilitative Services—These are headings in insurance policy manuals and CPT codebooks that contain the services provided by most manual therapists. Review your own insurance policy booklet, which is sometimes called the Certificate of Coverage and read the Schedule of Benefits. Under Physical Medicine (or Rehabilitative Services), read the description of covered services and excluded services. The list will include those who can provide the services, services that are allowed or excluded, whether or not a prescription is required, and a definition of **medical necessity**. For example:

> Rehabilitation services are covered . . . to restore or improve functional abilities following illness, injury, or surgery. . . . All services must be prescribed and provided by a rehabilitation team . . . that may include . . . medical, nursing, physical therapy, occupational therapy, massage therapy and speech therapy providers. . . . Such services are provided only when significant, measurable improvement to the Member's condition can be expected within a 60-day period. Excluded: . . . therapy for degenerative or static conditions when the expected outcome is primarily to maintain the level of functioning . . . recreational, life-enhancing, relaxation or palliative therapy.[3]

◆ ICD-9 codes—The initials refer to the International Classification of Diseases, Ninth Revision, which is a system of classifying diseases using specific diagnoses code numbers to describe a patient's health care condition. ICD-9 codes are updated annually and published by the World Health Organization (WHO). They are recommended for use in all clinical settings and are required when reporting diagnoses and diseases to the U.S. Public Health Service and the **Centers for Medicare and Medicaid Services (CMS)**. This organization was the **Health Care Financing Administration (HCFA)** until 2001. New, revised, and discontinued codes can be accessed via the CMS Web site at http://www.cms.hhs.gov/medlearn/icd9code.asp. Stanford University provides a free Web site that is fast and easy to use and does not require users to register before accessing codes. Go online to http://neuro3.stanford.edu/CodeWorrier/. For comprehensive listings, go to http://icd9coding.com/.

◆ CPT codes—These are standardized numerical codes and descriptions of clinical procedures developed by the American Medical Association (AMA) with the intent and spirit to accurately describe clinical procedures in a nonprovider-specific way so that personnel

180

HANDS HEAL:
COMMUNICATION,
DOCUMENTATION,
AND INSURANCE BILLING
FOR MANUAL THERAPISTS

in any specialty or discipline may use them.[4] CPT codebooks are updated annually and published by the AMA. The codes are available online at http://www.ama-assn.org (a fee is required to gain access to this site). An inexpensive way to stay current with these codes is to subscribe to a service and purchase only the codes you need. For an annual fee, you will be notified of code changes pertinent to your practice. A "Coders Club" is available at http://www.flashcode.com/ and at http://www.ama-assn.org.

◆ CCI or NCCI bundling—**Correct Coding Initiatives (CCI)** or **National Correct Coding Initiatives (NCCI)** are pairs of CPT codes that cannot be reimbursed when paired together on the same date of service. They must be bundled and submitted as a single code only. For example, CMS does not allow a practitioner to bill for manual therapy—97140—and massage therapy—97124—on the same date of service. Many private health insurers follow CMS guidelines, and even though you may not bill Medicare, you may still be bound by Medicare policies. To access these pairings, access the CMS Web site at http://www.cms.hhs.gov/medlearn/icd9code.asp.

Types of Insurance Coverage

Three common types of insurance coverage are personal injury coverage, workers' compensation, and private health insurance.

Manual therapists, whether they are licensed or unlicensed, are often able to have their bills reimbursed through a **personal injury** claim. When injuries are sustained because of the negligence of another, the **at-fault party** is financially responsible for the injured party's reasonable and necessary medical treatments at the conclusion of the case. These treatments generally include services intended to help the patient return to pre-injury status or to reach maximum medical improvement. When manual therapy is medically necessary, is prescribed by a primary HCP, and is performed by an HCP (or is under his or her supervision), it is covered under the at-fault party's liability insurance.

Many **workers' compensation** plans cover manual therapy services because in-house statistics support it as an inexpensive and effective way to return patients to work quickly. These state plans provide for manual therapy treatments for most on-the-job injuries and lead the way for inclusion in other health plans.[5]

Private health insurance, on the other hand, tightly defines the treatments and modalities that are reimbursable and the conditions under which they are covered. Insurance plans that cover manual therapy will often reimburse the treatment only when it is provided by physical therapists, nurses, or chiropractors. Few cover manual therapy provided by licensed massage therapists or certified bodyworkers. Increasingly, however, consumers are demanding that insurance carriers include CAM care in their plans, which includes massage therapy, acupuncture, naturopathy, and others. Some states, including Arkansas, Georgia, Indiana, Illinois, Kentucky, Minnesota, Virginia, and Wyoming, have what is called an **Any Willing Provider (AWP)** statute that allows willing providers to cover services for a predetermined fee that will be accepted by the health carrier. There are no networks to get into. Any provider willing to perform the services would simply bill the health carrier. In addition, states such as Washington are benefiting from a nondiscrimination statute indicating that insurers must contract with every category of health care provider. In this scenario, health care providers must be licensed or certified by the state's department of health and contracted by the insurance carrier, the patient's condition must be within the HCP's scope of practice to treat, and treatment must be within the provisions of the patient's insurance policy.

Before long, manual therapy will be a standard health care service covered in health plans across the United States.

Manual therapists in some states can bill all three types of coverage successfully. However, in other states, success may be obtained in only one or two of the three. Do your homework before providing the service.

PERSONAL INJURY INSURANCE*

Personal injury insurance is bundled into insurance policies such as car insurance, homeowners insurance, and commercial building insurance. Commonly, policyholders purchase medical coverage within these plans for personal injury, medical payments, and **liability coverage** (which includes bodily injury and property damage).

The most common type of claim for personal injury insurance is for injuries sustained in a motor vehicle collision (MVC). Each year, three to five million MVCs are reported to the police and to hospitals in the United States, and countless more go unreported.[6] Because of these staggering numbers, therapists in practice will frequently find themselves billing automobile insurance carriers.

Manual therapists need to be aware of five types of insurance coverage when treating patients involved in MVCs:

◆ Personal injury protection (PIP)
◆ Medical Payments (Med-Pay)
◆ Secondary PIP or Med-Pay insurance
◆ Third-party coverage or liability insurance
◆ Uninsured motorist (UM) protection

Personal Injury Protection

Personal injury protection is one component of automobile insurance coverage that can be purchased as part of any auto policy. Some states require drivers to purchase PIP; for other states, it is optional. In Washington State, for example, insurers are required to offer PIP to their policyholders, who have the right to refuse such coverage by signing a formal written "waiver" recognizing their understanding of the coverage and their decision to reject it. Benefits may include payment of medical and hospital fees, recovery of lost wages and loss of services (such as household help), and payment for funeral services. Payment of these benefits does not depend on any determination of who was at fault.

Various levels of PIP coverage can be purchased, and every company offers different options within those levels, including $5,000, $10,000, $25,000, $35,000 limits. A standard time provision on PIP coverage varies from one to three years. Therefore, it is important to know the provisions specific to each patient's plan before agreeing to bill directly to the insurance carrier. This will help ensure that the time limit has not expired or that coverage has not been exhausted by bills from other health care practitioners.

From a reimbursement standpoint, PIP is the most attractive type of coverage. Therapists do not have to wait for fault to be determined nor do they have to deal with health insurance policies that may not cover their treatment modalities. The primary requirement is that your documentation prove that your care is reasonable and necessary and that the treatment is for injuries sustained in the collision. Also, a referring HCP must have prescribed the treatment as medically necessary.

*This section is revised and reprinted with permission, all rights reserved. Adler, Giersch. Whiplash, Spinal Trauma, and the Personal Injury Case. Seattle: Adler◆Giersch PS, 2005.

182

HANDS HEAL:
COMMUNICATION,
DOCUMENTATION,
AND INSURANCE BILLING
FOR MANUAL THERAPISTS

Medical Payments

Medical Payments (Med-Pay) coverage is also a provision that can be purchased under the auto insurance policy. Again, the amount of coverage differs from state to state and from insurer to insurer. If there is no PIP coverage, Med-Pay may be available to cover manual therapy services. Med-Pay is generally available for a lower dollar amount than PIP and covers medical expenses only. As with PIP, payment does not depend on determining who was at fault.

Secondary PIP or Med-Pay Insurance

One or more PIP or Med-Pay policies may cover your patient for the same collision. For example, when Darnel was a passenger in his nephew's car, the nephew's PIP paid for Darnel's medical expenses as the **primary insurer**, even though Darnel had car insurance. If the nephew's PIP was exhausted, Darnel's PIP insurance coverage could kick in as the secondary PIP insurer if additional medical services were needed.

In other words, if Darnel did not have PIP or Med-Pay and the nephew's PIP had exhausted, Darnel's health insurance would become the **secondary insurer**.

Third-Party Coverage or Liability Insurance

Third-party coverage refers to the liability insurance coverage of the at-fault party. The driver of the truck that rear-ended Darnel is the at-fault party, and his insurance plan is the third-party or liability insurer. Billing the third-party insurance company is unproductive because the company is not required to pay bills until the injured party making the claim is ready to settle the entire claim at one time.

End-of-settlement cases are those in which the patient was not at fault and the patient's PIP or Med-Pay coverage (or secondary insurance) is insufficient or nonexistent and the provider of health services, such as a manual therapist, must wait until the claim against the at-fault party settles or a judge or jury issues a verdict before receiving payment for services. End-of-settlement cases can be risky. The patient may not be able to prove that he was not at fault. If Darnel, for example, had an attorney who was convinced that fault on the part of the truck driver could be established, the risk would be lessened. But, can you as a therapist in practice afford to wait until the case settles before getting paid? In many cases, months or even years will pass before a settlement is reached, depending on the statute of limitations and whether the case ever goes to trial. If the patient and the lawyer are willing to sign a contract guaranteeing your payment once the settlement ends, your risk will be reduced. A **health care lien**, filed in accordance with the requirements of your state, can lower the risk even further.

The positive side of an end-of-settlement case is that it becomes a savings account gaining simple interest monthly. Interest can be applied within the legal limit for health care services. For example, in the state of Washington, interest begins to accrue 45 days after no payment is made if you notify the patient at the beginning of treatment that interest will be charged (assuming payment is not made at the time services are provided). Some states also regulate how much time must pass before interest can accrue, which may be 45, 60 or 90 days. If you ensure adequate cash flow by limiting the number of end-of-settlement cases you carry at a time, and if you take precautions to reduce your risk, the occasional end-of-settlement case can enhance your cash flow (see Chapter 3 for information on reducing your risk by enhancing your relationship with the legal team).

In the event that the patient's insurance carrier pays for expenses up front, it will rely upon the subrogation provisions in the patient's insurance contract with the insurers. Under subrogation, the insurer will seek reimbursement of its health care payments from the injured party's third-party settlement. Subrogation is a complicated legal principle that has many exceptions and differences in implementation from state to state. Generally, subrogation means that a patient cannot have the same bill paid twice. This can happen when the PIP or health insurer pays a bill, and, during the third-party case, the patient has her attorney use the bill and her chart notes to demonstrate evidence of injury and economic loss. When the bill is used as evidence of damages and a settlement is reached involving that bill, it has been paid twice and the patient's insurer will assert a claim for reimbursement.

Uninsured Motorists

Uninsured motorist coverage protects the policyholder against MVC injuries inflicted by someone who does not have an active insurance policy or who flees the scene and remains unidentified. This coverage is also activated when the person who causes the collision has insurance but the injured person does not.

WORKERS' COMPENSATION

Workers' compensation is insurance that employers are mandated to purchase for all employees. These plans furnish medical and disability benefits for illnesses, injuries, disabilities, and death that result from job-related conditions and activities.

The primary intent of this coverage is to return the employee to full-duty work quickly and without recurrence of injury. Benefits vary from state to state. Often, limits apply on the services that are reimbursable, on who may perform those services, and on how many sessions are available. For example, fees allowed must be accepted as payment in full and health providers must agree to contracted provisions. Request a copy of the provider regulations for your profession and an application for a provider number, if applicable. Read the regulations thoroughly before determining whether you want to provide this service to your patients (see Appendix F for contact information).

Each state has an insurance plan available to employees through its Department of Labor and Industries or workers' compensation program. Employers pay fees according to job description, and funds are collected quarterly. Employers have the option of using the insurance provided by the state or, if their business is large enough, may choose to be **self-insured**. These self-insured plans must meet or exceed the coverage mandated by state law. For example, the U.S. government is self-insured. Rather than managing different plans that cover employees in every state, the federal government uses its own plan that meets or exceeds the requirements in each state. All federal claims, regardless of the state in which the employee works, are submitted to the same workers' compensation insurance carrier.

PRIVATE HEALTH INSURANCE

Private health insurance provides payment of benefits for covered illness and injury. Many types of health care reimbursement plans exist, with an array of companies to supply them, including:

◆ Managed care plans
◆ Indemnity plans or fee-for-service plans
◆ Major medical
◆ Medicare and Medicaid

184

HANDS HEAL:
COMMUNICATION,
DOCUMENTATION,
AND INSURANCE BILLING
FOR MANUAL THERAPISTS

The most widespread type of health insurance plan today is **managed care**, which is on the opposite end of the spectrum from traditional **indemnity plans** or **fee-for-service plans**.

Traditionally, people would go to their own doctor whenever they felt it was necessary. The doctor would do whatever he or she deemed necessary for the patient's health and would submit a bill to the insurance company for that visit. The insurance company would pay the doctor for the services provided. This is known as an indemnity plan, or a fee-for-service type of health care.

Because of an increase in accessibility of health care, the unrestricted use of reimbursement, and rising health care costs, insurance companies were driven to search for ways of managing health care costs. Managed care was created to limit:

◆ Coverage of services
◆ Supplier of those services
◆ Fees for those services

Major medical insurance covers the expense of major illness and injury. There are usually high benefit maximums and high deductibles, and the insurance company reimburses a percentage of the costs after the deductible.

Medicare and **Medicaid** provide public assistance to the aged and the financially challenged, respectively. These types of health insurance plans place restrictions on the techniques and modalities that are reimbursable.

Managed Care Plans

Managed care organizations manage costs by contracting with selected groups of providers who agree to receive predetermined rates. An administrator manages the patient's access to health care, assesses the patient's case from a financial and clinical perspective, develops a plan of care in conjunction with the referring HCP and other health care providers, determines medical necessity, and evaluates the quality of care provided. Managed care integrates the financing and delivery of health care services to covered individuals. Significant financial incentives are offered for members to use providers within the "network" and procedures associated with the plan.

Health Maintenance Organizations

Health Maintenance Organizations (**HMOs**) are a type of managed care organization. HMOs combine insurance reimbursement with the delivery of health care services and provide specified medical services to defined groups of individuals for a stated period of time at a fixed price.

HMOs vary in structure and in reimbursement methods. Some vary in their contracts with providers. For example, a group model contracts with a group of providers. An **independent practice arrangement (IPA)** contracts with providers in private practice. The point-of-service model allows the insured to use the contracted providers or receive services from outside the network. There are financial incentives to stay within the network of providers, however.

Reimbursement arrangements in HMOs include:

◆ Discounted fees for services
◆ Capped fees for services

- Bundling fees for all services provided
- Capitation

A **discounted fee** arrangement is a managed care approach in which the provider contracts with the insurance carrier to offer services to the insured at a discount. This is also known as an **affinity plan,** or **affinity network**. The patient pays the provider the discounted fee directly, and the provider accepts this fee as payment in full.

With a **capped fee**, the provider contracts with the insurance carrier for services at a reduced cost. The insurance carrier reimburses the provider for services at the capped rate—payment comes from the insurer—and the provider accepts this fee as payment in full. Bundling, or a **global fee** schedule, lumps all services provided into one fee. For example, Helena, Zamora's manual therapist, provides several services, including Rolfing (structural integration), hydrotherapy, and Polarity therapy. She bills each one at a different rate. With this reimbursement arrangement, all of her services are lumped into one CPT code—97124—and billed at the same rate.

Capitation is a fixed monthly payment made to a managed care insurer for contracted services during a specified period of time, regardless of how many times the member uses the services. Capitation is nearly impossible to apply to manual therapy practices because of the time required for delivering the service and the physical inability of the practitioner to provide more than a predetermined number of sessions per day.

Preferred Provider Organizations

Preferred Provider Organizations (PPOs) are similar to HMOs, except they primarily contract with independent providers and they share similarities with the traditional fee-for-service health plans. PPOs were developed as a bridge between managed care plans and indemnity plans as a response to concerns that services provided by HMOs could become inflexible, that patients' choice of providers could be eliminated, and that accelerating costs could make indemnity plans too expensive for employers and policyholders.

Becoming a Preferred Provider in a Managed Care System

Credentialing

Some insurance plans have a credentialing process for contracting with preferred providers. Other insurance carriers buy contracts from an insurance network. Networks credential providers and sell their contracts to insurance carriers for a user fee. The credentialing process varies among carriers and networks, but it generally consists of the following:

- Review of company standards, such as years in the profession, accessibility, and the like
- Completion of an application and acceptance of professional references
- Signed contract showing agreement to company policies and provider services, including a **hold harmless clause** in the event that the carrier becomes insolvent, to prevent health care providers, including manual therapists, from seeking payment from the patient
- Proof of licensure, certification, registration, or all three
- Proof of business license
- Proof of liability insurance
- Proof of education certificate, continuing education hours, current CPR training
- Proof of professional affiliations with organizations that enforce a code of ethics
- Background check for complaints and disciplinary actions

186

HANDS HEAL:
COMMUNICATION,
DOCUMENTATION,
AND INSURANCE BILLING
FOR MANUAL THERAPISTS

Plans often hire consultants from the profession to assist in developing credentialing criteria and procedures as more plans integrate manual therapy. However, once the criteria are in place, credentialing and peer reviewing are usually done by someone familiar with several professions, not just the one being reviewed. For example, a nurse might be hired to conduct a **peer review** for massage therapists, physical therapists, and occupational therapists.

Site inspections and reviews of patient records are common components of credentialing. Many insurance carriers will not credential practitioners who work at home, who do not provide handicap accessibility, or who do not maintain adequate patient records.

Specific continuing education courses in, for example, documentation and billing may be required as part of the credentialing process. Similarly, a **quality improvement program** may be mandatory for recredentialing on an annual basis. The manual therapist also agrees to comply with utilization management programs, which randomly audit practitioners to evaluate the effectiveness, appropriateness, and quality of services provided.

Contracts

Contracts vary among plans and among providers. Read all contracts carefully because they are legally binding. An article in the *Journal*, a publication of the American Massage Therapy Association (Washington Chapter), mentions paying close attention to the following sections of a contract[7]:

♦ Fee schedules
♦ Patient access
♦ Contract termination
♦ Records and documentation

By contracting with an insurance carrier, you exchange discounted services for marketing. Marketing can be expensive and time-consuming for small businesses. Many manual therapists are unprepared for the demands of self-employment and the responsibilities of marketing, which are in addition to providing services. Becoming a preferred provider may be a great boon to your business. Before agreeing to any discount, however, calculate your expenses, including additional office expenses for handling billing services, and determine your bottom line for each patient visit. Make sure the discount supports your business and does not become an unnecessary burden.

Some contracts may require you to keep a specified percentage of your practice open to their insureds. This can limit your ability to hold appointments open for cash patients. Other contracts require you to provide the agreed-upon discount to patients paying cash for wellness care if they are members of the plan, even though you are not billing the carrier for treatments. Some plans extend the discounted rate as payment in full to insureds involved in MVCs or on-the-job injuries, even if the worker's compensation or personal injury insurance reimburses at a higher rate. Read the patient access provision carefully and sign a contract only when you are willing to abide by it.

Consider how many days it takes to terminate a contract. Plans may require written notice from 30 to 120 days before the contract can be terminated without cause. If a plan reserves the right to revise the pay scale at any time, you may be bound to a rate that is unacceptable to you for months before you can terminate your contract. Most plans increase the fee schedule over time, but if the rates are reduced, it could cause you financial hardship.

Contracts will specify reasons for immediate termination. Read these carefully. Something as simple as not providing copies of patient records within three days can breach the contract and result in immediate termination. You should always learn what is expected of you and determine whether you are able to comply before signing any contract.

Inadequate documentation, as defined by some contracts, can allow the plan to refuse payment to you for your services. Find out the plan's definition of adequate documentation. Follow the guidelines presented in this book, and you will most likely meet or exceed the requirements.

Many contracts stipulate that copies of patient files must be provided upon request, free of charge within days of receiving the request. Contracting with an insurance plan may mean that you need to purchase a copier. Figure this expense into your bottom line when determining whether providing billing services for your patients is cost-effective for you.

Contracts may be amended if both parties agree to the changes. If the original contract is unworkable for your practice, but several of your patients are policyholders, request changes to the contract. The insurance carrier may be willing to negotiate with you. Your chances of successful negotiation become greater when several practitioners approach the company in an organized and professional manner. Use your membership affiliations to join forces, pay for counsel, and shape your relationships with carriers. Take care not to violate federal antitrust laws prohibiting providers from joining together to boycott a contract or to set fees. Hire legal counsel to ensure that all laws are followed. One time, the American Massage Therapy Association—Washington chapter (AMTA-WA) hired counsel to review insurance provider contracts and to advise them of changes to request as a group. The reviews were published in the *Journal*, which benefited hundreds of massage therapists who were considering the contract.

Approach the carriers from a position of cooperation and education, rather than animosity. You may feel insulted when they offer to pay you 75% of your customary fee, but an adversarial approach will not win you respect or give you an edge in negotiations. Every type of health care provider struggles with contracts, fee schedules, and reimbursement arrangements, and all try to negotiate a living wage. Be professional, educate the carriers about your profession, and try to understand the insurance company's position, as well as your own, during the negotiations.

▼

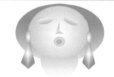

STORY TELLER
Every Provider Reduces Fees to Participate in Provider Lists

I had arthroscopic knee surgery recently. My jaw dropped when I received the Explanation of Benefits (EOB) statement from my insurance company. The surgeon's fee exceeded $3,000, but that wasn't the shocking news. My insurance company paid him $888 as payment in full! And I was upset about reducing my fees by 10 to 20%, depending on the insurance contract. My surgeon's fees had been reduced by more than 65%.

Guidelines for Insurance Documentation
PATIENT INFORMATION

Documentation for insurance personnel carries the same requirements as other forms of patient documentation. Everyone is interested in information that accurately reflects the patient's health and the treatment provided. The only thing to consider is that care can be

188

HANDS HEAL:
COMMUNICATION,
DOCUMENTATION,
AND INSURANCE BILLING
FOR MANUAL THERAPISTS

discontinued and payment reversed or denied based on the documentation.[8] Adequate documentation includes the following:

◆ Intake forms
◆ Prescription
◆ SOAP notes
◆ Progress reports

Recordkeeping must meet two goals for insurance reimbursement. First, you must justify care on that day. Second, you must justify the overall treatment plan.[8] To justify care on the day of service, document the following:

◆ Symptoms consistent with the condition covered by the insurance plan at the time treatment was provided
◆ Alteration of the patient's daily routine (at work, home, or recreational pursuits) because of the condition
◆ Positive objective findings within your scope of practice, including spasms, trigger points, postural deviations, and such

To justify the treatment, demonstrate that the techniques and modalities you use are positively affecting the patient's condition and improving the patient's quality of life:

◆ Present a treatment plan that identifies the goals of the sessions and shows how you and the patient will work to accomplish the goals.
◆ Perform periodic progress evaluations to assess the effectiveness and efficiency of the treatment plan. Also, identify the patient's progress toward accomplishing the stated goals using measurable changes in the patient's ability to perform daily activities (functional outcomes) and measurable changes in subjective and objective data.
◆ Adjust the treatment plan to respond to the individual needs of the patient, as determined by the progress evaluations and the goals accomplished.

Follow the guidelines presented in this book to help prepare yourself to produce documentation that meets insurance requirements for reimbursement.

INSURANCE INFORMATION

Make sure you have all the information necessary for insurance reimbursement before filing claims. The primary cause of payment delays is lack of information or inaccurate information on the billing form.[9] Because each insurer and each insurance plan have their own requirements for billing and reimbursement, you may need to confirm the billing and reimbursement information for each new patient and for each new occurrence or condition.

Two forms will help you identify the information necessary for insurance billing and reimbursement. The first, the billing information form, is one of the intake forms presented in Chapter 5 (see Appendix B for a blank form). This form provides information about the type of claim, contact information for the insurance company, and financial information regarding benefits, such as a **co-pay** or **deductible**.

The second, the insurance verification form, is completed by the practitioner (see Appendix B for a blank form). The form verifies the insurance coverage, identifies limitations or restrictions on the benefits, and confirms that reimbursement is authorized for your services. Verifying this information in advance greatly reduces the risk of having your claims denied after services have already been provided.

Any time information is verified over the phone, record the date, time, and name of the person you are speaking with directly on the insurance verification form and include notes on the conversation. Use a phone log for noting additional phone calls not pertaining to the insurance verification form. All conversations pertaining to patient information should be documented. It is easier to confirm information with the insurance carrier should something go awry when you can provide specific information about the date and time and the name of the person with whom you spoke.

Billing Information Form

Refer to Chapter 5 for details on filling out the billing information form. Use the form for every patient who requests insurance billing services. The information provided by the patient on the billing information form (see Figure 8-1) is necessary for verifying insurance benefits.

Send this form in advance of the patient's first session. If the completed form is not presented at the first appointment, request that the patient pay for the session in full to eliminate your risk. Do not extend billing services without having the patient verify coverage. Communicate your policy—payment is due at time of service until the form is completed and coverage has been verified—to prevent possible misunderstandings and to motivate the patient to come prepared to the initial visit.

Once the patient has verified coverage, call the insurance company to confirm the information and identify the services (techniques and modalities making up your treatment session) that are reimbursable. In an ideal setting, have your office personnel confirm the information during the treatment session and request authorization for services. If you work alone and are uncomfortable providing treatment before confirming coverage, call to authorize coverage while the patient is with you or ask the patient to fax the form back to you prior to the initial visit. Authorization can take time and interfers with the patient's treatment time. Establish the potential risk, and if acceptable, confirm the benefits and obtain authorization for your services prior to the second appointment.

Insurance Verification Form

The insurance verification form prompts the necessary information-gathering to confirm the patient's benefits, authorize your services, and record important billing information (see Figure 8-2).

Use the verification form in conjunction with the verification worksheet (see Figure 8-3). This worksheet provides space for listing common CPT codes that refer to techniques and modalities performed by manual therapists and prompts you to identify the specific limitations for each. The worksheet does not list every modality and therapeutic procedure found in the Physical Medicine and Rehabilitation section of the CPT codebook, but it is more than sufficient for most manual therapists across the country. Additional space is provided for more codes should one of your reimbursable services be missing from the form.

Complete a form for each new condition and for each recurrence of a previous condition.

Verify Patient Benefits

Contact the representative of the insurance company's provider service to verify that the specific treatment techniques and modalities you provide are covered. If, for example, you

FIGURE 8-1   Billing Information Form

〜〜〜〜〜〜〜〜〜〜〜〜〜〜〜〜〜〜

Insurance Information

Insurance plan name or program name: _____

Member ID#: _____ Group #: _____

Customer service phone #: _____ Date and time you called: _____

Name of customer service representative: _____

Insurance claim address: _____ State: _____ Zip: _____

Does the plan include a Physical Medicine and Rehabilitation benefit? ☐ Yes ☐ No

Who may provide the services? ☐ Massage Therapist ☐ Physical Therapist ☐ Other

Is pre-authorization required? ☐ Yes ☐ No   Who can authorize the services? _____

Is a prescription required? ☐ Yes ☐ No   Is a referral required? ☐ Yes ☐ No

Who may refer? ☐ MD ☐ DC ☐ ND ☐ PT ☐ Other _____

How often does the referral need to be updated to ensure continuous coverage? _____

Is there a Preferred Provider list for Manual Therapists? ☐ Yes ☐ No

Is _____ on the list? ☐ Yes ☐ No

〜〜〜〜〜〜〜〜〜〜〜〜〜〜〜〜〜〜

Provider _____

BILLING INFORMATION page 2

If this is a Workers' Compensation Claim, please fill out the following information:

Who is the attending HCP? _____ Phone: _____

Claim number: _____ Date eligibility began: _____

Number of visits authorized: _____ Number of visits remaining: _____

Dates of coverage: _____ Date claim closed: _____

If this is a Personal Injury Claim, please fill out the following information:

PIP policy amount: _____ Dates of coverage: _____ PIP available: _____

MedPay amount: _____ Dates of coverage: _____ MedPay available: _____

Liability amount: _____ Dates of coverage: _____ Liability available: _____

Uninsured/Underinsured (UMI) policy amount: _____ UMI available: _____

Has the PIP application been received? ☐ Yes ☐ No

Has an attorney been consulted? ☐ Yes ☐ No   Retained? ☐ Yes ☐ No

Name/Firm _____

Address _____ City _____ State _____ Zip _____

Phone _____ Fax _____

If this is a Private Health Insurance Claim, please fill out the following information:
(Or, if your Personal Injury claim defaults to secondary coverage, fill this out)

Maximum allowable benefit for Physical Medicine/Rehabilitation: _____

In network: $_____ # visits _____ Remaining $_____ # visits _____

Deductible: $_____ Satisifed to date: $_____ Co-Pay: $_____

Out-of-network: $_____ # visits _____ Remaining $_____ # visits _____

Deductible: $_____ Satisifed to date: $_____ Co-Insurance: $_____

Are these limits just for manual therapy? ☐ Yes ☐ No

If no, what other types of treatment do they include? _____
(i.e., chiropractic, physical therapy, occupational therapy, naturopathy, etc.)

〜〜〜〜〜〜〜〜〜〜〜〜〜〜〜〜〜〜

FIGURE 8-2 Insurance Verification Form

Provider _____

INSURANCE VERIFICATION

Patient Name _____ Date _____

Date of Injury _____ ID#/DOB _____

Verify and Authorize Patient Benefits

Company Name _____

Phone _____ Fax _____

Provider Service Rep _____

Date/time called _____

Check all verified:
☐ Physical medicine/rehab benfit
☐ I can provide services
☐ Covered services (from worksheet):
_____

Check all authorized:
☐ Number of visits _____
☐ Dates of coverage _____
Authorization # _____

Billing procedures:
☐ HCFA 1500 ☐ electronic ☐ other

Send with each bill:
☐ Prescription/referral ☐ Reports
☐ SOAPS ☐ License/certification

What is the expected turnaround time on claim reimbursement? _____
_____

Comments _____

Re-Authorize

Provider Service Rep _____

Date/time called _____

Check all authorized:
☐ Number of visits _____
☐ Dates of coverage _____
Authorization # _____

Total # of visits to date _____

Total $ spent to date _____

Comments _____

Re-Authorize

Provider Service Rep _____

Date/time called _____

Check all authorized:
☐ Number of visits _____
☐ Dates of coverage _____
Authorization # _____

Total # of visits to date _____

Total $ spent to date _____

Comments _____

Referring Health Care Provider Info

Name _____

Phone _____ Fax _____

Prescription received? ☐ Yes ☐ No

Dates of coverage _____

# of visits _____

Diagnosis (ICD-9 codes) _____
_____

Comments _____

Renewal

Date _____
Progress report sent? ☐ Yes ☐ No
Prescription received? ☐ Yes ☐ No

Dates of coverage _____

# of visits _____

ICD-9 codes _____

Comments _____

Renewal

Date _____
Progress report sent? ☐ Yes ☐ No
Prescription received? ☐ Yes ☐ No

Dates of coverage _____

# of visits _____

ICD-9 codes _____

Comments _____

Attorney Information (if applicable)

Name _____

Phone _____ Fax _____

Guarantee of Payment contract signed?
☐ Yes ☐ No

Date requested _____ Received _____

Medical Lien filed? ☐ Yes ☐ No

Date _____ Expires _____
Renewed _____ Expires _____
Renewed _____ Expires _____

Requests for patient files:

Date requested _____ Date sent _____
Authorization received? ☐ Yes ☐ No
Exclusive? ☐ Yes ☐ No Expires _____

Date requested _____ Date sent _____
Authorization received? ☐ Yes ☐ No
Exclusive? ☐ Yes ☐ No Expires _____

191

Provider _____

VERIFICATION WORKSHEET

Patient Name _____ Date _____

Date of Injury _____ ID#/DOB _____

Verify and Authorize Physical Medicine and Rehabilitation Services
(Common modality codes and procedure codes for manual therapists.)

Authorized?	Code #	Description	Restrictions	Max Rate
☐ Yes ☐ No	95831	Muscle testing, ROM, manual, with report		
☐ Yes ☐ No	97010	Hot or cold packs		
☐ Yes ☐ No	97012	Mechanical traction		
☐ Yes ☐ No	97039	Unlisted modality, Specify:		
☐ Yes ☐ No	97110	Therapeutic exercise		
☐ Yes ☐ No	97112	Neuromuscular reeducation		
☐ Yes ☐ No	97113	Aquatic therapy		
☐ Yes ☐ No	97116	Gait training		
☐ Yes ☐ No	97124	Massage therapy		
☐ Yes ☐ No	97139	Unlisted therapeutic procedure, Specify:		
☐ Yes ☐ No	97140	Manual therapy: eg, mobilization/manip., MLD, MFR, manual traction		
☐ Yes ☐ No	97050	Therapeutic procedure(s), group (2 or more)		
☐ Yes ☐ No	99056	Home/Hospital visit		
☐ Yes ☐ No	99075	Medical testimony		
☐ Yes ☐ No		Other:		
☐ Yes ☐ No		Other:		
☐ Yes ☐ No		Other:		
☐ Yes ☐ No		Other:		
☐ Yes ☐ No		Other:		
☐ Yes ☐ No		Other:		
☐ Yes ☐ No		Other:		

See CPT codebook for detailed descriptions of modalities and procedures listed above and for additional modalities and therapeutic procedures not listed on worksheet.

are a massage therapist in New York, several manual therapy procedural codes fall within your scope of practice. However, the patient's insurance plan may not reimburse for all the codes available to your profession. Check out each CPT code individually with every insurance plan. If you are a contracted provider for the plan, the reimbursable codes will be specified in the published fee schedule. If this is the case, simply fill in the spaces provided on the worksheet according to your contract. If not, verify coverage of the techniques and modalities you provide in your treatment sessions.

It is imperative to know the services that are reimbursable under each patient's plan and to clearly understand the restrictions on those services in order to submit clean claims and ensure prompt payment. For example, workers' compensation may include Swedish massage, neuromuscular reeducation, and cold packs as billable services, but may require that these be bundled under the single code 97124 for massage. Without understanding this information adequately, one might submit a bill with incorrect CPT codes—97112 and 97010—and the bill would be denied. Payment could be delayed 30, 60, or 90 days (perhaps longer) before the misunderstanding is resolved.

Before ending the call, confirm that bills will be submitted on an **HCFA 1500 form**. All insurance companies are obliged to accept HCFA 1500 billing forms, but some may prefer electronic billing or customized forms. Carriers that prefer electronic billing generally provide the software necessary to comply with their systems. A few companies prefer forms to be customized with their own bar code tracking system. Insurance carriers that require a special form generally provide them to you free of charge. Remember, once you transfer health care information electronically, you must comply with HIPAA regulations, which are addressed later in this chapter.

Find out whether copies of the patient's file should accompany the bills. If so, find out which records should be copied, such as SOAP notes, progress reports, prescriptions, and the like. Some contracts stipulate that the practitioner is to send copies of the patient's file upon request. The patient's signature authorizing the release of the file is not necessary in this case. If you are not under contract to provide the patient's information, make sure you have the patient's written consent before sending confidential information.

Ask about the expected turnaround time for payment. Inform the insurance representative of your fees, if they are not already determined by contract. Find out whether any further information would assist in ensuring timely payment. You might want to ask about common mistakes that delay payment and tips on how to avoid making those mistakes.

Send a confirmation letter verifying verbal authorization of benefits and services. Include a copy of the insurance verification form demonstrating that you have gathered all the necessary information (see sample in Figure 8-4). Verbal authorizations are sufficient for reimbursement, provided the claim is complete and accurate, but the confirmation letter ensures that the insurance carrier has the authorization documented and on file. On the verification form, record the date the letter was sent. Both you and the insurance carrier can refer to the date if complications arise.

Monitor Prescription Renewals

Once you have verified the insurance information and coverage, you are ready to provide treatment and billing for the services. Repeat the verification process with each request for ongoing services beyond the number of sessions and dates of service previously authorized. First, write a progress report to the referring HCP requesting a prescription for additional treatment. Once the prescription has been received, call the insurance representative to verify additional benefits necessary to cover the ongoing care and to authorize your services. Confirm that the ICD-9 codes provided on the new prescription are covered under the

FIGURE 8-4 Confirmation Letter

Helena LaLuna, CR
123 Sun Moon and Stars Drive
Capitol Hill, WA   98119
Tel   206 555 4446   •   Fax   206 555 4447   •   Email   laluna@email.com

Dear _Aziz Amaden_____ :

Thank you for the opportunity to provide services to _Zamora Hostetter_____.

This letter confirms that:

1. Manual therapy is a covered benefit for the following diagnosis: _724.2_____

__723.1, 840.9, 728.85, 784.0_____

2. The following CPT codes are authorized for the following rate: _97140 @____

__28.78 per unit maximum 4 units per tx_____

3. _6_____ sessions are authorized to be completed between _4-1 → 5-1-01____.

4. The patient's co-pay/co-insurance amount of $ __0___ will be collected from the patient at the time of service.

5. ☒ Prescription   ☐ SOAPs   ☒ Progress reports   ☐ License/Certification

will accompany each billing statement.

6. Payment is anticipated within _30___ days of receipt of a clean claim.

7. If ongoing care is deemed necessary by the referring HCP, re-authorization will be requested by _4-24-01_ to ensure no break in care fo the patient.

8. All claims will be sent to: _WA. Dept. of L & I_____

Attn: _claims department_____   Address _PO Box 323 Olympia WA 98055_

If you have any questions, please call. If I do not hear from you within 24 hours of receipt of this letter, I will assume that reimbursement for services is confirmed.

Sincerely,

Helena La Luna, CR

patient's plan and that they warrant your services. Record the second authorization on the original insurance verification form.

Use the form to log that a prescription has been obtained, as required for all adjunctive services, and to monitor the prescriptions. Ensure that the prescriptions cover the dates of treatments. Gaps in prescriptions can be costly to you and your patient. Darnel's physician wrote a prescription for six treatments in a four-week period beginning on April 4. Only four treatments were provided in the time allotted, with the additional two provided the following week. The new prescription was dated May 16. The two treatments provided between May 4 and May 16 are not covered by either prescription and therefore may not be reimbursable by the insurance company. Avoid costly mistakes by tracking the prescriptions on the insurance verification form.

Record the diagnoses from the prescription on the insurance verification form to ensure that the information is available when you speak with insurance representatives. Provide the diagnosis to the insurance representative to verify eligibility. Confirm whether an ICD-9 code is required on the billing form or whether the bill can be processed with a description of the diagnosis instead. The referring HCP may have written "low back pain" on the prescription, for example, without providing an ICD-9 code. If the insurance company insists on an ICD-9 code identified on the billing form for reimbursement, contact the referring HCP and ask for the proper code for the diagnosis.

Monitor Attorney Contracts, Liens, and Requests for Records

If the patient has retained an attorney for a personal injury case, log and monitor all pertinent information regarding payment contracts, liens, and requests for medical records. If PIP, Med-Pay, or other secondary coverage is exhausted or nonexistent, file liens on the case with copies mailed to the insurer, patient, and attorney per the requirements of state law. For example, in the state of Washington, health care liens must be renewed yearly from the date filed. Health care liens may need to be renewed prior to expiration dates; note the date filed and the dates renewed. Note the date the contractual guarantee was requested from the attorney and the date it was returned and filed. On the insurance verification form, note the expiration dates of authorizations to release medical information and ensure (by monitoring) that requests for records fall within the authorized dates. Log the date the requests were received and the date the information was mailed.

If the insurance coverage is not straightforward and the patient was not able to complete the billing information form to your satisfaction, ask the attorney to complete the insurance status form (see Appendix B). Consult the attorney to verify coverage and to authorize services.

Guidelines for Insurance Billing
THE HCFA 1500 BILLING FORM

The **HCFA 1500** (Health Care Financing Administration) **form** is the standard billing form approved by the American Medical Association (see Figure 8-5). The insurance information form and the insurance verification form provide information necessary to complete the form, which is divided into two parts: patient and insured information and provider information. It is fairly self-explanatory, but some sections can be confusing or do not apply to manual therapists. Each section is numbered and corresponds with the explanation that follows it.

Box 1.   Check the box that applies to the type of insurance for the patient. For health insurance, check the Group Health Plan box and write either the patient's social security number or the insurance identification number (box 1a). For personal injury cases or worker's compensation cases, check the Other box and write the claim number (box 1a).

FIGURE 8-5 HCFA 1500 Billing Form

PLEASE
DO NOT
STAPLE
IN THIS
AREA

← CARRIER →

HEALTH INSURANCE CLAIM FORM

PICA

| | PICA |

1. MEDICARE MEDICAID CHAMPUS CHAMPVA GROUP HEALTH PLAN FECA BLK LUNG OTHER   1a. INSURED'S I.D. NUMBER   (FOR PROGRAM IN ITEM 1)

(Medicare #) (Medicaid #) (Sponsor's SSN) (VA File #) (SSN or ID) (SSN) [X] (ID)   **C98-7654321**

2. PATIENT'S NAME (Last Name, First Name, Middle Initial)   3. PATIENT'S BIRTH DATE MM DD YY   SEX   4. INSURED'S NAME (Last Name, First Name, Middle Initial)

Hostetter Zamora   **05 22 80** M [ ] F [X]   **same**

5. PATIENT'S ADDRESS (No., Street)   6. PATIENT RELATIONSHIP TO INSURED   7. INSURED'S ADDRESS (No., Street)

63 18TH Ave W   Self [X] Spouse [ ] Child [ ] Other [ ]

CITY   STATE   8. PATIENT STATUS   CITY   STATE

Capitol Hill   **WA**   Single [X] Married [ ] Other [ ]

ZIP CODE   TELEPHONE (Include Area Code)   ZIP CODE   TELEPHONE (INCLUDE AREA CODE)

98119   **(206) 555-1221**   Employed [X] Full-Time Student [ ] Part-Time Student [ ]   ( )

9. OTHER INSURED'S NAME (Last Name, First Name, Middle Initial)   10. IS PATIENT'S CONDITION RELATED TO: 11. INSURED'S POLICY GROUP OR FECA NUMBER

Same

a. OTHER INSURED'S POLICY OR GROUP NUMBER   a. EMPLOYMENT? (CURRENT OR PREVIOUS)   a. INSURED'S DATE OF BIRTH MM DD YY   SEX

555-63-1819   [X] YES [ ] NO   M [ ] F [ ]

b. OTHER INSURED'S DATE OF BIRTH MM DD YY   SEX   b. AUTO ACCIDENT? PLACE (State)   b. EMPLOYER'S NAME OR SCHOOL NAME

M [ ] F [ ]   [ ] YES [X] NO   **Howling Moon Cafe**

c. EMPLOYER'S NAME OR SCHOOL NAME   c. OTHER ACCIDENT?   c. INSURANCE PLAN NAME OR PROGRAM NAME

Howling Moon Cafe   [ ] YES [X] NO   **WA Dept. L & I**

d. INSURANCE PLAN NAME OR PROGRAM NAME   10d. RESERVED FOR LOCAL USE   d. IS THERE ANOTHER HEALTH BENEFIT PLAN?

Health Co Selections   [X] YES [ ] NO *If yes, return to and complete item 9 a-d.*

READ BACK OF FORM BEFORE COMPLETING & SIGNING THIS FORM.
12. PATIENT'S OR AUTHORIZED PERSON'S SIGNATURE I authorize the release of any medical or other information necessary to process this claim. I also request payment of government benefits either to myself or to the party who accepts assignment below.

SIGNED **signature on file**   DATE **4-4-01**

13. INSURED'S OR AUTHORIZED PERSON'S SIGNATURE I authorize payment of medical benefits to the undersigned physician or supplier for services described below.

SIGNED **signature on file**

14. DATE OF CURRENT: ILLNESS (First symptom) OR INJURY (Accident) OR PREGNANCY(LMP) MM DD YY   15. IF PATIENT HAS HAD SAME OR SIMILAR ILLNESS. GIVE FIRST DATE MM DD YY   16. DATES PATIENT UNABLE TO WORK IN CURRENT OCCUPATION MM DD YY FROM TO

03 31 01

17. NAME OF REFERRING PHYSICIAN OR OTHER SOURCE   17a. I.D. NUMBER OF REFERRING PHYSICIAN   18. HOSPITALIZATION DATES RELATED TO CURRENT SERVICES MM DD YY FROM TO

Manda Rae Yuricich, DC

19. RESERVED FOR LOCAL USE   20. OUTSIDE LAB? $ CHARGES

[ ] YES [ ] NO

21. DIAGNOSIS OR NATURE OF ILLNESS OR INJURY. (RELATE ITEMS 1,2,3 OR 4 TO ITEM 24E BY LINE)   22. MEDICAID RESUBMISSION CODE ORIGINAL REF. NO.

1. **724.2**   3. **840.9**

2. **723.1, 784.0**   4. **728.85**

23. PRIOR AUTHORIZATION NUMBER

24.	A					B	C	D		E	F	G	H	I	J	K
	DATE(S) OF SERVICE					Place of Service	Type of Service	PROCEDURES, SERVICES, OR SUPPLIES (Explain Unusual Circumstances)		DIAGNOSIS CODE	$ CHARGES	DAYS OR UNITS	EPSDT Family Plan	EMG	COB	RESERVED FOR LOCAL USE
	From MM DD YY		To MM DD YY					CPT/HCPCS	MODIFIER							
1	4 4 01		4 4 01			11	9	97140		1,2,3,4	25 —	1				
2	4 4 01		4 4 01			11	9	97140		1,2,3,4	25 —	1				
3	4 4 01		4 4 01			11	9	97140		1,2,3,4	25 —	1				
4	4 4 01		4 4 01			11	9	97140		1,2,3,4	25 —	1				
5																
6																

25. FEDERAL TAX I.D. NUMBER SSN EIN   26. PATIENT'S ACCOUNT NO.   27. ACCEPT ASSIGNMENT? (For govt. claims, see back)   28. TOTAL CHARGE   29. AMOUNT PAID   30. BALANCE DUE

91-1777771 [ ] [X]   [ ] YES [ ] NO $ **100** — $ **0** $ **100**

31. SIGNATURE OF PHYSICIAN OR SUPPLIER INCLUDING DEGREES OR CREDENTIALS (I certify that the statements on the reverse apply to this bill and are made a part thereof.)

SIGNED **Helena La Luna, CR** DATE **4-4-01**

32. NAME AND ADDRESS OF FACILITY WHERE SERVICES WERE RENDERED (If other than home or office)

33. PHYSICIAN'S, SUPPLIER'S BILLING NAME, ADDRESS, ZIP CODE & PHONE #

Helena La Luna, CR
123 Sun Moon and Stars Dr.
Capitol Hill, WA 98119
PIN# **(206) 555-4446** GRP#

FORM HCFA-1500 (12-90)   *PLEASE PRINT OR TYPE*   FORM OWCP-1500 FORM RRB-1500 APPROVED OMB-0938-0008
NORTHWEST BUSINESS FORMS (206) 728-8181   (APPROVED BY AMA COUNCIL ON MEDICAL SERVICE 8/88)

PATIENT AND INSURED INFORMATION

PHYSICIAN OR SUPPLIER INFORMATION

Boxes 2–7.   Fill in the patient's name, address, and telephone number (boxes 2, 3 and 5). If the patient is also the insured, record "Same" as the insured's name (box 4). If the insured is someone other than the patient, fill in the insured's name, address, and phone number (boxes 4 and 7). For example, Darnel's nephew was the owner of the car in which Darnel was riding when the accident occurred. Therefore, you would fill in the nephew's name, address, and phone number as the primary insured. The nephew's insurance is first in line to cover Darnel's medical expenses. A common situation in which the insured is not the patient occurs when the spouse is insured through work and the insurance policy covers the patient. Check the box that signifies the patient's relationship to the insured (box 6).

Box 8.   Self explanatory.

Box 9.   Other Insured refers to second-party coverage. For example, this may be the patient's car insurance if the primary coverage is someone else's, or it may be the patient's health insurance if the car insurance does not provide PIP. Darnel's other insured, or secondary coverage, is his own automobile insurance. If the patient does not drive and does not carry auto insurance, his health insurance is considered the other insured.

Box 10.   Self explanatory.

Box 11.   Fill in the insured's applicable policy number. This might be the group insurance number or the plan number, whichever identifies the type of plan carried by the insured. Fill in the date of birth and sex (11a). The name of employer or school (11b) is necessary only when the insurance plan is provided through one of them. Personal injury cases do not require this information unless the injury occurred while the patient was working. Fill in the plan name (11c) and answer the question regarding secondary insurance coverage (11d).

Box 12.   The patient is required to authorize the release of any medical information necessary to process the claim. The patient does not have to sign every billing form if he has signed a release on file in the chart. This release is included on the billing information form. Make sure the patient signs the release when he fills out the form and note "Signature on File," rather than having the patient sign every bill. The date for this section should reflect the date the patient signed the insurance information form.

Box 13.   Here, the patient's signature authorizes the insurance company to pay the health care provider directly. Payment will be written and mailed to the provider shown in box 33, which is also included on the billing information form. Again, rather than requiring the patient to sign every bill, recording "Signature on File" will suffice (when the patient's signature is on the intake form).

Boxes 14 and 15.   Self explanatory.

Boxes 16 and 18.   These may not apply to adjunctive care and can be left blank.

Box 17.   Fill in the referring HCP's name and provider number, if applicable.

Box 19.   Leave blank.

Box 21.   Most insurance carriers require a diagnosis to reimburse for services, regardless of your ability to diagnose. If diagnosing is not within your scope of practice, simply transfer the diagnosis from the prescription to the HCFA 1500. Filling in the diagnosis code (ICD-9) on an HCFA 1500 form will not be construed as acting outside your scope of practice, as long as a

198

HANDS HEAL:
COMMUNICATION,
DOCUMENTATION,
AND INSURANCE BILLING
FOR MANUAL THERAPISTS

referring HCP provided the codes for you and the prescription is on file. If the patient is self-referred—no HCP is overseeing your treatments—and the insurance company requires an ICD-9 code before payment will be authorized, complete this section with ICD-9 codes that are symptomatic in nature, such as a code for pain (see Appendix E for ICD-9 codes to use with self-referred patients).

Boxes 22 and 23.   Leave blank.

Box 24.   The date(s) of service column displays a From section and a To section (box 24A) in which you are record the date (or dates) on which you provided the service (repeat the same date in both sections). The codes in the place of service column (box 24B) vary among carriers and may be found in the company's billing manual. Some use numbers:

1. Inpatient Hospital
2. Outpatient Hospital
3. Office
4. Residence
5. Emergency Room
6. Other Medical/Surgical Facilities
7. Nursing Home
8. Other Location

Or

11. Office
12. Home
21. Hospital
22. Outpatient Hospital
24. Ambulatory Surgical Center
25. Birthing Center
33. Custodial Care Facility
34. Hospice

Others use letters:

AC—Ambulatory Surgical Center
ER = Emergency Room
HM= Patient's Home
HS = Hospice
IH   = Inpatient Hospital
NH = Nursing Home
OH = Outpatient Hospital
OF = Practitioner's Office

Check with the insurance representative for the preferred codes or request a billing manual to ensure accurate billing. The type of service column also varies among insurance carriers (box 24C). The following is one example of a carrier's code list:

01. Medical Care
02. Surgery
03. Consultation
04. Diagnostic X-ray

05. Diagnostic Labs
06. Radiation Therapy
07. Anesthesia
08. Surgical Assistant
09. Other Medical Services

Again, check with the insurance carrier for its preferred codes. The services you bill for must be listed by CPT code unless state regulations dictate otherwise (box 24D). ABC codes, mentioned in Chapter 5, are experimental and require the manual therapist to register with participating insurance companies and obtain separate authorization before billing with these service codes. CPT codes are the standard according to the AMA and are typically required for insurance reimbursement for health care services. Refer to the list on the insurance verification worksheet for each patient and use the codes that describe your services, that are within your scope of practice, and that are reimbursable within the patient's plan.

The diagnosis codes are numbered in box 24E. Fill in the number that corresponds to the diagnosis of the conditions that you treated in the session. For example, the patient might have two conditions—low back pain and cervical subluxation—and two diagnosis codes listed for each condition. Last Tuesday, you treated the low back pain only and did not have time to treat the neck condition. For that session, you would fill in the numbers 1 and 2 (shown as 1, 2 in column). This Monday you were able to address both conditions and put 1, 2, 3, 4 in the column.

Charges should reflect the total amount for the line item (box 24F). A common mistake is to give the value of one unit of service rather than the total for all units of service. If, for example, you provided four units of the service listed and each unit is billed at $25 per unit, the total charges would be $100.

Days or units (box 24G) refers to a designated period of time or a single, specified procedure. Each CPT code lists a unit of time in the description. Some are 15-minute units; others are 30-minute units. If no unit of time is provided in the description, the CPT code refers to the procedure as a single unit, independent of the amount of time it takes to perform the procedure. For example, hot and cold packs may be applied as a procedure undefined by time; whereas neuromuscular reeducation is billable in 15-minute units and an extended new patient office visit is defined as a 45-minute unit. Refer to the CPT codebook for the definition of units to ensure accurate billing for your services.

Boxes 24H, I, J, and K.   Leave blank.

Box 25.   Self explanatory.

Box 26.   Giving this information is optional. If you organize your office records by assigning your patients numbers, put the patient's number here to assist you in filing the bills.

Box 27.   Leave blank.

Box 28.   Total all the charges for each line item.

Box 29.   Fill in any payments paid by the patient.

Box 30.   Fill in the balance due.

Box 31.   Self explanatory.

200

HANDS HEAL:
COMMUNICATION,
DOCUMENTATION,
AND INSURANCE BILLING
FOR MANUAL THERAPISTS

Box 32.   Increasingly, insurance companies are requesting that this box be completed even when it is the same address as in box 33. Make sure this address is the physical location where services were performed and not a post office box or the billing address of a billing service that submits the bills and collects the payments.

Box 33.   Make sure this information is legible. Checks will be made payable to the name listed here and sent to the address listed here. Include your phone number. If there are any questions regarding the bill, a bill processor may prefer to call you before denying the bill or sending it back in the mail.

TIMING

Submit the HCFA 1500 billing form immediately after the first session. If there are any problems with the billing procedures, it is best to work out the glitches early in the reimbursement process. The most common delay in billing is a simple lack of information, such as failure to attach a copy of the prescription or providing an inappropriate diagnosis code. Once complete and accurate information is provided, the billing usually proceeds smoothly.

Bill as often as you are comfortable billing. Many computerized billing programs make it easy to bill after each session. Other practitioners designate one day each week or so for office work and to do all their billing, report writing, and correspondence. Whichever approach you choose, make sure you bill treatment dates within the same month. It is easier on the other end to organize and track reimbursement when all dates of service fall within a calendar month. This may be stipulated in your contract under billing procedures.

Do your billing frequently to avoid reimbursement delays, especially on high dollar amounts, which often require additional signatures or higher authority to authorize payment.

Re-bill every 30 days for the balance due. Stamp the HCFA 1500 form with the notation: COPY—RESUBMITTED (provide date of resubmission). Attach an invoice adding interest charges, if applicable, and state the new balance. If you are a preferred provider under contract with the carrier, check your contract for stipulations regarding interest. Also, check for state regulations regarding interest charges on medical services. For example, the state of Washington limits interest on medical services to 12% simple interest annually, or one percent per month applied only to the treatment amount. In other words, practitioners may not apply interest to interest. Typically, providers will accrue interest 90 days after the billing date. Provide the patient and the insurance company 30 days' notice before assigning interest and calculate the interest according to state regulations.

PAYMENT LOGS

Create a payment log for each patient (Figure 8-6) to help you track billing dates, reimbursement dates, and payment amounts. File all payment logs in a three-ring binder in alphabetical order. Go through the binder twice monthly to determine whom to re-bill at 30-day intervals.

Enter all payments into the logs before depositing funds. Verify the dates of service for each reimbursement check. This is a critical step. Each check will specify the dates of service to which the payment applies on the Explanation of Benefits (EOB) statement. Sometimes, the payment for one bill may not follow the previous payment. For example,

FIGURE 8-6 Payment Log

Helena LaLuna, CR
123 Sun Moon and Stars Drive
Capitol Hill, WA   98119
TEL 206 555 4446

PAYMENT LOG

Name _Zamora Hostetter_ Date _6-18-04_

Date of Injury _3-31-04_ ID#/DOB _C98-7654321_

Insurance Company _____ Phone _____

Billing Date: _5-18-04_ Total Billed: $ _100_

Patient Paid: $ _0_ Insurance Paid: $ _0_ Total Paid: $ _0_

If Total Paid does NOT equal Total Billed, complete below for each date of service (from lines 1-6, Section 24 of HCFA 1500)

Line 1, Initial Billing
Treatment Date: _5-18-04_ Bill Date: _5-18-04_
Charges: _100_ Adjustments: _0_ Amount Billed: _100_
Due from patient: _0_ Due from Insurance: _100-_
Patient Paid: _0_ Insurance paid: _0_

Line 1, Rebilling
Rebill Date: _6-18-04_ Rebilled to: _Ins._
Outstanding: _100-_ Interest: _0_ Amount Billed: _100-_
Rebill Date: _7-18-04_ Rebilled to: _Ins._
Outstanding: _100-_ Interest: _1%_ Amount Billed: _101-_

Line 2, Initial Billing
Treatment Date: _____ Bill Date: _____
Charges: ____ Adjustments: ____ Amount Billed: _____
Due from patient: _____ Due from Insurance: _____
Patient Paid: _____ Insurance paid: _____

Line 2, Rebilling
Rebill Date: _____ Rebilled to: _____
Outstanding: _____ Interest: _____ Amount Billed: _____
Rebill Date: _____ Rebilled to: _____
Outstanding: _____ Interest: _____ Amount Billed: _____

Line 3, Initial Billing
Treatment Date: _____ Bill Date: _____
Charges: ____ Adjustments: ____ Amount Billed: _____
Due from patient: _____ Due from Insurance: _____
Patient Paid: _____ Insurance paid: _____

Line 3, Rebilling
Rebill Date: _____ Rebilled to: _____
Outstanding: _____ Interest: _____ Amount Billed: _____
Rebill Date: _____ Rebilled to: _____
Outstanding: _____ Interest: _____ Amount Billed: _____

Line 4, Initial Billing
Treatment Date: _____ Bill Date: _____
Charges: ____ Adjustments: ____ Amount Billed: _____
Due from patient: _____ Due from Insurance: _____
Patient Paid: _____ Insurance paid: _____

Line 4, Rebilling
Rebill Date: _____ Rebilled to: _____
Outstanding: _____ Interest: _____ Amount Billed: _____
Rebill Date: _____ Rebilled to: _____
Outstanding: _____ Interest: _____ Amount Billed: _____

Line 5, Initial Billing
Treatment Date: _____ Bill Date: _____
Charges: ____ Adjustments: ____ Amount Billed: _____
Due from patient: _____ Due from Insurance: _____
Patient Paid: _____ Insurance paid: _____

Line 5, Rebilling
Rebill Date: _____ Rebilled to: _____
Outstanding: _____ Interest: _____ Amount Billed: _____
Rebill Date: _____ Rebilled to: _____
Outstanding: _____ Interest: _____ Amount Billed: _____

Line 6, Initial Billing
Treatment Date: _____ Bill Date: _____
Charges: ____ Adjustments: ____ Amount Billed: _____
Due from patient: _____ Due from Insurance: _____
Patient Paid: _____ Insurance paid: _____

Line 6, Rebilling
Rebill Date: _____ Rebilled to: _____
Outstanding: _____ Interest: _____ Amount Billed: _____
Rebill Date: _____ Rebilled to: _____
Outstanding: _____ Interest: _____ Amount Billed: _____

202

HANDS HEAL:
COMMUNICATION,
DOCUMENTATION,
AND INSURANCE BILLING
FOR MANUAL THERAPISTS

Helena sent three billing statements to HealthCo. The first bill was for treatment provided on April 12, 2001. The second bill was for treatments on April 15, 2001; April 18, 2001; and April 21, 2001. The third bill was for treatment on May 1, 2001. The first payment received was for the April 21 treatment. The second payment received was for the May 1 treatment. Helena erroneously applied the second payment to the second treatment that appeared chronologically on the payment log. After Helena resubmitted a modified bill for the second billing statement and a copy of the third bill, HealthCo informed her that she had been paid already for services provided on May 1, 2001, and the company refused to pay the third bill. Helena received only partial payment for the second bill because of the modified statement and no payment for the third bill, and she cannot contest the situation successfully until she resolves the misapplied amount.

Strategies for Managing Reimbursement Challenges

Private health insurance companies are required by law to respond to a designated number of claims within a specified amount of time. (This does not include personal injury insurance or workers' compensaiton.) For example, Washington state law requires 95% of clean claims to be paid within 30 days and 95% of unclean claims to be paid or denied within 60 days.[10] **Clean claims** are insurance claim bills submitted with complete and accurate information for services that are covered for the patient and that the practitioner is authorized to provide. **Unclean claims** lack information or contain disputable information, such as a procedure that is not authorized for the diagnosis.

Ask for clarification whenever a diagnosis code is denied. Sometimes, a code is too specific and, as a result, is not listed in the insurance manual as an authorized diagnosis for your service. Instead, a general ICD-9 code describing the same diagnosis will authorize the treatment. For example, at HealthCo., lumbar pain is an acceptable diagnosis (724.2) for manual therapy reimbursement, but lumbar subluxation (839.20) is not covered for manual therapy services. If a code is denied, ask the insurance representative for a list of the allowable codes for the condition. Then, contact the referring HCP and request that a different diagnosis code be recorded on the prescription. This practice is acceptable as long as it does not misrepresent the patient's diagnosis. Reimbursement for unclean claims can be delayed, denied, or reversed. Most unclean claims are returned to the practitioner for clarification or correction and must be returned clean within a designated time frame to prevent further delay in payment. Other claims require investigation from a **utilization management program** or review board. Peer reviews determine whether or not treatment and cost of care were:

◆ Appropriate for the condition
◆ Effective—resulting in improved quality of life for the patient
◆ Reasonable

Peer reviewers determine whether claims meet these requirements by studying patient files and looking for answers to the following questions:

◆ Did the provider deliver the promised services?
◆ Did the provider deliver the promised services in the agreed upon time?
◆ Did the intervention deliver the expected outcome?
◆ Did the provider charge **usual, customary, and regular** (**UCR**) fees for services?

Denied claims may result in partial payment, no payment, or a reversal in payment. Denial resulting in partial payment is often because of:

◆ Treating outside the diagnosis. Raphael treated a patient diagnosed with an ankle sprain by administering manual therapy both to the upper extremities and the lower extremities. The insurance claims processor determined that the treatment was not consistent with the diagnosis and awarded a partial payment. Sixty percent of the treatment was designated appropriate treatment and 40% was deemed unnecessary treatment. The partial payment reflected 60% of the total fee for all treatments. Appeals of this type can be successful if the therapist can prove the necessity of care and, in this case, can explain the necessity of treating the upper extremities to benefit the injured ankle.

◆ Treating outside the time frame authorized for treatments. If authorization was obtained for six sessions within 30 days and the sixth treatment was given on day 32, be aware that appeals caused by scheduling negligence rarely succeed. Become aware of time limitations as they pertain to your services.

◆ Treating beyond the standard of care for the condition. If 10 sessions are the maximum allowable for low back pain and 13 were provided, expect only partial payment. This can be easily avoided by verifying the number of sessions authorized before administering the treatment.

Denial resulting in no payment is common when the practitioner:

◆ Bills for treatment outside his or her scope of practice
◆ Bills for services not authorized for the diagnosis
◆ Bills for two or more similar modalities provided on the same day. If the patient receives physical therapy *and* massage therapy on the same day, the practitioner who submits the claim first usually will be the only one reimbursed.

Denial resulting in reversal of payment occurs when the practitioner is found guilty of using fraudulent or abusive billing practices, such as charging for procedures that were not performed, billing for services in addition to those actually performed, charging for medically unnecessary services, submitting claims with misleading diagnostic codes so as to receive benefits for an excluded service, or billing at a higher rate than would be charged in the absence of third-party reimbursement.

It is illegal to charge different rates for the same service to different people or organizations. It is appropriate, however, to charge different fees for different services or to offer reasonable discounts for payment on the day of service, as long as the discount is offered to all patients equally. For example, if a patient pays cash but is submitting the bill to an insurance carrier for reimbursement, he or she must be offered the same discount at the time of service as any other patient would be offered. Acceptable discounts range between 5% and 15%, depending on state regulations. Consistent across insurance carriers is the fact that billing an insurance company at one rate and cash patients at another is considered fraudulent and abusive, particularly when the cash patient seeks reimbursement at the higher rate.

During peer reviews involving fraudulent billing, all of the provider's files are seized and reviewed for consistency. If, for example, the massage therapist clearly charges one fee for relaxation massage and one fee for treatment massage, the difference in fees is justified. But if the review board finds that the practitioner's primary techniques—manual

204

HANDS HEAL:
COMMUNICATION,
DOCUMENTATION,
AND INSURANCE BILLING
FOR MANUAL THERAPISTS

lymphatic drainage and neuromuscular reeducation, for example—are performed equally among relaxation patients and insurance patients, the different fee schedules are not justifiable. The practitioner may be required to reimburse insurance payments retroactively for up to seven years, depending on the laws of the state.

▼

STORY TELLER
Usual and Customary Fees

A local physical therapist was found guilty of using fraudulent billing practices and was required to reimburse the Department of Labor and Industries (L&I) more than $4,800 in back payments plus interest and penalties. She was not a dishonest person but had misinterpreted the fee schedule provided by L&I for treating workers' compensation cases. The fee schedule stated that the maximum payable amount for manual therapy was $76 per visit. She assumed that L&I was offering to pay her that amount for her services, regardless of her usual and customary fee. She charged patients who pay out-of-pocket and the health insurance plans $65 per visit. The contract she signed with L&I, however, stipulated that she was to charge her usual and customary fee *up to* $76. Her negligence in not reading the contract carefully resulted in financial hardship, and she was forced to relocate her practice.

Insurance billing can be risky, and billing challenges are unavoidable. Staying on top of outstanding bills is imperative. Successful strategies for managing insurance reimbursement are covered in the following sections.

PROVIDE COMPLETE AND ACCURATE INFORMATION

Patient information and insurance information must be complete and accurate to avoid delays in payment. Follow these guidelines to avoid challenges regarding patient documentation:

♦ Record a comprehensive history of each patient.
♦ Keep SOAP charts on every session.
♦ Make sure the treatments noted reflect the procedures and modalities billed.
♦ Document measurable subjective and objective data that validate the treatment provided.
♦ Set goals that reflect measurable progress in the patient's everyday activities.
♦ Create a treatment plan to accomplish the patient's functional goals.
♦ Evaluate patient progress regularly (every 30 days or 6 to 8 sessions).
♦ Make adjustments to the treatment plan to meet the patient's changing needs.
♦ Date all forms and SOAP charts.
♦ Make sure treatment dates correspond accurately with billing dates.
♦ Write monthly progress reports.
♦ Make sure the progress reports reflect information in the SOAP charts.
♦ Write legibly.
♦ Stamp *your* name, address, and phone number on every page in the patient's file.
♦ Take notes that are spontaneous and unique to each individual patient.

Follow these guidelines to make sure the insurance information you provide is complete and accurate:

◆ Have the patient fill out a billing information form.

◆ Review the completed billing information form with the patient to verify content.

◆ Make sure the patient and insured's information, especially the patient's insurance identification number or birth date and insurance policy numbers, is accurately transposed onto the billing form.

◆ Require a prescription from the patient's primary HCP.

◆ In case of an incomplete prescription, provide a prescription form for the referring HCP to complete (or gather necessary information over the phone).

◆ Complete the insurance verification form with assistance from the verification worksheet (see Figures 8-2 and 8-3).

◆ Verify insurance coverage for your services, given your professional scope.

◆ Verify patient eligibility for the services, given the diagnosis.

◆ Inform the insurance representative in advance of your fee, unless dictated by contract.

◆ Double-check the provider information on the billing form to eliminate most mistakes, such as transposing numbers, giving inaccurate procedure codes, or providing an incomplete diagnosis.

◆ Make sure the treatment dates on the HCFA 1500 billing form correspond with the SOAP notes.

◆ Know what information should accompany the billing form and send it as required, including SOAP notes, progress reports, and prescriptions.

STAY WITHIN DESIGNATED TIME LIMITS

Specific requirements must be met by the patient and the practitioner to ensure payment. Many of the requirements revolve around time. Stay within designated time limits when providing treatments, submitting bills, and seeking reimbursement:

◆ Provide treatment within the time period authorized.

◆ Make sure prescriptions cover all dates of treatment.

◆ Submit bills in a timely fashion. Never wait more than 30 days to submit a bill.

◆ Monitor the time frames for deductibles—when they are satisfied and when they are renewed—and collect appropriate fees at the time of service.

◆ Record the names, dates, and times of all phone conversations with insurance representatives.

◆ Resubmit bills after 31 days of no payment. Stamp each bill with the rebilling date and follow up with a phone call.

◆ Resubmit bills after 61 days of no payment. Include the following statement: "This claim is more than 60 days past due. If this claim is not paid or denied within 30 days, a written complaint will be submitted to the insurance commissioner's office." (See Appendix F for contact information regarding insurance commissioners.) Follow up with a phone call.

◆ Return unclean claims with the requested information as soon as possible.

◆ Appeal all denied claims within the time limit specified.

◆ Monitor expiration dates of medical liens and authorizations for release of medical records.

◆ Know the statute of limitations for filing a lawsuit.

206

HANDS HEAL:
COMMUNICATION,
DOCUMENTATION,
AND INSURANCE BILLING
FOR MANUAL THERAPISTS

PROVE MEDICAL NECESSITY

Practitioners must be able to prove that the treatment provided was medically necessary. Follow these guidelines to avoid disputes over medical necessity:

◆ Make sure prescriptions communicate that the adjunctive care is integral to the treatment plan.

◆ Prove progress specific to the patient's daily activities.

◆ Treat within the diagnosis. For holistic treatments, ensure that the prescription requests treatment to structures outside the diagnosis, and if denied, you can justify full-body treatment with confidence.

◆ Document active *and* passive care. Educate patients in self-care, which includes self-massage, breathing exercises, application of hot and cold packs, stretching and strengthening exercises, ergonomics and movement mechanics, and increased awareness of aggravating activities.

◆ If a formal **appeal** is necessary, educate the reviewer on the necessity of treatment and the benefits of manual therapy. Some insurers will see CAM care as experimental treatment and not reimbursable. Be prepared to send research articles and to write letters detailing the benefits of manual therapy.

FILE LIENS ON PERSONAL INJURY CASES

Medical or health care liens are used to guarantee payment for treatments provided to people who have sustained a personal injury. The intent is to place a hold on the patient's claim until satisfying the outstanding medical bills. Depending on state law, the health care provider must file the lien in a specified way. For example, in Washington, the lien must be filed with the county auditor—the county in which the services were performed, not the county where the MVC occurred—before settlement and payment have been made to the injured party.

File medical liens on all personal injury cases in which payment has been deferred. Send copies of the lien to the patient, to the patient's and the at-fault party's insurance company, and the patient's attorney, if applicable.[8]

MISCELLANEOUS REIMBURSEMENT TIPS

These tips address topics and procedures to help minimize delays in reimbursement.

◆ Establish positive, cooperative relationships with insurance representatives. Your attitude may affect the reimbursement results.

◆ Read insurance contracts carefully. Follow the contractual language of the policy.

◆ Correctly apply all payments according to the dates of treatment stated on the EOB.

◆ Be prepared. Know the standard billing practices and procedure codes for your profession for each type of insurance before agreeing to provide billing services.

◆ Type the information onto the HCFA 1500 form or use computerized billing. Handwritten bills are difficult to read and will often result in delays.

◆ Ask the patient to intervene. If the insurance company is delaying payment, a phone call from the patient can speed up claims processing.

◆ Ask the attorney to intervene. A letter or a phone call can be very effective in prompting payment.

◆ If necessary, send a request to the insurance commissioner's office (OIC) to intervene. A formal complaint to the OIC reflects badly on the insurance company and often results in an investigation, the results of which will remain in an insurance carrier's file for several years.

◆ Require contracts guaranteeing payment from attorney liens or medical liens for all personal injury cases. If the attorney refuses to sign the letter guaranteeing payment from the settlement, stop deferring payment immediately, file a medical lien, and require the patient to make regular payments on the outstanding balance.

State regulatory agencies, such as the Office of the Insurance Commissioner (OIC), may provide additional assistance to manual therapists and patients. Generally, the OIC investigates formal complaints against insurance carriers and assists with writing, interpreting, and implementing rules that providers and insurers must follow. These regulations offer support and protection for both the health care providers and their patients. Additionally, staff members can be strong advocates for patients and providers, by helping patients receive appropriate levels of benefits based on the insurance packages purchased and supporting providers in receiving fair treatment and prompt payment by insurers. Individual provider assistance varies from state to state, so you should become aware of options in your state (see Appendix F about contacting state agencies).

Appealing Claims Denials

Claims can be denied before treatment is provided, during treatment (with the frequent result of discontinued care), or after the services have been provided. There is no financial risk to the practitioner or the patient when a claim is denied before treatment is provided or when the denial simply prevents ongoing care. However, when a claim is denied after the service has been delivered, the practitioner has financial motivation to appeal the denial to ease the financial hardship not only for himself or herself, but ultimately for the patient.

Financial hardship is not the only reason to appeal a claim. You may have a great deal of emotional investment in getting the patient the needed care. You can be successful in appealing denials if a lack of treatment can result in harm to the patient. The process of appealing becomes an opportunity to educate the insurance representatives about the benefits of manual therapy and the patient's level of need.

The denial may be the result of a simple mistake that can be corrected and the denial reversed, or it may be a valid response to an infraction of policy undeserving of an appeal. However, an appeal is warranted if a denial is issued when treatment is critical for the health of the patient and the denial is a result of the insurance carrier's failure to cover the needs of the patient or of the insurance representative's failure to understand the patient's condition and need for care. Appeals are commonly needed for chronic conditions or conditions poorly understood by health professionals and claims managers, such as lymphedema and fibromyalgia. Plans rarely cover chronic conditions because insurers consider treatment for these conditions to be preventative or palliative—symptoms do not subside—even though a lack of treatment may result in a substantial decrease in the patient's ability to function and ultimately may leave the patient predisposed to serious acute flare-ups.

Appeals must be written so that they validate treatment based on the patient's specific condition and prove that such care is neither preventive nor palliative and is necessary for the patient's ability to function in everyday activities. Without the treatment, the quality

208

HANDS HEAL:
COMMUNICATION,
DOCUMENTATION,
AND INSURANCE BILLING
FOR MANUAL THERAPISTS

of the patient's life is diminished. For information on resolving disputes related to ICD-9 coding, visit http://www.appeallettersonline.com/int_icd.htm (download sample letters free of charge).

Appeals must be filed within a specified time frame or the appeal does not have to be heard. Level 1 appeals are conducted by a peer review panel. Your peers may not be representative of your profession, but typically include nurses or physical therapists—professionals who subsume your scope of practice and oversee all HCPs who fall under physical medicine. If your appeal is denied, you may petition for a Level 2 review. An internal grievance and appeals committee will consider your case at this level. Your final opportunity for a favorable outcome is a Level 3 review, which is conducted by an external review agency. Every insurance company conducts its appeals a little differently. Refer to your provider contract for rules regarding appeals processes.

▼

STORY TELLER
Winning Appeals

Karin was pregnant. She had injured her low back at work and was coming to Lakeside Massage Clinic for manual therapy treatments to ease the pain and muscle spasms in her low back and supporting musculature. Her pregnancy made it difficult to treat the muscles of her anterior lumbar spine and hip flexors. I used foot reflexology to address the structures I could not treat directly and safely. The insurance company paid for only 68% of the amount billed and refused to pay for foot massage, which the company considered palliative. I filed an appeal, did my research, and wrote a letter explaining the patient's condition and the need for indirect treatment in response to the patient's overriding safety concerns. I also defended my decision to treat the opposing flexors as well as the extensors that were directly injured and provided documentation of the effectiveness of reflexology techniques. I was paid the remaining 32% within two weeks of submitting the appeal to the peer review panel.

Insurance companies have internal quotas regarding claims denials. It is common knowledge that employees are instructed to deny a minimum percentage of claims to ensure reserve funds for the company and to discourage ongoing treatment. Their hope is that the patient or the practitioner will give up on seeking reimbursement. As a result, you will inevitably come face to face with a reimbursement challenge. The best thing to do is stay on top of unpaid claims and limit the financial risk to your patient and yourself. Follow these guidelines when you find yourself faced with a denied claim for necessary treatment after the service has been provided:

- Identify the cause for the denial.
- Submit a written request outlining your objection to the denial.
- Write a detailed request for reconsideration, including the patient's situation and the benefits of the treatment provided.
- Cite references from the insurance carrier's policy manual to support your case.
- Cite applicable state law (particularly in disputes over scope of practice).
- Request support from the referring HCP and enclose any supportive statements or reports.

- Cite research on the efficacy of the treatment provided.
- Provide photocopies of articles and other documents that may help the claims investigation.
- Cite references from the patient's SOAP charts and progress reports, if applicable, to demonstrate the treatment planning and the progress resulting from the treatment.

Select your appeals wisely. Insurance billing often involves an ethical dilemma: When is it the insurance company's responsibility to pay for treatment and when is care the patient's responsibility? When have we finished treating the condition and begun providing palliative or preventative care?

Once you have identified worthy cases, arm yourself with applicable facts, knowledge, and a desire to educate. Take a positive approach and assume the review board has the patient's best interest in mind and simply does not have the information necessary to come to the appropriate conclusion. Provide the board with more information than necessary to reverse the decision. Be honest and thorough and communicate respectfully.

HIPAA Regulations for Electronic Billing

The **Health Insurance Portability and Accountability Act (HIPAA) Administration Simplification**, the section that has the most impact on manual therapists, was signed into law in 1996. Its purpose is to simplify the transfer and storage of information so that all health care providers who transmit health information electronically or use a billing service or clearinghouse to do this use the same set of codes, data content, and data formats and keep patient information safe and secure throughout the process.[11] **Electronic transactions** refer to exchanges of protected health information between computers.

Compliance with HIPAA regulations has been challenging. Certainly, confusion was common when CPT codes and ICD-9 codes were first introduced. The intent was to create a universal language for services and diagnoses in order to standardize billing procedures and expedite reimbursement. Though not without limitations, the codes have served their purpose. In time, the benefits of these regulations should become apparent.

Since HIPAA regulations became law, many attempts have been made to interpret compliance: To whom does HIPAA apply? What is required for compliance and how should practitioners meet these requirements? The following section briefly addresses these questions and provides a few basic tools to point you in the right direction for obtaining the additional help you may need regarding HIPAA regulations and compliance.

- For help demystifying the complexities of HIPAA regulations, read *HIPAA Plain & Simple: A Compliance Guide for Health Care Professionals* by Carolyn P. Hartley and Edward Jones, published by the AMA (2004).
- Access the official Web site of the Centers for Medicare and Medicaid Services (CMS) at http://www.cms.hhs.gov/hipaa/hipaa2 or e-mail your questions to askhipaa@cms.hhs.gov.
- Visit the official Web site of the U.S. Department of Health and Human Services at http://www.hhs.gov/ for HIPAA updates. Once there, type *administrative simplification* in the Search bar (a list of resources will appear) or go directly to http://aspe.os.dhhs.gov/admnsimp/index.shtml for information on administrative simplification in the health care industry.
- Download free HIPAA-compliant forms from a variety of Web sites and customize them to meet your needs. Many sites provide basic forms for use by HCPs. These forms

210

HANDS HEAL:
COMMUNICATION,
DOCUMENTATION,
AND INSURANCE BILLING
FOR MANUAL THERAPISTS

must be tailored to each particular practice and should be reviewed by a competent legal professional familiar with HIPAA requirements. Because HIPAA is still in a state of flux, these forms may become outdated and require revisions. For forms and information specific to the state of Washington, visit http://www.peick-usa.com/forms.htm. For Colorado, visit http://www.cdhs.state.co.us/HIPAA/hipaa_forms.htm. For forms applicable to your state, use a search engine to find your state's department of human services. Forms used in chiropractic and manual therapy practices can be found online at http://www.worldchiropracticalliance.org/hipaa/introduction.htm.

Three sets of standards from the HIPAA Administrative Simplification section are addressed in this chapter. They are:

1. Privacy issues
2. Security issues
3. Transactions and code sets

DOES HIPAA APPLY TO ME?

Health care providers who transmit confidential patient information electronically or use a third-party billing service or clearinghouse to transmit information electronically are required to comply with HIPAA regulations. Electronic transactions include:

◆ Claims or patient encounter information, such as patient files and billing information
◆ Patient eligibility requests
◆ Referrals, prescriptions, and authorizations
◆ Claims status inquiries

If you conduct all of your business activities and health care transactions on paper, by phone, or a dedicated fax (as opposed to faxing from a computer), HIPAA does not apply to you. However, you may be required to comply with state regulations that dictate health care privacy standards. Regardless of state and federal law, it is good business to protect your patients' confidential health information. Inform your patients of their rights regarding their health information, explain your privacy practices, and describe how you intend to use and disclose their health information. Secure patient information in your office so that only you and authorized staff members have access to it.

The **U.S. Department of Health and Human Services (HHS)** has developed a "covered entity decision tool" for providers to help you determine whether you should be HIPAA compliant. Visit http://www.cms.hhs.gov/hipaa/hipaa2 to access this tool (under General Information) and other educational materials.

HIPAA PRIVACY ISSUES

Privacy is an important issue for people. All health care providers should take adequate measures to protect their patients' confidential information. The HIPAA **Privacy Rule** section takes a common sense approach applicable to all practitioners. It has garnered a considerable amount of attention in health care practices because it is nontechnical and deals mainly with administrative policies and procedures. Simply stated, patient information must be protected at rest (i.e., storage) or in motion (i.e., spoken communication), as well as in electronic, oral, or written forms. The privacy rule also includes safeguard measures to control the unauthorized **disclosure** of, access to, and use of **protected health information (PHI)**.[11]

To adequately protect your patient's PHI, identify all the places in your office, home, or other location in which patient information can be found, such as your appointment book, patient sign-in sheets, patient files, and address book. Then, identify privacy risks, such as anyone who may have access to this information or whether patient files, your address book, or appointment book are ever left unattended while you are, for example, in the treatment room. Next, come up with a system for protecting this information, such as locking these items in a file cabinet, putting away all files between patients, and using first names only in your appointment book if it is ever visible to patients. Create policies that are HIPAA compliant and require your staff (if any) to follow them.

Map out how PHI flows through your office. If you use an outside billing service, how is information transferred? If you take client files home because you don't have a computer in your office for writing reports, who has access to this computer? Where do you store patient files when you travel from office to office? When you have conversations about patients with officemates, such as chiropractors or fellow therapists, in hallways or other public areas, how do you keep the information confidential? The HIPAA privacy rule allows patients to access their health information, so where do you log the content of your discussions so your patients can gain access to it?

Next, write and implement a **Notice of Privacy Practices (NPP)**. This notice must describe the **use and disclosure** of patient health information and how patients can access this information. Review several NPPs from various practices and develop one that works for you. Search online or access the Web sites mentioned earlier for privacy statements that you may download and use to create your own practice policies. Conduct an online search of HIPAA and its privacy regulations. An effective NPP will:

◆ Describe the health information you intend to protect, including medical records, conversations among health care providers, billing information, and patients' name and other identifying information such as contact information.

◆ State how you will protect your patients' health information. For example, explain when you will require patients' authorization to use and disclose their information and how you will limit access to that information. For example, state that patient health information may be shared for the following reasons and in the following ways:

—For treatment, health information may be shared within the office and outside the office with members of the health care team

—For education and research to improve quality of care

—For administrative functions, such as staff training

—For setting appointments and contacting patient for health-related communications

—For judging the practitioner's quality of care, information may be shared with the patient's health plan

—For payment, eligibility, and claims purposes

◆ List the six patients' rights provided by HIPAA:

—Access and right to copies of medical records

—Request for amendment to designated record set

—Request for accounting of disclosures

—Request to be contacted at an alternate location

212

HANDS HEAL:
COMMUNICATION,
DOCUMENTATION,
AND INSURANCE BILLING
FOR MANUAL THERAPISTS

—Request for further restrictions on who has access

—Right to file a complaint

The **Office for Civil Rights (OCR)** has been designated by HHS to enforce the HIPAA privacy rules. The patient may also contact a consumer advocate group, the state's attorney general, or the American Civil Liberties Union. If a complaint has been filed against you, your office will be asked to produce significant records documenting your privacy efforts.[11] The NPP for your office, the forms shown in the following list, and your implementation procedures will be your first line of defense in demonstrating your compliance to HIPAA.

Determine how you will respond to and manage patient requests and develop and implement the following forms for patients to use:

◆ Acknowledgment of Notification of Privacy Practices—This form shows patients' signatures acknowledging that they have received your privacy practices and have read them.

◆ Patient Consent Form—This form gives the HCP permission (patients' consent) to communicate with those necessary to facilitate safe treatment and expedite reimbursement. Some things can be spelled out, such as how you may contact the patient and with whom (on the health care team) you may share information. It is intended for general purposes without which you will be unable to provide care for the patient. If a patient does not sign the form, you should not provide treatment. Consent statements can be found on the billing information form and the health information form (see Appendix B) and can be binding for up to seven years unless otherwise noted or revoked in writing.

◆ Patient Authorization for the Use and Disclosure of Protected Information—This form is very specific to the kind of information that may be shared, with whom, and for what purpose. The authorization has a short life span and typically expires in 90 to 120 days, which should be stated on the form.

◆ Revocation of Authorization—You must provide patients with explicit instructions on how they may revoke their authorization to release medical information.

Finally, determine how you will protect your patients' rights. After you have gone through the steps of identifying where patient PHI can be found in your office, how it travels through your office, and what your patients' rights are regarding that information, outline the steps you will take to protect them. It could be as simple as printing a confidential statement on fax cover sheets, tracking who you share information with and why (use the insurance verification form to log and monitor this information), and using the suggested forms to obtain your patients' consent or authorization to share their PHI. Whatever your plan, write it down and follow it.

Here is a sample statement to print on the bottom of your fax cover sheet:

> The documents accompanying this transmission may contain confidential health information that is legally protected. This information is intended only for the use of the individual or **covered entities** named above. The authorized recipient of this information is prohibited from disclosing this information to any other party unless permitted by law or regulation.
>
> If you are not the intended recipient, you are hereby notified that any use, disclosure, copying, or distribution of these documents is strictly prohibited. If you have received this information in error, please notify the sender immediately and arrange for the return or destruction of these documents.[12]

Protect transmitted information further by verifying the accuracy of all fax numbers before sending documents.

Some **incidental use and disclosure** of health information is permitted. For example, discussions can take place to coordinate care in person or on the phone if you speak in a low voice and away from listeners. You can leave messages on patients' answering machines or with family members if you only provide the minimum information necessary. You may ask patients to sign in and you may call their name in the waiting area as long as the reason for the visit is not disclosed.

Safeguard your patients' PHI—you cannot have privacy without security. Take the necessary precautions, such as locking your cabinets and doors and limiting access to patient records. Review your privacy practices and forms annually. Evaluate the status of patients' rights. Stay abreast of the updates by accessing HIPAA Web sites regularly and making changes as necessary.

HIPAA SECURITY ISSUES

Security and privacy go hand in hand. Security is about controlling access to electronically transmitted PHI, and privacy is about controlling how electronic, oral, and written PHI is used and disclosed.[11] The biggest difference between these rules is that security only applies to electronic PHI. These are the types of safeguards you must have in place to be compliant with HIPAA:

◆ Physical safeguards—rooms and storage facilities with locks or other safeguards to control access

◆ Administrative safeguards—policies and procedures that define authorized access to information, including user IDs and passwords and actions that will be taken if violations occur.

◆ Technical safeguards—encryption of electronic data and use of passwords to verify use and to track users who have logged onto the system.[11]

Unless your office has a staff of 10 or more people, your security issues will be minor. Purchase and install a sufficient firewall for your hardware and secure all access to your computer.

TRANSACTIONS AND CODE SETS

This section focuses on the HIPAA processes of electronic transactions from patient eligibility through claim for payment. Proper use of correct code sets is key for success in the payment process. Although most of these HIPAA regulations refer to the coders and the payers, they have to be able to receive your standardized transactions. There are four transaction standards:

1. Health care claims or equivalent encounter information—a request from an HCP to a payer for reimbursement for health care services, including submission of a bill
2. Eligibility for a health plan—a request from an HCP to a payer to verify benefits
3. Referral certification and authorization—communication between a primary HCP and a specialist, such as a manual therapist, who is confirmed by the payer
4. Health care claim status—an inquiry to determine the status of a claim, such as whether a claim has been paid or is pending and in need of additional information

214

HANDS HEAL:
COMMUNICATION,
DOCUMENTATION,
AND INSURANCE BILLING
FOR MANUAL THERAPISTS

These transactions can be time consuming when done over the phone or by fax, but they can be done quickly by electronic means. Follow these guidelines for collecting the information necessary for conducting electronic transactions:

- Gather all the necessary contact information for the patient and the insured
- Gather insurance information
- Take a thorough health history
- Gather the necessary diagnostic codes (ICD-9) from the referring HCP
- Determine the appropriate procedure and modality codes (CPT) for your services

With the proper information and codes, verifying the insurance benefits with the payer and authorizing your services can be fast and easy.

SUMMARY

Insurance billing has it benefits and its risks. Limit the risks by familiarizing yourself with the various types of insurance, by following the billing strategies presented, and by educating yourself on common billing practices specific to your state and profession. Reap the benefits of an increased patient load, a variety of patients offering accelerated learning opportunities, and the satisfaction of influencing the health care community.

Three types of insurance commonly reimburse for manual therapy:

- Personal injury insurance
- Workers' compensation
- Private health insurance

Each plan has its own billing protocols and reimbursement methods, but use a standard billing form and universal procedure codes and diagnostic codes. All plans require alert claims management and tenacious follow-through to ensure payment. Follow these strategies for successful insurance reimbursement:

- Provide accurate and complete patient documentation and insurance information.
- Stay within designated time limits when providing treatment, billing for services, and appealing claims denials.
- Be prepared to prove medical necessity by obtaining prescriptions for services, documenting patient progress, and providing effective treatment.
- File attorney liens or medical liens on all personal injury cases.
- Maintain accurate payment logs.
- Communicate with insurance representatives professionally, respectfully, and cooperatively.

REFERENCES

1. Hands On: The Newsletter of the American Massage Therapy Association 2000;XVI #4.
2. Owens C. Managed Care Organizations: Practical Implications for Medical Practices and Other Providers. Los Angeles: PMIC, 1996.
3. AlliantPlus Health Plan. c22389 CA-119202a. GroupHealth Options, Inc. Seattle, 2004.
4. Mootz RD. Advances in Chiropractic, Vol. 4. Mosby-Year Book, Inc., 1997.
5. Dolan DW. Insurance Reimbursement and Specialty Physician Referrals. Jacksonville: American Health Press, 1998.

6. Foreman SM, Croft AC. Whiplash Injuries: The Cervical Acceleration/Deceleration Syndrome. 2nd Ed. Baltimore: Lippincott Williams & Wilkins, 2001.

7. Grigsby B, Rosen S. Some contracts are not worth signing. The Journal: A Publication of the American Massage Therapy Association–Washington Chapter 2000;16 #1:1–6.

8. Adler RH, Whiplash, Spinal Trauma, and the Personal Injury Case. Seattle: Adler◆Giersch PS, 2004.

9. Alternáre Health Network Seminar, Seattle, 1997.

10. WAC 284-43-321: Provider Contracts—Terms and Conditions of Payment. (See http://www.leg.wa.gov/WAC/index.cfm?section=284=43=322&fuseaction=section)

11. Hartley CP, Jones ED. HIPAA Plain and Simple: A Compliance Guide for Health Care Professionals. AMA, 2004.

12. Vanderbilt University Medical Center, HIPAA Forms (See http://www.mc.vanderbilt.edu/root/vumc.php?site=hippaprivacy&doc=1671)

CHAPTER 9

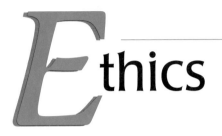

*E*thics

CHAPTER OUTLINE

After just six additional sessions, Sandee is able to garden, play with her grandson, and clean her house. She even took up bike riding this summer! She has enjoyed all this activity without acute flare-ups of her chronic low back pain. She stretches daily, adding warm-up and cool-down exercises with more strenuous activities, and she stops and rests when her body becomes stiff or achy. She has learned that when she doesn't exercise and rest, the ensuing pain and stiffness limits her activities for several days.

If you remember from Chapter 4, Sandee had nearly given up on her massage therapist, Holly. But after reviewing her SOAP charts, Sandee decided to recommit to Holly's treatment plan, albeit with alterations. Together, they set and accomplished goals and reviewed clinical and functional progress frequently. Sandee's awareness of her body's needs increased, and she learned to identify effective self-care exercises in response to those needs. Sandee's healing curve rose dramatically with her renewed commitment and enhanced communication skills.

Now Sandee is faced with another dilemma. Her insurance company has notified Holly that Sandee has reached **maximum benefit** and coverage is no longer available. Sandee feels that care is being terminated prematurely. She is not yet pain free and without ongoing care, she and Holly both fear that the symptoms could return.

Sandee's insurance policy defines reasonable and necessary care as care provided to correct the presenting condition, bringing it to maximum improvement. The policy clearly states that therapy for chronic conditions is not covered when the treatment outcome is primarily to maintain the patient's level of function. Maintenance, relaxation, and wellness care are not covered benefits and are the financial responsibility of the patient. Holly knows that Sandee may never be completely pain free, and she feels that Sandee *is* managing her chronic pain successfully. Should Holly support Sandee in fighting for coverage until she is pain free, or should she support the insurance company in its decision to discontinue coverage?

Faced with this dilemma, Holly reaches out to her peers for support. She invites three fellow manual therapists over for dessert. All share a passion for chocolate, and all have experience with various insurance companies. Holly explains her patient's situation (respecting patient confidentiality by not mentioning Sandee's name), and the four friends share experiences and opinions. They imagine an ideal world in which the patient's health always takes precedence over profits, and they discuss actions that would best serve the patient's long-term health in the real world.

In the end, they all agree on one thing: The patient *is* successfully managing her chronic pain, a condition that has plagued her for many years. At this point, it is more important to celebrate the success of the treatments and instill confidence in the patient and in her ability to manage her health than to prove to the insurance company that she still suffers from chronic pain.

Holly's friends also agree that now is not the time to withdraw all support. Old habits are easy to fall into. Sandee may not be able to afford ongoing care weekly nor does she need that level of care anymore, but monthly treatments for three months will maintain progress and monitor any potential flare-ups. It is important for Sandee to realize that preventive care is available and affordable. After three months of treatments, Sandee could choose to continue treatments with Holly on a monthly or quarterly basis to maintain her progress or to schedule appointments as needed.

As a result of their discussion, Holly and her friends recognized that they typically treat patients until the prescription runs out or until the insurance benefit is depleted. Preventive health care is the sensible approach; but is it ethical to provide maintenance care when the insurance company clearly states that prevention and maintenance are not covered? Is it ethical to continue care just because the prescription has not been fulfilled or the benefit has not been exhausted? What if the patient has an acute flare-up or suffers from an unrelated trauma later in the year and has no benefits remaining? Together, they agree to consider the question "When is treatment finished?" They want to celebrate when patients accomplish their goals ahead of schedule and educate their patients on the importance of prioritizing regular preventive care in their budgets and on their schedules.

Introduction

Webster's defines ethics as the study of standards of conduct and moral judgment. Ethics comes from the Greek word *ethos*, which means the characteristic and distinguishing attitudes, habits, and beliefs of an individual or a group. By definition, manual therapists are students of right and wrong, striving to be moral and just and to respect and uphold the standards of the profession.

With few written guidelines and a great desire to be of service, we learn how to conduct ourselves professionally by taking risks. Life is our classroom; our pursuit of excellence provides the lessons. Obstacles that challenge our sense of fairness and test our integrity serve to develop our beliefs and shape our character.

As students, we learn by engaging in debates with our peers, questioning our teachers, and consulting our mentors. Through these activities, our visceral and intellectual understanding of right and wrong expands; and our ability to speak honestly, act without fear and greed, and express compassion without prejudice matures. Eventually, we become role models to others and our learning expands through interactions with those who seek guidance from us.

As health care providers, we care deeply for our patients and strive to nurture and heal their bodies and souls. In our efforts to be successful, we are influenced by fears, needs, desires, and spiritual longings. Ethical dilemmas are unavoidable. It is critical that we take steps to encourage personal and professional growth and protect those we intend to serve by setting standards for our business practices, evaluating these practices regularly, and discussing ethical beliefs with others. For example:

- Define your ethical standards. Write them down. If your professional organization has a code of ethics, frame it and hang it in your office. Read it often.
- Create office policies, distribute them to your patients, and stick to them.
- Join a supervision group. If you cannot find one, form your own.
- Evaluate your business practices and professional relationships monthly.
- Invite others to review your business practices annually.
- Establish a relationship with a mentor.
- Mentor others.

This chapter first presents several current ethical dilemmas for manual therapists in the areas of documentation and insurance billing, treatment practices, and relationships with other health care professionals. It then recommends steps for building and maintaining an ethical practice and includes a sample code of ethics, a self-evaluation tool for reviewing your business practices and relationships, and an outline for organizing and participating in supervision groups and mentoring. Be a role model to your peers, patients, and other health care providers.

Ethical issues involving emotional and physical relationships between the practitioner and the patient, such as dual relationships and patient confidentiality, are not discussed in

220

HANDS HEAL:
COMMUNICATION,
DOCUMENTATION,
AND INSURANCE BILLING
FOR MANUAL THERAPISTS

this chapter because of the enormous scope of this subject matter. Many books are dedicated to such topics. A resource list of books on ethical issues in the practitioner-patient relationships is provided in Figure 9-1.

Current Ethical Dilemmas: Billing and Documentation Practices

RESPONSIBILITY FOR PAYMENT

Sandee's story poses an interesting dilemma concerning when treatment is finished and when maintenance or wellness care begins? A fine line exists between the two, especially when the condition is chronic. If we can identify guidelines for delineating treatment versus wellness care, we can ethically apply those standards to the insurance issue: Who is responsible for paying for care?

The insurance issue is often clouded by our beliefs and experiences. We may believe that insurance policies or case managers too often limit access to manual therapy and prevent patients from receiving the number of treatments necessary to recover from their injuries. Therefore, in the seemingly few situations in which authorized treatment exceeds the number of sessions necessary for healing, we often feel we are justified in continuing to provide care. Certainly, the patients are willing to continue. After all, manual therapy feels good and is effective. Continuing it makes sense because, of course, an ounce of prevention is worth a pound of cure.

According to standard insurance definitions, treatment is warranted until the condition is corrected or maximum functional improvement is made. These definitions also state that treatment must provide the patient with appropriate instruction for follow-up, self-care, and prevention of future occurrences. All maintenance and wellness care are the financial responsibility of the patient unless otherwise specified by the insurance plan. Given those parameters, how do we determine when treatment ends and maintenance care begins?

Sometimes, it becomes obvious when the patient has reached maximum healing. He or she is pain free and fully functional. At other times, as with chronic pain, things are not so clear. In such cases, wellness is determined by the patient's ability to manage pain and successfully modify activities. The focus is not on living pain free, but on the patient's quality of life—the ability to participate in everyday activities. Use the following guidelines to determine when treatments are no longer necessary for resolving the patient's condition:

◆ The patient is able to function normally or functional progress has peaked.
◆ The patient has no significant symptomology or clinical progress has peaked.
◆ The patient demonstrates self-awareness by identifying situations, activities, or emotions that exacerbate his or her condition.

FIGURE 9-1   Books on Ethics

1. Benjamin BE, Sohnen-Moe C. The Ethics of Touch. Tucson, AZ: SMA Inc, 2001.
2. McIntosh N. The Educated Heart: Professional Guidelines for Massage Therapists, Bodyworkers, and Movement Teachers. Memphis, TN: Decatur Bainbridge Press, 1999.
3. Taylor K. The Ethics of Caring: Honoring the Web of Life in Our Professional Healing Relationships. 2nd ed. Santa Cruz, CA: Hanford Mead Publishers, 1995.

◆ The patient applies self-care techniques to limit exacerbations and to remedy the exacerbations when they do occur.

Test your findings by discontinuing care for a predetermined length of time. If, for example, after four weeks without treatment, Darnel is sufficiently symptom free and active, care can be reduced to a monthly (or maintenance) level of care. If Darnel experiences an exacerbation or acceleration of the condition, in spite of performing his self-care routines, ongoing treatment is warranted.

Most patients who reach maximum improvement for their conditions would benefit from wellness care. Encourage the patient to return monthly for wellness care for three months after terminating treatment. During that time, provide care as needed and fine-tune the patient's self-care instructions. If his or her health deteriorates without regular care, you have a case for the reinstatement of insurance coverage. If the patient is able to administer appropriate self-care and maintain his health status, celebrate his accomplishments and invite him to continue participating in monthly or quarterly wellness sessions, or you can refer him to someone who specializes in wellness care.

PREFERRED PROVIDER STATUS

Insurance carriers contract with health care providers in an attempt to limit what the providers of health care services do and the amount they reimburse for those services. The carriers either contract with providers directly or purchase provider contracts through an **insurance network**. The insurance carrier then provides incentives to motivate insureds to seek health care services from preferred providers. Incentives may include reduced co-pays or waived deductibles.

Insurance networks and insurance carriers can support only a limited number of providers. Set numbers of providers are credentialed for a given area based on the number of insureds or **lives** that reside in that area. As the number of covered lives changes in a given area, the network or panel may open up to new providers until the ratio of lives to providers is considered adequate.

Only credentialed manual therapists are permitted to bill under the preferred provider contract. It is unethical and often illegal for noncredentialed practitioners to bill for services under the license of the credentialed provider.

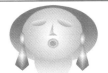

STORY TELLER
One Preferred Provider in a Clinic of Many

Rosie owns a manual therapy clinic in a bustling urban setting. The trendy neighborhood has a reputation for being health conscious, and it boasts a well-worn walking trail, several juice bars and cafés, a health club, day spas, and wellness centers. Rosie is an excellent practitioner, and her services are in high demand. She has added a dozen other manual therapists to her staff over the years to meet the demand. She and her staff receive referrals from the various health care providers in the area, as well as walk-in traffic.

(Continued)

222

HANDS HEAL:
COMMUNICATION,
DOCUMENTATION,
AND INSURANCE BILLING
FOR MANUAL THERAPISTS

STORY TELLER *(Continued)*

A large insurance network provides manual therapy contracts to most insurance carriers in the area. Rosie was able to get on the preferred provider list several years ago. Because the neighborhood is densely populated with manual therapists, it has become difficult to get new providers credentialed. Rosie is the only practitioner in her clinic with preferred provider status. As a result, she has had to refer her steady cash-paying patients to her staff so that she can accommodate the large number of insurance patients referred to the clinic.

Rosie and her regular patients are upset at the turn of events. Rosie wants to be able to see her cash-paying patients, and her regulars miss her care. She decides to have her staff treat the insurance patients, and she signs the charts and bills under her name. They are her employees, after all—this must be permissible. She promises to check it out with the insurance network, but she never gets around to it.

During a random audit, the insurance company uncovers Rosie's fraudulent billing practices. Company policy states that only the credentialed provider may deliver the health care services unless the provider is on vacation and notifies the company in advance of the dates during which her staff will be taking over her patients. As a result, her provider status is revoked and her staff is barred from contracting with the company as preferred providers. In addition, the company filed a complaint with the state regulatory body requesting disciplinary action against all practitioners involved.

FEE SCHEDULES

Ethical billing practices include charging reasonable and consistent fees for services provided. It is tempting to charge higher fees to insurance companies because of the time and paperwork required for billing. However, it is unethical and, if proven fraudulent, illegal to charge insurance companies higher rates than you charge patients who do not have insurance coverage, a practice commonly referred to as payer discrimination.

Every patient should be charged the same rate for the same service, regardless of who is paying for the service. Establish fees based on the type of service you provide. For example, it requires more education and experience to provide rehabilitation services for treating specific injuries and illnesses than it does to provide a wellness massage for a healthy person. Make a list of all the therapeutic procedures and modalities you provide—use the CPT codes to differentiate services—and assign fees accordingly.

Insurance carriers often will refer to the **Relative Value Unit** (**RVU**) when establishing fee schedules. Units are calculated taking into account the degree of difficulty of the work as performed by a physician, the cost of overhead, and the malpractice risk. The **Resource-Based Relative Value Scale** (**RBRVS**) is available for CPT codes online at http://www.icd9coding.com. You may consult the published values for your services, but take into account that a physician's overhead and malpractice risk are greater than a manual therapist's.[1] Start by researching common practices in your area to determine competitive rates for your services. Consider your level of experience, effectiveness of care, investment in continuing education, quality of supplies, office location, and style of professional dress as you develop your fee schedule—those are all things your patients will be assessing as well.

Once you have established your fee schedule for each service you offer, consider the cost of providing a billing service. It is more costly to delay payment and bill for services than to accept payment at the time of service. The issue is whether or not you must provide billing services for the patient, not who is being billed. The billing service costs the same whether you send the bills to the patient or to the insurance company. Therefore, it makes sense to offer a cash discount to all patients who pay at the time services are rendered and to penalize all patients who opt for delaying, regardless of who is responsible for payment. The ethical solution is to offer a modest cash discount as an incentive to patients to pay at the time of service.

What is an ethical discount for payment at the time of service—5%, 10%, or even 50%? Excessive cash discounts are also considered discriminatory and may provoke an audit by the insurance company. Therefore, it is important to be able to justify the discount by comparing it with the actual expense of billing. Billing agencies generally charge between 7 and 15% of the amount collected. An office providing the service in-house can usually perform the service for less than an outside agency would charge. A discount for payment at the time of service that does not exceed the expense of billing is an ethical discount.

Some forms of payer discrimination are considered ethical, such as senior discounts, student discounts, and considerations for financial hardship. List eligibility specifics on your fee schedule, such as income bracket for hardship. Check with a local attorney to make sure that your fee schedule is legal.

Unethical billing practices also arise when services are chosen because they cost more than other equally appropriate services or when a practitioner bills for services that pay higher rates than the services actually performed. This course of action is known as **up-coding**. Upcoding is tempting when insurance fee schedules delineate different fees for different manual techniques, as though one technique was better than another. For example, Health R Us published a fee schedule that pays $20 per unit for therapeutic massage, $25 per unit for manual therapy, and $28 per unit for energetic therapeutic touch. It is unethical to bill for four units of energetic therapeutic touch if other techniques were also performed. It is also unethical to use only energetic techniques when other techniques would be equally or more effective.

The key to an ethical fee schedule is in its application. Follow these steps to be consistent and not discriminatory.

◆ Apply the same fee for the same service to everyone, regardless of the type of payer.
◆ Provide the service that is most appropriate to the patient, regardless of the reimbursement rate for the service.

The consequences of ignoring fee schedule guidelines can be severe. Health care fraud is both a state and federal crime. HIPAA extends the reach of federal fraud and abuse statutes, as well as enforcement, to all private health care plans. In addition to possible civil claims and professional sanctions, you could be facing a federal prosecutor.[2]

▼

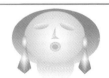

STORY TELLER
Consequences of Fraudulent Billing

"Two chiropractic doctors learned this lesson the hard way last year and spent 10 months in a federal maximum security prison, in addition to six-figure income losses resulting from defense costs, fines, and the loss of their practice. On top of all that, they faced professional discipline charges.

224

HANDS HEAL:
COMMUNICATION,
DOCUMENTATION,
AND INSURANCE BILLING
FOR MANUAL THERAPISTS

TIMELY DOCUMENTATION

Unethical charting practices occur when a patient's chart is filled in weeks, months, or years later because of a request for charts, payment has been denied, or rebilling requires copies of all treatment notes. Charting should be done in a timely fashion. It is difficult to remember a particular session after several other sessions have blurred the details. The best time to chart is during or immediately after the session. Everyone has days, however, when the charts pile up and note are not taken until the next morning. It is stressful but possible to recreate the session 24 hours later. However, few of us can record a session accurately weeks, months, or years later.

▼

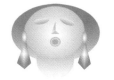

STORY TELLER
Carbon-Dating?

At a billing seminar, an attorney told a story of a chiropractor whose notes were carbon-dated—a test that establishes the time frame of a record. His patient had been injured in a car accident and the attorney for the at-fault party suspected tampering with the treatment notes, so he ordered the tests. Test results showed that the health care provider had filled in the chart notes 2 to 3 years after the treatments had been provided. The patient's case was adversely affected.

Current Ethical Dilemmas: Treatment Practices

TREATMENT EXPECTATIONS

At times, patients form expectations of their therapist based on hearsay. Patients' healing time and abilities vary in many ways, including condition, past history, genetics, emotional complications, daily physical demands, and the like. As the therapist, we may or may not be able to live up to the stories our patients have been told by their friends and family. It is critical to represent our abilities honestly and refrain from committing to specific results or time limits for healing.

▼

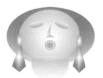

STORY TELLER
Promises Promises

Annie experienced what anyone would call a miraculous recovery. She had a long history of head and neck trauma, and after a summer of painting the exterior of her house and working long hours at the computer, she ruptured a disk in her neck. The pain was so intense that she could not lift her head high enough to gaze across the horizon, nor could she hold her head up long enough to eat at the dinner table. The numbness and weakness in her right arm was so great that she could not butter her toast or brush her teeth.

(Continued)

STORY TELLER   *(Continued)*

Annie's doctor scheduled an MRI. In the meantime, Annie began seeing her Feldenkrais practitioner, John. The first few visits were house calls because riding in a car was excruciating for Annie—she had to hold her head in her hands and apply traction so the bumps in the road wouldn't cause more pain than necessary. By the time the results of the MRI came back and the neurosurgeon met with Annie to discuss treatment options, she was pain free, driving to her own appointments and working part-time. One month from the date of injury, she was working full time and had full mobility in her neck.

John's phone started ringing off the hook. Annie worked in health care and her peers, amazed by Annie's progress, began referring their patients, friends, and family members to John. But not everyone responded to John's care as Annie had, and several were disappointed when they were not symptom-free in two weeks.

Annie took care of herself in more ways than John knew and in more ways than she told her peers at the clinic. She took naps after every session, limited her activities, and received acupuncture, Tui Na, Polarity, and lymph drainage. She even had a healing session with a Tibetan lama. She began her treatment immediately and aggressively after her injury, getting daily care for the first week and three times a week for the following three weeks. She had the resources and knowledge to seek treatment that was effective for her, whether or not it was prescribed by her doctor or covered by her insurance. Annie was willing to do whatever it took to get well; she acted quickly and she never lost sight of her belief that she could heal instantaneously.

John is a brilliant practitioner. He serves all patients equally to the best of his abilities, given each patient's unique situation. The only thing lacking in his sessions has been the conversation about each person's unique healing cycle. Although he had made no promises about the results of his treatments, he neglected to address the patient's expectations. He, too, had been carried away by his success with Annie. This experience not only increased his skills for working with disk injuries, but also reminded him of the need to communicate clearly with his patients; that is, to hear their expectations and cautiously discuss possible outcomes based on individual circumstances.

Many factors influence healing. As health care providers, we can only try to find the right combination of therapeutic procedures and modalities, communication techniques, and referrals for each patient. Don't take it upon yourself to meet the expectations of everyone who comes to you for help. Instead, talk with them, find out about their expectations, tell them what you can honestly predict—which is often nothing more than possibilities—and ask for their help in discovering the best treatment plan.

Educate yourself on the state regulations for your profession. Know what claims are legal for your scope. For example, in New York, claims regarding the benefits of massage therapy must be qualified with a statement that massage therapy "may" reduce inflammation, or "may" improve range of motion. The only concrete claim permissible is that massage therapy increases circulation.

SCOPE OF PRACTICE

Manual therapy encompasses many professions and techniques. Much cross-training occurs, often without knowledge of the licensing laws for each profession in each state.

226

HANDS HEAL:
COMMUNICATION,
DOCUMENTATION,
AND INSURANCE BILLING
FOR MANUAL THERAPISTS

workshop on a manual technique may be taught by an osteopath and may include chiropractors, nurses, physical therapists, dentists, and massage therapists as students. Remember that you may be taught techniques that are outside your scope of practice. Receiving training in a technique does not automatically license you to perform it in your practice.

▼

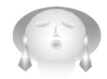

STORY TELLER
Do the Right Thing

Leisha is a massage therapist in Oregon. To escape the cold winter rains, she travels to Hawaii every January for Lomilomi training in the home of an elder Lomi master. Leisha lives there for four weeks every year and adheres to a rigorous schedule of fasting, taking cleansing herbs, and giving and receiving treatments. She learns to harvest the herbs, make cleansing tonics, perform thrust adjustments on the extremities, and apply vigorous manual techniques to increase the circulation. After four years of training, she received the blessing of the elder to provide this healing ritual to others.

Leisha is confident of her skills but knows that Oregon law does not permit her to perform joint manipulations with a thrusting force. Several months go by without temptation. Then, one day, Leisha treats a 40-year-old woman with gnarled, stiff, and painful toes. Leisha knows that the joint manipulations she learned in her Lomi training would benefit this woman, who is prematurely losing mobility in her toes and feet. What should she do?

If the laws that dictate your profession's scope of practice do not adequately represent the skill and training of those licensed, then work to update the laws. Until the laws change, resist the temptation to provide services outside your scope. Create a list of practitioners who can provide those services and refer out when necessary.

Current Ethical Dilemmas: The Health Care Team
COMMUNICATING WITH REFERRING HEALTH CARE PROVIDERS

As health care is currently structured, physicians and possibly naturopaths or chiropractors (depending on the insurance policy and the state regulations) are considered primary health care providers (HCPs). It is the primary HCP's responsibility to diagnose the patient's problem, orchestrate treatment, and refer to adjunctive therapists, such as massage therapists.

Many of our patients are self-referred, and their HCP may or may not know they are receiving massage therapy. It is imperative to receive permission from patients before communicating with their HCP to avoid any embarrassment or conflict between them and their HCP. If you are working under the direction of the referring HCP but not under his supervision, good communication is required. In either case, provide the HCP with clear, complete information so that he or she can give the patient the best possible treatment.

Occasionally, you may find yourself disagreeing with the referring HCP about a patient's condition or treatment. Do not express this disagreement to the patient. Instead, state your views to the referring HCP—calmly, professionally, tactfully—with all the supporting evidence you can provide. If your input is not considered or if you find that you can't endorse the prescribed treatment, your best choice may be to withdraw from the case. However you choose to handle the situation, remember that the referring HCP is the final authority and that it is unethical for the manual therapist to undermine the relationship between the referring HCP and the patient. If the patient approaches you with complaints about the referring HCP's approach to the treatment plan, support the patient in addressing the issues directly with the referring HCP.

PERMISSION TO CONSULT WITH THE HEALTH CARE TEAM

The health information form contains a request for permission to exchange information with the other members of the patient's health care team. In many cases, practitioners do not need the patient's consent to speak with referring providers—state health care privacy laws permit open communication between referring HCP and adjunctive care and HIPAA regulations don't apply because the HCP does not bill or transfer patient information electronically. Regardless, it is a good idea to inform the patient that information will be shared and with whom it will be shared. HIPAA privacy rules make good sense for all HCP and their patients (see Appendix B for blank forms). An authorization for releasing protected health information is valid and meets HIPAA regulations when it contains the following core requirements:

◆ A description of the information to be disclosed
◆ The name of the person authorized to make the disclosure
◆ The name of the person to whom the disclosure may be made
◆ A description of each purpose of the requested disclosure, such as "at the request of the individual" when an individual initiated the authorization
◆ An expiration date or event for the authorization as it relates to the individual or the purpose of the disclosure
◆ Signature of the authorizing individual and the date of signing
◆ Statement about the right of the individual to refuse to sign the authorization and to revoke any authoization given in writing and a brief explanation of how to do so
◆ The potential for information disclosed under the authorization to be redisclosed by the recipient and no longer protected by the act
◆ The authorization must be written in plain language[3]

When providing information to other practitioners, respect the patient's confidentiality and limit those conversations to information pertinent to the patient's condition. Omit your personal opinions about the patient and any gossip or details that have no bearing on the case. Refrain from discussing patient cases in public, where others who are not bound by HIPAA confidentiality regulations might overhear sensitive information. Follow the guidelines for protecting patient's health information detailed in Chapter 8, regardless of your status with HIPAA compliance. Your patients will appreciate it.

PAYMENT FOR REFERRALS

As health care providers, we are responsible for serving the patient to the best of our ability. Accepting payment for referrals can cloud that ability and compromise our ethics. In all cases, this creates a conflict of interest. In many cases, it is illegal.

228

HANDS HEAL:
COMMUNICATION,
DOCUMENTATION,
AND INSURANCE BILLING
FOR MANUAL THERAPISTS

The practice of accepting payment for referrals, or referring to clinics or laboratories in which the provider has a financial interest, is known as **rebating**. Severe penalties can be placed on practitioners who violate laws of this nature.

It is appropriate to refer within a health system network or preferred provider list. It is not appropriate when the referral is based on the prospect of financial gain.

▼

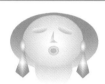

STORY TELLER
Who Is Best for the Patient?

Helena's office is centrally located in town. As a result, several HCPs from around the area refer patients to her. One chiropractor on the north end has expanded his office and needs more patients to meet his expenses. He offers Helena $25 for every patient she refers to him. Typically, Helena provides a list of chiropractors to patients in need of chiropractic services and highlights those who are located conveniently for the patient and who specialize in the area of need. After the chiropractor's offer, Helena begins passing out his card to every patient, regardless of which end of town they live and work in or what their special needs for care are.

Steps Toward an Ethical Practice
CODE OF ETHICS

Hang your code of ethics in your office. This code should be one you strive to abide by—one that reflects your beliefs and professional behavior. Many professional organizations have a code of ethics and a disciplinary body to enforce it. Displaying ethical standards instills confidence in patients that their practitioner cares for them, observes a high standard of behavior, and is accountable for his or her actions.

▼

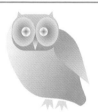

WISE ONE SPEAKS
Code of Ethics

The following is the official code of ethics of the American Massage Therapy Association:

This code of ethics is a summary statement of the standards by which massage therapists agree to conduct their practice and is a declaration of the general principles of acceptable, ethical, professional behavior.

- Demonstrate commitment to provide the highest quality massage therapy/body-work to those who seek professional service.
- Acknowledge the inherent worth and individuality of each person by not discriminating or behaving in any prejudicial manner with patients and/or colleagues.
- Demonstrate professional excellence through regular self-assessment of strengths, limitation, and effectiveness by continued education and training.

(Continued)

WISE ONE SPEAKS   *(Continued)*

- **Acknowledge the confidential nature of the professional relationship with patients and respect each patient's right to privacy.**
- **Conduct all business and professional activities within their scope of practice, the law of the land, and project a professional image.**
- **Accept responsibility to do no harm to the physical, mental, and emotional well-being of the self, patients, and associates.**
- **Refrain from engaging in any sexual conduct or sexual activities involving their patients.**

Reprinted with permission from the American Massage Therapy Association, Evanston, 2000. All rights reserved.

SELF-EVALUATIONS AND PEER EVALUATIONS

Take time to review your business practices and professional relationships. Regular self-evaluations help identify and resolve difficult situations before problems arise. When you open a new business, establish office policies and a fee schedule, list your services and office hours, and provide copies to all patients. Setting clear boundaries and business parameters helps you treat all patients fairly and equally and provides a comfortable working environment for you and your patients. Review your business guidelines monthly and keep them current. Patients become confused and frustrated when they are given policies that no longer apply or are no longer enforced.

As part of your monthly self-evaluation, take 10 minutes to consider a few questions. If your answers to them highlight a problem situation or motivate a call to action, describe the specific situation in writing. Clarify your role in the situation honestly and compassionately. Seek counsel from your peers when necessary. Identify possible actions and consider the consequences. Determine the timeline for the appropriate action, then follow through.[4]

- Did I conduct myself ethically and legally in all my professional affairs?
- Did I maintain the confidentiality of my patients?
- Did I maintain good boundaries with my patients?
- Was I uncomfortable enforcing any office policies? If so, did the situation warrant flexibility, or did fear dictate my decision to bend a policy?
- What are my strengths and limitations? What action can I take to improve?
- What steps have I taken to ensure my well-being?
- Are there any issues on which I should seek counsel from my peers?

Annually, review your fee schedule, office policies, and business practices with a peer or a mentor. Review your billing and accounting practices with a professional. Implement changes when appropriate.

CONSULTATION GROUPS

Consultation groups, also known as peer supervision or co-vision groups, consist of people who have a common interest who meet regularly to share ideas, solve problems, and build a community. Common interests may be as broad as manual therapy or as specific as therapists who treat AIDS patients.

230

HANDS HEAL:
COMMUNICATION,
DOCUMENTATION,
AND INSURANCE BILLING
FOR MANUAL THERAPISTS

Individuals join consultation groups to get support and information, to form professional relationships, and to gain skills. Not only do the people who participate in the consultation groups benefit from the results, but so do their patients, the community, and the profession.

Ethics are difficult to learn out of a book. They must be experienced, experimented with, discussed, and hotly debated. By participating in consultation groups, we can study ethical dilemmas from a variety of perspectives and differing levels of experience, sorting out the possible consequences before our patients can be harmed by our actions. The group members hold one another accountable for telling the truth, express compassion and respect for all involved, and offer advice about difficult or confusing issues.[4]

Follow these guidelines for establishing a consultation group in your area:

◆ Define goals for establishing a group.
◆ Identify parameters, including how many people to involve, how often to meet, length of the meetings, and such.
◆ Create a list of individuals who have similar goals or needs for a group.
◆ Check the list for individuals you respect and from whom you can learn. It is important to include those who share similar opinions but also people who can offer diversity to the group.
◆ Select a date for the first meeting. Explain your vision for the group with those on your list and invite them to join you. If you are lacking in numbers, ask those who are interested in being part of the group to invite others who may also share the same vision.
◆ Get names and phone numbers of those interested, call back to confirm dates and times, and ask for assistance when necessary.

At the first meeting:

◆ Confirm the dates, locations, and times of the meetings. If it is important to the cohesiveness of the group, get a commitment from everyone to attend four consecutive meetings.
◆ Clarify the goals of the group.
◆ Identify the topics to be covered the first few meetings.
◆ Find out whether a mediator, provocateur, or educator is desired for any of the meetings.
◆ Decide whether you want to rotate responsibilities, such as hosting, providing snacks, facilitating the discussion, monitoring the time, and such.
◆ Identify guidelines for group interaction, such as maintaining one another's confidentiality, communicating with respect, and speaking honestly.
◆ Identify guiding principles that suggest ethical behavior without mandating specific rules.

For information on identifying guidelines for such occasions, Margaret Wheatly offers guiding principles in her book, *Leadership and the New Science: Take Care of Yourself, Take Care of Each Other, and Take Care of This Place*.[5] Kylea Taylor, in *The Ethics of Caring*, defines ethical behavior as reverence for life demonstrated by right relationship and offers Buddha's concepts for right relationship: What I do affects you, what you do affects me, and what I do to you ultimately affects me.[6]

◆ At the end of the meeting, evaluate the outcome. Did you meet your goals? Did you have fun? Make adjustments when necessary to ensure the success of future meetings.

STORY TELLER
A Call to Action

Barb works for a natural foods grocery chain that provides seated massage to customers. There are five stores in her town, and each store employs 4 to 5 manual therapists. Barb discovers that providing massage in front of the checkout lines in a grocery store presents problems that she never had to deal with in her private practice, such as maintaining confidentiality. She can tell that her coworkers are also struggling with the same issues, but she knows it is not appropriate to discuss them at work. She decides to call the practitioners from the stores and try to stir up interest in meeting together and helping one another with the problems inherent in the work environment.

Barb finds 10 people interested in meeting. She secures a meeting room at the community center and invites one of her teachers from massage school to facilitate the group discussion. She asks a few people to bring snacks and drinks and someone else to make confirmation calls.

Eight of the 23 massage employees attend the meeting. Barb welcomes everyone and introduces the facilitator. The facilitator leads the group in defining the goals for the meeting and identifying topics for discussion. She suggests some guidelines and creates a safe environment for discussion. The group agrees to communicate respectfully and to use a round-robin format to ensure that everyone has the opportunity to speak. The facilitator explains her purpose at the meeting as being one to provide organization and keep the discussion moving in a positive direction, not one of offering her opinion. She begins with a story.

MENTORING

One-on-one consultation lacks the diverse perspectives available in consultation groups, but allows for more spontaneous interactions, more personal attention, and a safe environment for those who find it difficult to speak openly in groups.

Mentors influence and shape us by sharing who they are, not just what they know. The study of ethics is about learning how to live and grow and contribute as a human being, as well as a professional. Select a mentor who is not afraid of sharing his or her mistakes, as well as personal and professional successes. A role model is not a perfect human being, but rather someone who is very much like yourself. Marsha Sinetar, in *The Mentor's Spirit,* says, "Show me your mentor and I'll show you yourself."[7]

Select a mentor who:

◆ Is available weekly by phone
◆ Is available monthly in person
◆ Has more professional experience than you
◆ Is committed to your growth
◆ Has qualities important to you, such as compassion, wisdom, and an ability to confront

232

HANDS HEAL:
COMMUNICATION,
DOCUMENTATION,
AND INSURANCE BILLING
FOR MANUAL THERAPISTS

SUMMARY

Create an ethical business. Review and revise your business practices regularly.

◆ Set standards for identifying when treatment is complete and wellness care begins, then bill appropriately.

◆ Charge reasonable and consistent fees for services.

◆ Provide appropriate treatment and bill for the services provided.

◆ In your charts, do not misrepresent the patient's health or the treatment performed.

◆ Chart patient sessions in a timely fashion.

◆ Represent your services accurately. Discuss treatment outcomes honestly and realistically.

◆ Provide services within your scope of practice. Refer out for services that are outside your scope.

◆ Discuss disagreements about the treatment plan or patient care directly with the referring HCP, never with the patient.

◆ Support the patient in addressing conflicts with other providers directly.

◆ Request permission from the patient to discuss the case with other members of the health care team.

◆ Limit all conversations with the health care team to information pertinent to the patient's condition.

◆ Be an active student of ethics.

◆ Develop your ethical beliefs through discussion with peers and mentors.

◆ Consult your peers and mentors when problems arise in your professional relationships.

◆ Mentor others.

▼

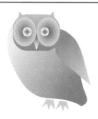

WISE ONE SPEAKS
Discover What Lies Within

I leave you with the following as an inspiration to be in relationship: It is during interactions with others that we discover what lies within us. That is the gift of our profession—the gift we offer our patients through our listening and the gift we give ourselves through mentoring.

"We usually look outside ourselves for heroes and teachers. It has not occurred to most people that they may already be the role model they seek. The wholeness they are looking for may be trapped within themselves by beliefs, attitudes, and self-doubt. But our wholeness exists in us now. Trapped though it may be, it can be called upon for guidance, direction, and most fundamentally, comfort. It can be remembered. Eventually we may come to live by it."

Reprinted with permission from Remen RN. Kitchen Table Wisdom: Stories That Heal. New York: Riverhead Books, 1996.

1. Madison-Mahoney V. Setting your fees: Important factors to consider. Washington Massage Journal Sept/Oct 2003:10–11.

2. Peick JC. Are You Committing Billing Fraud and Didn't Know It? Washington Massage Journal Jan/Feb 2005:35.

3. Miale-Gix B. Legal memo: Setting the record straight on HIPAA. What is and is not required in a medical authorization. The Advocate July 2003:1–2.

4. Sohnen-Moe CM. Business Mastery: A Guide for Creating a Fulfilling, Thriving Business and Keeping It Successful. 3rd Ed. Tucson: Sohnen-Moe Associates, Inc., 1997.

5. Wheatley MJ. Leadership and the New Science: Learning about Organization from an Orderly Universe. San Francisco: Berrett-Koehler Publishers, Inc., 1994.

6. Taylor K. The Ethics of Caring: Honoring the Web of Life in Our Professional Healing Relationships. 2nd Ed. Santa Cruz: Hanford Mead Publishers, 1995.

7. Sinetar M. The Mentor's Spirit: Life Lessons on Leadership and the Art of Encouragement. New York: St. Martin's Griffin, 1999.

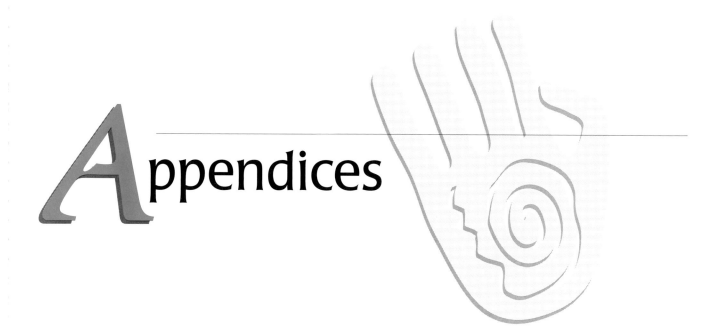

Appendices

APPENDICES OUTLINE

Glossary

active listening communication tool that demonstrates to the speaker that he or she is being understood and respected; nonverbal attendance to the speakers' tone, body language, facial expressions, and the like

Advanced Billing Concepts (ABC) codes comprehensive coding system that supports research, management, and commerce in the fields of alternative medicine, nursing, and other forms of integrative health care

affinity plan, affinity network contractual agreement between the provider and the network or carrier to provide a substantial discount directly to the members of the plan

analog scale method of measurement that uses a continuum and places one extreme on one end and the opposite extreme on the other end

Any Willing Provider (AWP) statute that allows any provider willing to provide services to be accepted by the health carrier. The AWP law is currently in effect in Arkansas, Georgia, Idaho, Indiana, Illinois, Kentucky, Minnesota, Virginia, and Wyoming.

appeal legal request for a higher court or reviewing body to review a decision made by a lower court or reviewing body regarding issues of law or policy, including denial of a claim

at-fault party individual who causes harm to another individual or damages property

Attorney Lien written agreement between patient and health care provider guaranteeing payment in full to the patient's health care providers upon settlement of a personal injury case; also known as *Guarantee of Payment*

audit a formal and often periodic examination of accounts, financial records, or claims to verify correctness of documentation

body language the nonverbal behavior of a person, including facial expressions, postures, gestures, and other actions; a primary means of emotional expression

bundling type of reimbursement arrangement that combines two or more health care procedures under one procedure code and establishes a flat fee to pay for all health care services performed under the single code; see *global fee*

capitation individual monthly payment made in advance to a managed care insurer for contracted services. The insurance provider agrees to provide specified services to eligible members at a fixed, predetermined payment during a specified period of time, regardless of how many times the member uses the services.

capped fee predetermined discounted fee allowed for a particular procedure

Centers for Medicare and Medicaid Services (CMS) a federal agency within the U.S. Department of Health and Human Services (HHS) responsible for programs such as Medicare, Medicaid, State Children's Health Insurance Program, HIPAA, and Clinical Laboratory Improvement Amendments; formerly, the Health Care Financing Administration (HCFA), which became CMS in 2001

238

HANDS HEAL:
COMMUNICATION,
DOCUMENTATION,
AND INSURANCE BILLING
FOR MANUAL THERAPISTS

clean claim insurance claim bill submitted with complete and accurate information for services that are covered for the patient and that the practitioner is authorized to provide

co-insurance provision that the insured and the carrier share losses in agreed proportion; also known as *percentage participation*. In managed care, it refers to the portion of the cost of care for which the individual is responsible, usually determined by a fixed percentage. This often applies after a deductible is met.

complementary and alternative medicine (CAM), complementary and alternative health care (CAHC) medical and clinical services that typically are not taught at conventional medical institutions (also includes practitioners whose services are not typically covered by traditional insurance programs)

complimenting communication tool used to reinforce behavior, such as a positive reaction or evaluation by the practitioner in response to the patient or a question that indirectly implies something positive about the patient

co-pay patient's share of a health care bill, usually a small amount per office visit

Correct Coding Initiatives (CCI) pairs of CPT codes that cannot be used together in the same claim and is an attempt to control costs by preventing providers from unbundling services from one treatment session for reimbursement purposes

covered entities health care providers, health plans, or clearinghouses through which health information is transmitted electronically in connection with a HIPAA transaction

Current Procedural Terminology (CPT) codes descriptive terms and identifying codes for reporting health care services and procedures performed by health care providers

deductible part of the insured's expenses or loss that must be paid before the insurer begins to pay on a claim

deposition discovery procedure whereby the attorney calling for the deposition asks questions of witnesses and experts while the individuals are under oath

disability percentage overall rating of a physical handicap as determined by scoring the revised Oswestry Low Back Pain and Disability Index or the Vernon-Mior Neck Pain and Disability Index

discharge SOAP notes final summary of the patient's progress, health status, and subsequent course of action to be taken

disclosure release, transfer, provision of, access to, or divulgence of information by an entity to persons or organizations outside that entity

discounted fee reimbursement arrangement in which an insurance carrier contracts with a provider for health care services at a predetermined and often considerably lower fee

door openers communication tool used as an invitation to talk; open-ended questions

electronic transactions, covered transactions electronic exchanges of information between two covered entities using HIPAA-defined electronic data interchange transaction standards

end-of-settlement personal injury case in which the provider of health services must wait until the claim against the at-fault party is settled or a judge or jury issues a verdict before receiving payment for services

Every Category of Provider (ECP) nondiscrimination statute that requires health insurance carriers to allow different provider categories to compete to provide services within their scope to perform and allows every insured access to the category of provider of his or her choice. The ECP law is currently only in effect in the state of Washington.

Explanation of Benefits (EOB) report from an insurance company to the patient and provider explaining the benefits paid, reduced, or denied

fee schedules maximum allowable charges; amounts set by the insurer as the highest amounts to be charged for particular services

fee-for-service plans traditional payment method in the U.S. health care industry in which patients pay doctors, hospitals, and other providers for services rendered at the time of service (and are charged according to a fee schedule set for each service or procedure provided). Typically, the patient seeks reimbursement for those costs from a private insurer or government program, such as Medicare.

following skills communication tools, usually open-ended questions, used to discover how a patient views a situation, including how he or she feels about something in life, how he or she views an event, and who or what the patient feels is important

functional goals short-term and long-term goals for health based on daily activities that the patient is having difficulty performing

functional outcomes goals for which a client's progress toward improved health creates an increased ability to participate in daily activities

functional outcomes reporting style of charting that addresses (1) client's ability to function in everyday activities, (2) goal setting, and (3) treatment design to improve function and motivate increased client participation

Functional Rating Index (FRI) a self-reporting instrument consisting of 10 items, each with five possible responses that express graduating degrees of disability. The Functional Rating Index combines the concepts of the Oswestry Low Back Disability Questionnaire and the Vernon-Mior Neck Disability Index and seeks to improve on clinical utility, such as the time required for administration.

global fee type of reimbursement arrangement that combines two or more health care procedures under one procedure code and establishes a flat fee to pay for all health care services performed under the single code; see *bundling*

good faith provisions requirements that insurers address matters with their insured members to satisfy the obligations of a contract, regulation, or law

HCFA 1500 form standard billing form approved by federal health and financing agencies

Health Care Financing Administration (HCFA) formerly the U.S. Department of Health and Human Services that administers federal health financing and related regulatory programs, principally Medicare, Medicaid, and Peer Review Organization programs, now known as the Centers for Medicare and Medicaid Services (CMS)

health care lien health care provider's legal claim or lien on the patient's personal injury claim intended to guarantee that the provider's bills will be paid once the case is settled

Health Insurance Portability and Accountability Act (HIPAA) legislation that provides rights, protections, and assurances of portability and continuity of health coverage to participants in group health plans

Health Insurance Portability and Accountability Act (HIPAA) Administrative Simplification Title II, Subtitle F that gives the U.S. Department of Health and Human Services the authority to mandate the use of standards for the electronic exchange of health care data; to specify what medical and administrative code sets should be used within those standards; to require the use of national identification systems for health care patients, providers, payers (or plans), and employers (or sponsors); and to specify the types of measures required to protect the security and privacy of personally identifiable health care information

Health Maintenance Organizations (HMOs) legal entities that provide health care in a geographic area and accepts responsibility for providing (directly or by contract) an agreed-upon set of health services to a defined, voluntarily enrolled group of individuals. HMOs are reimbursed through a pre-determined, fixed, periodic prepayment made by or on behalf of each subscriber without regard to the amount of actual services provided. In many states, HMOs are synonymous with managed care.

hold harmless clause legal concept commonly used among insurance carriers and in managed care contracts whereby the HMO and its providers do not hold one another liable for malpractice or corporate malfeasance if the other is found liable in a dispute. State laws require such a clause for the purpose of prohibiting health care providers from billing patients if the managed care company becomes insolvent.

ICD-9 codes acronym for International Classification of Diseases, Ninth Revision; a statistical classification system that arranges diseases and injuries into groups according to established criteria (revised approximately every 10 years by the World Health Organization and published annually by the Health Care Financing Administration)

incidental use and disclosure permissible use or disclosure of protected health information (PHI), such as announcing a name in a waiting room or having a sign-in sheet at the front desk. Sign-in sheets may not contain any PHI other than the patient's name.

240

HANDS HEAL:
COMMUNICATION,
DOCUMENTATION,
AND INSURANCE BILLING
FOR MANUAL THERAPISTS

indemnity plans insurance plans that provide benefits paid to the insured at a predetermined amount in the event of a covered loss (automobile insurance policies are based on indemnity principles)

Independent Practice Arrangement (IPA) HMO contract with a physician organization that, in turn, contracts with individual physicians to provide health services to its members. IPA physicians practice in their own offices and see fee-for-service patients. The IPA is reimbursed on a capitated basis and may reimburse its physicians on a capitated or modified fee-for-service basis when physicians charge agreed-upon rates to the HMO patients, then bill the IPA.

initial reports summaries following the first visit (written in letter format) of the findings and plan for treatment

initial SOAP notes comprehensive notes recording the patient's first visit with a practitioner for a particular condition, including exam, findings, treatment, and treatment plan regarding the patient's health and current situation

insurance companies for-profit businesses primarily engaged in selling indemnification policies to individuals or groups to cover a defined set of benefits in the event of a loss

insurance medical exam (IME), independent medical exam examination of a patient, his or her health care records, or both; often used in personal injury cases to determine reasonable and necessary care and to support the insurer's decision to deny, limit, or terminate an insured's health benefits

insurance network company that contracts with two or more independent group practices or solo practices to provide health services to various insurance carriers' members

insurance plan, insurance policy specific benefit package offered by an insurer

insured, member party to an insurance agreement to whom, or on behalf of whom, the insurance company agrees to indemnify for losses, provide insurance benefits, or render service (preferred to *policyholder*). In pre-paid hospital service plans, the insured is called the *subscriber*.

liability coverage insurance plan that pays for and renders service on behalf of an insured for loss resulting from the insured's negligence toward others as imposed by law or assumed by contract

lives number of insureds in a given area

major medical type of health insurance that provides benefits for most types of medical expenses incurred up to a high limit and expenses that occur in and out of the hospital—often subject to a large deductible

managed care philosophy of health care coverage that streamlines health services and creates a health care system that includes both the financing and delivery of services to the consumer. It also assumes greater responsibility for maintaining subscribers' health beyond just curing them once they are sick. Managed care lowers costs by matching the patient with appropriate care as efficiently as possible. Different insurance carriers use different kinds of managed care and often are differentiated by their reimbursement methods.

manual therapists health care providers, such as massage therapists, chiropractors, physical therapists, and somatic educators who primarily rely on a manual means of providing health care services

maximum benefit limit of benefits paid to the injured party

Medicaid state program that provides public assistance to persons, regardless of age, whose incomes and resources are insufficient to pay for health care

medical necessity, medically necessary terms referring to health care services that, in order to be covered by insurance, are performed in order to preserve the health status of a patient in accordance with the area's standards of medical practice

Medical Payments (Med-Pay) coverage insurance provision that allows benefits to be paid for medical expenses

Medicare federal hospital insurance system and supplementary medical insurance coverage for the aged; created in 1965 by an amendment to the Social Security Act

morning pages practice of writing three pages each morning of "whatever comes to mind"

narrative reports summaries written in letter form of a patient's injuries, treatment, and progress throughout the entire course of treatment

National Correct Coding Initiatives (NCCI) pairs of CPT codes that cannot be used together in the same claim and is an attempt to control costs by preventing providers from unbundling services from one treatment session for reimbursement purposes

network adequacy basis upon which a carrier determines the number of providers necessary to provide services to the lives. The formula used considers a combination of the number of lives within a geographic location and time and distance traveled to the provider. Requirements are determined by the insurer and available to the Department of Insurance.

no-fault insurance benefits provided regardless of responsibility or liability of party

Notice of Privacy Practices (NPP) legal document stating the actions and policies a given practice will provide to protect its patients' rights (developed by the individual health care practice and its legal counsel)

Office for Civil Rights (OCR) enforcement agency for the HIPAA Privacy Rule

peer review mechanism to control health care utilization and quality of care; an internal peer review process used to evaluate the quality of care provided and to assess medical necessity

personal injury bodily injury resulting from the negligence of another person

Personal Injury Protection (PIP) coverage insurance provision that allows benefits to be paid for medical and hospital costs, loss of wages and services, and funeral expenses

Physician's Desk Reference (PDR) resource manual of drugs and medications, including information on generic terms, doses, and side effects

pre-existing conditions injuries, illnesses, or symptoms that existed prior to the onset of the current injury or condition

Preferred Provider Organizations (PPOs) companies that offer a health care arrangement between purchasers of health care, such as employers and insurance companies, and providers, to manage benefits and provide them at a reasonable cost and with incentives, such as lower deductibles and co-pays, to motivate members to use providers within a selected network. Use of out-of-network, or nonpreferred, providers involves higher costs. Preferred providers must agree to specified fee schedules and are required to comply with certain utilization and review guidelines.

preferred provider status contracted, licensed, health care providers who provide specified health care services for a predetermined fee

prescriptions formal referrals for adjunctive services. Prescriptions infer medical necessity, provide patient information (such as diagnosis and ICD-9 codes), and define treatment parameters.

primary care first care a patient receives, either from a family physician, nurse, paramedic, or other health care provider, depending on the situation (often the level at which managed care systems try to resolve health problems)

primary care status health care providers who are authorized to manage a patient's care, as determined by individual health care programs; status is often limited to physicians, but may include naturopaths and nurses

primary insurer patient's main source of insurance coverage; the company primarily responsible for providing benefits

Privacy Rule HIPAA Administrative Simplification section mandating that information identifying a patient is to be protected and that the transmission of protected information is to be kept secure. The Privacy Rule includes safeguard measures to control the unauthorized disclosure of, access to, and use of protected health information (PHI) and grants patients six rights, including the right to gain access to and have more control over the use and disclosure of their PHI. The rule also requires personnel in medical practices to respect those rights.

private health insurance insurance coverage against loss resulting from sickness or bodily injury

problem-oriented medical record (POMR) documentation system, introduced by Dr. Lawrence Weed in the 1960s, that lists the patient's problems at the front of the chart and allows the practitioner to write a SOAP note to address each problem

progress reports summaries of patient progress and suggested additions or changes to the treatment plan submitted in letter format to the referring HCP every 30 days

242

HANDS HEAL:
COMMUNICATION,
DOCUMENTATION,
AND INSURANCE BILLING
FOR MANUAL THERAPISTS

progress SOAP notes comprehensive notes for recording reevaluation and reexamination sessions

protected health information (PHI) information that can be used to identify an individual because it contains the patient's name, social security number, telephone number, zip code, e-mail address, or other identifiers. The HIPAA Privacy Rule states that PHI must be protected whether it exists in written, spoken, or electronic form. Health information that has been stripped of patient identifiers is not considered PHI.

proximate cause initial act that sets off a sequence of events that produces injury, which, in the absence of the initial act, would not have resulted

quality improvement program internal peer review process used to audit the quality of care provided and often includes an educational mechanism to identify and prevent discrepancies in care

range of motion (ROM) a movement test to access the available motion allowed by the shape of the joint and the soft tissue surrounding it.

reasonable and necessary a standard insurance and legal term found in automobile and health care insurance policies governing the basis for paying or denying treatment claim expenses

rebating practice of accepting payment for referrals or referring to clinics

referring health care providers (HCPs) health care providers who prescribe adjunctive care; often the primary care provider or provider with diagnostic scope authorized to manage the patients' health care

reflecting communication tool using parroting, paraphrasing, or summarizing the information and feelings the patient has expressed verbally or nonverbally

Relative Value Unit (RVU) unit calculated and proposed by the AMA and refined and approved by the HCFA using RBRVS methodology

Resource-Based Relative Value Scale (RBRVS) process methodology developed at Harvard University to assess physician work, overhead cost, and malpractice risk for individual CPT codes

Revised Oswestry Low Back Pain and Disability Index type of pain questionnaire used to evaluate injuries to the low back and lower extremities

scope of practice law defining the standards of competence, practice areas, and conduct of a health care provider

secondary insurer insurance that becomes active after primary coverage is exhausted or expires

self-care the patient's active participation in the healing process. Includes remedial exercise, hydro-therapy, self-message, diaphragmatic breathing, and referrals to other practitioners, self-help groups, or exercise programs.

self-insured, self-insurance practice of an employer or organization to assume the responsibility for health care losses of its employees. Usually, a fund is established and claims payments are drawn against it. Claims processing is often handled through an administrative services contract with an independent organization, usually an insurer.

silence communication tool that allows a patient to sort out thoughts, take a short breather from the work at hand, or search deeper for answers to the practitioner's questions

SMART goals acronym for Specific, Measurable, Attainable, Relevant, Time-Bound; a system for creating well-defined functional goals

SOAP charting acronym for Subjective, Objective, Assessment, and Plan; a process for providing a standard health care format for charting and documenting treatment sessions. Information is organized into four categories: S = data provided by the client, O = practitioner findings, A = functional outcomes and diagnoses, and P = treatment recommendations.

statute of limitations, statutory time limits provisions within laws that govern the time frame within which a lawsuit must be brought (otherwise the claim will be barred or dismissed); statutes of limitations differ from state to state and according to the nature of the claim

stipulation request for medical records containing the patient's and patient's attorney's consent to authorize release

subpoena court-ordered, written command requiring a person to appear at a specific time and place to give testimony on a specific matter. A *subpoena duces tecum* is a written command requiring a witness to produce documents in his or her possession or control that are pertinent to the issues.

subrogation a legal principle that generally means that a patient cannot have the same bill paid twice.

subsequent SOAP notes brief notes addressing the patient's immediate concerns for the day's session

Team Therapy Model paradigm for approaching the interview and information-gathering process; a combination of a medical model and intervention-free model of solution building

third-party coverage liability insurance coverage of the at-fault party or the uninsured/underinsured coverage of the patient

treatment plan formal description of how a patient will be treated; a list of functional goals and treatment goals, including the techniques, modalities, and specific ways that treatment will be applied, as well as the frequency and duration of treatment sessions and homework and self-care education

unclean claims insurance claim bills that lack information or contain disputable information

uninsured motorist component of automobile insurance coverage that protects an insured driver from losses that should be the responsibility of the other driver who is not carrying liability insurance to cover losses

upcoding fraudulent practice of increasing the value of a procedure code from lower to higher that results in a large reimbursement amount

U.S. Department of Health and Human Services (HHS) the regulatory agency that implements HIPAA

use and disclosure refers to the sharing of protected health information inside a medical office (use) and the releasing, transferring, or accessing of protected information outside the medical office (disclosure)

usual, customary, and regular (UCR) refers to fees that health insurance plans will pay to a health care provider when deemed reasonable and do not exceed usual amounts customarily charged by local health care providers and others; also called *usual and customary*

utilization patterns of use of a service or type of service within a specified time. Usually expressed in rate per unit or population-at-risk for a given period. Utilization experience multiplied by the average cost per unit or service delivered equals capitated costs.

utilization management program a systematic process to review and control patients' use of medical services and quality of care through data collection, review, or authorization, especially for services involving specialists and use of an emergency department or hospital

Vernon-Mior Neck Pain and Disability Index type of pain questionnaire used to evaluate injuries to the neck and upper extremities

Wellness charting charting method for recording treatments and tracking results to create individualized, effective treatment plans

workers' compensation insurance coverage that includes medical and disability benefits for illnesses, injuries, disabilities, and death resulting from job-related conditions and activities (employers are mandated by law to purchase for all employees)

Blank Forms

246

HANDS HEAL:
COMMUNICATION,
DOCUMENTATION,
AND INSURANCE BILLING
FOR MANUAL THERAPISTS

Description of Forms

1. Health Information: Every patient with a health concern completes this two-page form annually, more frequently if the patient's health condition changes rapidly. Healthy patients seeking wellness care may fill out the health information section of the Wellness chart in lieu of this form. When charting sports massage at events, the questions can be asked orally, and only positive answers need recording.

This information is useful for designing a safe and effective treatment plan (and provides contact information).

Attach your logo, name, and contact information to the top of page 1. Include your provider number if applicable. Photocopy the two-page form front to back. File completed forms in the patient's chart.

2. Injury Information: Every workers' compensation and personal injury patient completes page 1 of this form. Every patient whose injury is the result of a motor vehicle accident completes page 2 of this form. Complete a new form for each incident. This information is useful for designing a safe and effective treatment plan and for providing proof of significant injury.

Attach your logo, name, and contact information to the top of page 1. Include your provider number if applicable. Photocopy this form front to back. Mark a line through page 2 if it does not apply. File completed forms in the patient's chart.

3. Billing Information: If you offer billing services, each patient who requests direct billing to his or her insurance company fills out this form. The patient should complete a new form for each incident because billing information can change based on the type of health condition or situation. This information is useful for completing the Insurance Verification form.

Attach your logo, name, and contact information to the top of the page. Include your provider number if applicable. Photocopy this form front to back. File completed forms in the patient's chart.

4. Prescription: Send a pad of these forms with your logo, name, and contact information at the top to every potential referring health care provider. HCPs do not have to use your form. If the form they use does not provide the pertinent information, gather the necessary information and attach it to the prescription provided.

Update as needed. If the patient's insurance is paying for care, every session must be medically necessary and accounted for on the prescriptions. File in the patient's chart.

5. Health Report: The patient reports on his or her current condition. This form has multiple uses:

◆ The patient completes the form before the session every 30 days as a subjective record of ongoing progress.

◆ The patient completes the form before and after the session every 30 days as a subjective record of immediate treatment results and ongoing progress. This requires a two-sided form: Side one is completed before the session; side two is completed after the session.

◆ The health report can be used as a substitute for a Wellness chart. The patient completes side one before the session and side two after the session, as above. The manual therapist records the findings, treatment, and plan in the comments section.

Attach your logo, name, and contact information to the top of the page. Include your provider number if applicable. Photocopy front to back, when applicable. This form is available in female, male, and non–gender-specific versions to use at your discretion. File completed forms in the patient's chart.

248

HANDS HEAL:
COMMUNICATION,
DOCUMENTATION,
AND INSURANCE BILLING
FOR MANUAL THERAPISTS

6. **Pain Questionnaires**: Every patient with a complaint of pain resulting in a loss of function completes the applicable form. The Neck Pain Index can be used for the neck as well as any upper extremity pain; the Low Back Pain Index can also be used for any lower extremity pain. The Functional Rating Index can be used for any condition. Update the form every 30 days, or until the patient's functional status stabilizes. If the form is used in lieu of a pain diary, the patient completes the form daily or weekly, as recommended by the attorney or HCP.

Attach your logo, name, and contact information to the top of the page. Include your provider number if applicable. The form stands alone, but may be piggybacked with the health report and photocopied front to back, when applicable. File completed forms in the patient's chart.

7. **Initial Report Without Treatment**: This is the only acceptable fill-in-the-blank report completed by the practitioner. All other reports should be typed and written in paragraph form. Use this form when you receive a referral or prescription but the patient does not receive a treatment from you.

8. **Soap Charts**: A SOAP note should be written for each curative treatment session. There are two types of SOAP charts used for recording SOAP notes:

◆ Long Version: Use the full-page SOAP chart for initial notes, progress notes, discharge notes, or at any time additional space is required.

◆ Short Version: Use the half-page SOAP chart for subsequent notes or for health conditions that do not require extensive space for recording information.

Attach your logo, name, and contact information to the top of each page. Include your provider number if applicable. Photocopy the long version as page 1 and the short version as page 2. Also photocopy the short version back to back. This chart is available in female, male, and non–gender-specific versions to use at your discretion. File completed forms in the patient's chart.

9. **Wellness Charts**: A Wellness note should be written for each wellness session. Three types of Wellness charts are provided, any of which can be modified to enhance specific charting needs.

◆ Standard Wellness: This is useful for table work, as the human figures are in a standing position.

◆ Seated Wellness: This is useful for on-site sessions, as the figures are in a seated position.

◆ Sports Chart: This is useful for sporting events. The intake questions are designed for the treatment of athletes before and after competition. Treatments are general and rarely require additional notation.

Attach your logo, name, and contact information to the top of each page. Include your provider number if applicable. The Standard and Seated Wellness charts have a page 2 for ongoing care. Photocopy page 1 and page 2 back-to-back. Page 2 can also be photocopied back-to-back, as the intake form only needs to be completed annually or biannually. The Sports Chart only has one page and can be photocopied back-to-back.

Patients receiving ongoing care should have individual files. File charts for events by event and date, rather than by patient's name.

10. **Range of Motion**: Use this for ease in charting range of motion tests. Space is provided for pre-treatment and post-treatment assessment, for up to three joint assessments. You may use one form for up to three sessions when you are only assessing the motion of one joint by writing the treatment date next to each test. If you photocopy back-to-back, one piece of paper can be used for up to six treatment sessions. File completed forms in the patient's chart.

Attach your logo, name, and contact information to the top of the page. Include your provider number if applicable. File completed forms in the patient's chart.

11. Release of Health Care Information: Before sending any personal health care information outside the office, have the patient sign one of these. The release from the attorney expires in 90 days, and the HIPAA release form expires after 6 months, so update them as needed. File completed forms in the patient's chart.

12. Insurance Status—Personal Injury: If the patient has retained an attorney as counsel in a personal injury case, the attorney completes this form. Send this form with a letter of introduction, a request for information, and a self-addressed, stamped envelope. Complete a new form for each incident. This information is useful for completing the Insurance Verification form.

Attach your logo, name, and contact information to the top of the page. Include your provider number if applicable. This form stands alone. File in the patient's chart.

13. Guarantee of Payment: If the patient has retained an attorney as counsel in a personal injury case and there is no PIP, Med-Pay, or UIM coverage or the policy limit has been reached, have the patient and his or her attorney sign and date this form. File in the patient's chart.

14. Insurance Verification: Complete this form using the information provided on the Billing Information form or Insurance Status—Personal Injury form. Gather the remaining information from an insurance representative. Verify coverage and authorization of services. Before providing additional services, complete the Reauthorization/Verification section. For multiple reauthorizations, use the Reauthorization/Verification form. Track the prescriptions on the same form to ensure all treatments provided are covered by a prescription.

Complete a new form with each incident. This form is useful for reducing the risk involved in billing the patient's insurance company.

Attach your logo, name, and contact information to the top of page one. Include your provider number if applicable. Photocopy front-to-back. File in the patient's chart.

15. Payment Log: Complete this form each time the payment does not match the amount billed. Attach to the corresponding HCFA 1500 form. File in billing binder earmarked for rebilling. Follow through with phone calls and resending bills every 30 days until payment matches the amount billed.

HEALTH INFORMATION

Patient Name _____ Date _____

Date of Injury _____ ID#/DOB _____

A. Patient Information

Address _____

City _____ State ____ Zip _____

Phone: Home _____

    Work _____ Cell _____

Employer _____

Work Address _____

Occupation _____

Emergency Contact _____

Phone: Home _____

    Work _____ Cell _____

Primary Health Care Provider

Name _____

Address _____

City/State/Zip_____

Phone: _____ Fax _____

I give my massage therapist permission to
consult with my health care providers
regarding my health and treatment.

Comments _____

Initials _____ Date _____

B. Current Health Information

List Health Concerns Check all that apply

Primary _____
☐ mild ☐ moderate ☐ disabling
☐ constant ☐ intermittant
☐ symptoms ↑ w/activity   ☐ ↓ w/activity
☐ getting worse ☐ getting better ☐ no change
treatment received _____

Secondary _____
☐ mild ☐ moderate ☐ disabling
☐ constant ☐ intermittant
☐ symptoms ↑ w/activity   ☐ ↓ w/activity
☐ getting worse ☐ getting better ☐ no change
treatment received _____

Additional _____
☐ mild ☐ moderate ☐ disabling
☐ constant ☐ intermittant
☐ symptoms ↑ w/activity   ☐ ↓ w/activity
☐ getting worse ☐ getting better ☐ no change
treatment received _____

List Daily Activities Limited by Condition

Work _____
_____

Home/Family _____
_____

Sleep/Self-care _____

Social/Recreational _____

List Self-Care Routines

How do you reduce stress? _____
_____

Pain? _____
_____

List current medications (include pain relievers
and herbal remedies) _____
_____
_____
_____

Have you ever received massage therapy
before? _____ Frequency? _____

What are your goals for receiving massage
therapy?_____
_____
_____

C. Health History

List and Explain. Include dates and treatment
received.

Surgeries _____
_____
_____

Injuries _____
_____

Major Illnesses _____
_____
_____

250

Check All Current and Previous Conditions Please Explain

General

current   past   comments
- ☐ ☐ headaches _____
- ☐ ☐ pain _____
- ☐ ☐ sleep disturbances

  _____
- ☐ ☐ fatigue _____
- ☐ ☐ infections _____
- ☐ ☐ fever _____
- ☐ ☐ sinus _____
- ☐ ☐ other _____

Skin Conditions

current   past   comments
- ☐ ☐ rashes _____
- ☐ ☐ athlete's foot, warts _____
- ☐ ☐ other _____

Muscles and Joints

current   past   comments
- ☐ ☐ rheumatoid arthritis

  _____
- ☐ ☐ osteoarthritis _____

  _____
- ☐ ☐ osteoporosis _____
- ☐ ☐ scoliosis _____
- ☐ ☐ broken bones _____
- ☐ ☐ spinal problems_____

  _____
- ☐ ☐ disk problems _____
- ☐ ☐ lupus _____
- ☐ ☐ TMJ, jaw pain _____
- ☐ ☐ spasms, cramps

  _____
- ☐ ☐ sprains, strains

  _____
- ☐ ☐ tendonitis, bursitis

  _____
- ☐ ☐ stiff or painful joints _____
- ☐ ☐ weak or sore muscles

  _____
- ☐ ☐ neck, shoulder, arm pain

  _____
- ☐ ☐ low back, hip, leg pain

  _____
- ☐ ☐ other _____

Nervous System

current   past   comments
- ☐ ☐ head injuries, concussions

  _____
- ☐ ☐ dizziness, ringing in ears

- ☐ ☐ loss of memory, confusion

  _____
- ☐ ☐ numbness, tingling

  _____
- ☐ ☐ sciatica, shooting pain

  _____
- ☐ ☐ chronic pain _____
- ☐ ☐ depression _____
- ☐ ☐ other _____

Respiratory, Cardiovascular

current   past   comments
- ☐ ☐ heart disease_____

  _____
- ☐ ☐ blood clots _____
- ☐ ☐ stroke _____
- ☐ ☐ lymphadema _____
- ☐ ☐ high, low blood pressure

  _____
- ☐ ☐ irregular heart beat

  _____
- ☐ ☐ poor circulation_____
- ☐ ☐ swollen ankles_____
- ☐ ☐ varicose veins _____
- ☐ ☐ chest pain, shortness of
      breath _____
- ☐ ☐ asthma _____

Allergies

current   past   comments
- ☐ ☐ scents, oils, lotions _____
- ☐ ☐ detergents _____
- ☐ ☐ other _____

Digestive/Elimination System

current   past   comments
- ☐ ☐ bowel problems _____

  _____
- ☐ ☐ gas, bloating _____
- ☐ ☐ bladder/kidney/prostrate

- ☐ ☐ abdominal pain _____
- ☐ ☐ other _____

Endocrine System

current   past   comments
- ☐ ☐ thyroid _____
- ☐ ☐ diabetes _____

Reproductive System

current   past   comments
- ☐ ☐ pregnancy_____

  _____
- ☐ ☐ painful, emotional menses

- ☐ ☐ fibrotic cysts_____

Cancer/Tumors

current   past   comments
- ☐ ☐ benign_____
- ☐ ☐ malignant _____

Habits

current   past   comments
- ☐ ☐ tobacco _____
- ☐ ☐ alcohol _____
- ☐ ☐ drugs _____
- ☐ ☐ coffee, soda _____

Contract for Care

I promise to participate fully as a member of my health care team. I will make sound choices regarding my treatment plan based on the information provided by my manual therapist and other members of my health care team, and my experience of those suggestions. I agree to participate in the self care program we select. I promise to inform my practitioner any time I feel my well-being is threatened or compromised. I expect my manual therapist to provide safe and effective treatment.

Consent for Care

It is my choice to receive manual therapy, and I give my consent to receive treatment. I have reported all health conditions that I am aware of and will inform my practitioner of any changes in my health.

Signature _____   Date _____

Manual Therapist

WELLNESS CHART-F

Name _____ ID#/DOB _____ Date _____

Phone _____ Address _____

1. What are your goals for health, and how may I assist you in achieving your goals? _____
   _____

2. List typical daily activities—work, exercise, home. _____
   _____

3. Are you currently experiencing any of the following? If yes, please explain.

   pain, tenderness   ☐ No ☐ Yes: _____   stiffness ☐ No ☐ Yes: _____
   numbness or tingling   ☐ No ☐ Yes: _____   swelling   ☐ No ☐ Yes: _____
   allergies   ☐ No ☐ Yes: _____

4. List all illnesses, injuries, and health concerns you have now or have had in the past 3 years.
   (Examples: arthritis, diabetes, car crash, pregnancy) _____
   _____

5. List medications and pain relievers taken this week. _____

6. I have provided all my known medical information. I acknowledge that massage therapy is
   not a substitute for medical diagnosis and treatment. I give my consent to receive treatment.

   Signature _____ Date _____

   Tx: _____
   _____

   C: _____

Legend:

ℭ TP	• TeP	○ ℗	✳ Infl	≡ HT	≈ SP	initials _____
✕ Adh	≋ Numb	◯ rot	╱ elev	⊱⊰ Short	⟷ Long	

252

Copyright © 2005 Lippincott Williams & Wilkins

WELLNESS CHART-M

Name _____ ID#/DOB _____ Date _____

Phone _____ Address _____

1. What are your goals for health, and how may I assist you in achieving your goals? _____
   _____

2. List typical daily activities—work, exercise, home. _____
   _____

3. Are you currently experiencing any of the following? If yes, please explain.

pain, tenderness	☐ No ☐ Yes: _____	stiffness ☐ No ☐ Yes: _____
numbness or tingling	☐ No ☐ Yes: _____	swelling ☐ No ☐ Yes: _____
allergies	☐ No ☐ Yes: _____	

4. List all illnesses, injuries, and health concerns you have now or have had in the past 3 years.
   (Examples: arthritis, diabetes, car crash) _____
   _____

5. List medications and pain relievers taken this week. _____

6. I have provided all my known medical information. I acknowledge that massage therapy is
   not a substitute for medical diagnosis and treatment. I give my consent to receive treatment.

   Signature _____ Date _____

   Tx: _____
   _____

   C: _____

Legend:

℮ TP	• TeP	○ ⓟ	⁕ Infl	≡ HT	≈ SP	initials _____
✕ Adh	≋ Numb	↻ rot	⁄ elev	⪤ Short	↔ Long	

253

Manual Therapist

WELLNESS CHART

Name _____ ID#/DOB _____ Date _____

Phone _____ Address _____

1. What are your goals for health, and how may I assist you in achieving your goals? _____
   _____

2. List typical daily activities—work, exercise, home. _____
   _____

3. Are you currently experiencing any of the following? If yes, please explain.

pain, tenderness	☐ No ☐ Yes: _____	stiffness ☐ No ☐ Yes: _____
numbness or tingling	☐ No ☐ Yes: _____	swelling ☐ No ☐ Yes: _____
allergies	☐ No ☐ Yes: _____	

4. List all illnesses, injuries, and health concerns you have now or have had in the past 3 years.
   (Examples: arthritis, diabetes, car crash, pregnancy) _____
   _____

5. List medications and pain relievers taken this week. _____

6. I have provided all my known medical information. I acknowledge that massage therapy is
   not a substitute for medical diagnosis and treatment. I give my consent to receive treatment.

   Signature _____ Date _____

   Tx: _____
   _____

   C: _____
   _____

Legend:

℮ TP	● TeP	○ Ⓟ	✳ Infl	≡ HT	≈ SP	initials _____
✕ Adh	≋ Numb	⟲ rot	╱ elev	⊱─⊰ Short	⟷ Long

Manual Therapist

WELLNESS CHART—SEATED

Name _____ ID#/DOB _____ Date _____

Phone _____ Address _____

1. What are your goals for health, and how may I assist you in achieving your goals? _____

    _____

2. List typical daily activities—work, exercise, home. _____

    _____

3. Are you currently experiencing any of the following? If yes, please explain.

    pain, tenderness   ☐ No ☐ Yes: _____   stiffness ☐ No ☐ Yes: _____

    numbness or tingling   ☐ No ☐ Yes: _____   swelling ☐ No ☐ Yes: _____

    allergies   ☐ No ☐ Yes: _____

4. List all illnesses, injuries, and health concerns you have now or have had in the past 3 years.
   (Examples: arthritis, diabetes, car crash, pregnancy) _____

    _____

5. List medications and pain relievers taken this week. _____

6. I have provided all my known medical information. I acknowledge that massage therapy is
   not a substitute for medical diagnosis and treatment. I give my consent to receive treatment.

    Signature _____ Date _____

    Tx: _____

    _____

    C: _____

    _____

initials _____

Legend: ℮ TP   ● TeP   ○ Ⓟ   ⁕ Infl   ≡ HT   ≈ SP

          ✕ Adh   ≷ Numb   ◯ rot   ╱ elev   ⊶ Short   ⟷ Long

255

INJURY INFORMATION

Patient Name _____ Date _____

Date of Injury_____ Insurance ID# _____

A. General Injury Information

1. How did the accident occur?
   ☐ Auto   ☐ On-the-Job   ☐ Other _____

2. Was a police report filed?   ☐Yes   ☐ No
   Was a work incident report filed?
   ☐Yes   ☐No

3. Describe your injury and how it occurred:
   _____
   _____
   _____
   _____
   _____
   _____

4. Describe how you felt during and immediately after the injury:
   _____
   _____
   Later that same day: _____
   _____
   The next day: _____
   _____
   _____
   The next week: _____
   _____
   The next month: _____

   Describe any bruises, cuts, or abrasions as a result of the injury:
   _____
   _____

5. Are your symptoms ☐ getting better
   ☐ getting worse   ☐ no change
   What makes them better? _____
   _____
   _____
   _____
   Worse? _____
   _____
   _____
   _____

6. Did you return to work on the day of the injury? ☐ Yes   ☐ No
   Have you lost time from work since the injury? ☐ Yes   ☐ No

7. What are your work responsibilities?
   _____
   _____
   Which work activities are affected by this injury? _____
   _____
   Have your work responsibilities changed as a result of this injury?   ☐ Yes   ☐ No
   Explain _____
   What other daily activities are affected by this injury? _____
   _____

8. Did you go to the emergency room?
   ☐ Yes   ☐ No
   Were you hospitalized?   ☐ Yes   ☐ No
   List the health care providers who have treated you for this injury, the type of treatment provided, and their diagnosis.
   _____
   _____
   _____
   _____

9. Have you ever had this type of injury before? ☐ Yes   ☐ No
   Explain _____
   _____
   Did you have any physical complaints before the injury? ☐ Yes   ☐ No
   Explain _____
   _____
   Do you have any illnesses or previous injuries that may have been affected by this injury? ☐ Yes   ☐ No
   Explain _____
   _____

Signature _____Date _____

B. Motor Vehicle Accident Information

1. Did the police arrive at the accident?
   ☐ Yes ☐ No

2. How was your vehicle hit?

   ☐ Rear end ☐ Head on ☐ Side swipe

   OR Did your vehicle hit another vehicle/object?

   ☐ Rear end ☐ Head on ☐ Side swipe

   If you were hit from behind, was your vehicle pushed forward upon impact?
   ☐ Yes ☐ No If yes, how much?

   _____

   Did your vehicle hit anything else after the initial impact? ☐ Yes ☐ No

   Explain _____

   _____

   _____

   _____

3. Were you at a stop or moving at the time of impact? ☐ Stopped ☐ Moving
   If you were stopped, was your foot on the brake? ☐ Yes ☐ No
   If you were moving, were you:
   ☐ Increasing speed
   ☐ Decreasing speed
   ☐ Traveling at a steady speed

   Was the other vehicle moving at the time of impact? ☐ Yes ☐ No
   If yes, was it: ☐ Increasing speed
   ☐ Decreasing speed ☐ Traveling at a steady speed

4. Where were you seated in the vehicle?

   _____

   _____

   _____

5. Which way was your head facing upon impact?

   _____

   _____

   _____

6. Were you aware of the approaching vehicle or did the impact catch you by surprise?
   ☐ Aware ☐ Surprise

7. Did you lose consciousness?
   ☐ Yes ☐ No

8. Were you wearing a seat belt? ☐ No
   ☐ Lap belt ☐ Shoulder harness ☐ Both

9. Is your vehicle equipped with an airbag?
   ☐ Yes ☐ No
   Did it activate? ☐ Yes ☐ No

10. Is the top of your head rest:
    ☐ Above your head ☐ Below your head
    Does your head touch the head rest?
    ☐ Yes ☐ No
    If no, how far in front of the head rest is your head?

    _____

11. What were the road conditions?
    ☐ Wet ☐ Dry ☐ Icy ☐ Oily

12. What type of vehicle were you in? (make, model, year)

    _____

    What type of vehicle hit you? (make, model, year)

    _____

13. Did any part of your body come into contact with the vehicle? ☐ Yes ☐ No
    Explain _____

    _____

    _____

    Did any parts of the vehicle break?
    ☐ Yes ☐ No
    Explain _____

    _____

    _____

14. Check all of the following symptoms that you have experienced since the accident:
    ☐ Loss of memory _____
    ☐ Loss of balance _____
    ☐ Visual disturbances _____
    ☐ Hearing difficulties _____
    ☐ Difficulty breathing _____
    ☐ Sleep disturbances _____

15. Anything else you want to tell me about the accident or how you feel?

    _____

    _____

    _____

Patient Signature _____ Date _____

Provider _____   **BILLING INFORMATION**

Patient Name _____   Date _____

Date of Injury _____   ID#/DOB _____

Billing Policy

Our office is set up to receive direct payment from insurance companies. For the best chance of reimbursement from your insurance carrier, <u>we ask that you:</u>

• Contact your insurance company to determine your manual therapy coverage and provider stipulations. Coverage depends on your insurance company and the specific plan you have chosen. We have provided a list of questions for you to ask your insurance representative or attorney that will help determine your eligibility for our billing service.

• You will need a current prescription for manual therapy from a primary health care provider, such as a physician or a chiropractor in order to submit your claim. Referrals are current for 90 days unless otherwise specified.

It is important that you understand your insurance policies in order for you to budget for your manual therapy services. You are personally responsible for all charges incurred in our office. We expect payment in full until your insurance coverage has been verified.

We realize that the completion of this form is an added burden to you as a consumer, and we thank you very much for your assistance. This completed form will provide both you and our billing department with important information regarding your manual therapy insurance benefits, and enable us to process your claim in a timely fashion.

Patient Information

Is patient's condition related to:

☐ auto collision—In what state? _____
☐ other accident _____
☐ employment ☐ illness

Patient status: ☐ male ☐ female
☐ single ☐ married/partnered ☐ other

Patient relationship to insured
☐ self ☐ spouse/partner ☐ child ☐ other

Insured's Information (if other than patient)

Name _____
Address _____
City _____ State ____ Zip _____
Phone: _____
Date of birth _____
Sex: ☐ Male ☐ Female
Employer's Name or School Name _____
_____

Insurance Information

Insurance plan name or program name: _____

Member ID#: _____   Group #: _____

Customer service phone #: _____   Date and time you called: _____

Name of customer service representative: _____

Insurance claim address: _____   State: _____ Zip: _____

Does the plan include a Physical Medicine and Rehabilitation benefit? ☐ Yes ☐ No

Who may provide the services? ☐ Massage Therapist ☐ Physical Therapist ☐ Other

Is pre-authorization required? ☐ Yes ☐ No   Who can authorize the services? _____

Is a prescription required? ☐ Yes ☐ No   Is a referral required? ☐ Yes ☐ No

Who may refer? ☐ MD ☐ DC ☐ ND ☐ PT ☐ Other _____

How often does the referral need to be updated to ensure continuous coverage? _____

Is there a Preferred Provider list for Manual Therapists? ☐ Yes ☐ No

Is _____ on the list? ☐ Yes ☐ No

258

If this is a Workers' Compensation Claim, please fill out the following information:

Who is the attending HCP? _____ Phone: _____

Claim number: _____ Date eligibility began: _____

Number of visits authorized: _____ Number of visits remaining: _____

Dates of coverage: _____ Date claim closed: _____

If this is a Personal Injury Claim, please fill out the following information:

PIP policy amount: _____ Dates of coverage: _____ PIP available: _____

MedPay amount: _____ Dates of coverage: _____ MedPay available: _____

Liability amount: _____ Dates of coverage: _____ Liability available: _____

Uninsured/Underinsured (UMI) policy amount: _____ UMI available: _____

Has the PIP application been received? ☐ Yes ☐ No

Has an attorney been consulted? ☐ Yes ☐ No   Retained? ☐ Yes ☐ No

Name/Firm _____

Address _____ City _____ State _____ Zip _____

Phone _____ Fax _____

If this is a Private Health Insurance Claim, please fill out the following information:
(Or, if your Personal Injury claim defaults to secondary coverage, fill this out)

Maximum allowable benefit for Physical Medicine/Rehabilitation: _____

In network: $_____ # visits _____ Remaining $_____ # visits _____

Deductible: $_____ Satisifed to date: $_____ Co-Pay: $_____

Out-of-network: $_____ # visits _____ Remaining $_____ # visits _____

Deductible: $_____ Satisifed to date: $_____ Co-Insurance: $_____

Are these limits just for manual therapy? ☐ Yes ☐ No

If no, what other types of treatment do they include? _____
(i.e., chiropractic, physical therapy, occupational therapy, naturopathy, etc.)

Assignment of Benefits

My signature below authorizes and directs payment of medical benefits for services billed to my health care provider: _____

Release of Medical Records

My signature below authorizes the release of my medical records including intake forms, chart notes, reports, and billing statements to my attorneys, health care providers, and insurance case managers, for the purpose of processing my claims. (I will inform my practitioner immediately upon signing any exclusive Release of Medical Records with my attorney.)

Financial Responsibility

It is my responsibility to pay for all services provided. In the event that my insurance company denies payment or makes a partial payment, I agree to be and remain responsible for the balance. It is also my understanding and agreement that if you have contracted with my insurance company at a discount rate and the agreed-upon fee has been satisfied, the balance owed on those specific visits will be waived.

Signature _____ Date _____

Manual Therapist   **PRESCRIPTION**

Patient Name _____ Date _____

Date of Injury _____ ID#/DOB _____

A. Diagnosis

(Include ICD-9 codes that specifically
address Manual Therapy Treatment)

_____

_____

_____

_____

Condition is related to

☐ Auto Accident
☐ Work Injury
☐ Illness
☐ Other: _____

_____

_____

B. Medically Necessary Treatment: Implement Plan as Prescribed Below

Application (Primary & Secondary)

☐ Head _____
☐ Neck _____
☐ Chest _____
☐ Shoulders _____
☐ Abdomen _____
☐ Back _____
☐ Lowback/Hips _____
☐ Upper extremities _____
☐ Lower extremities _____
☐ All of the above _____
☐ Other: _____

Frequency & Duration

☐ 1× wk for _____ wks
☐ 2× wk for _____ wks
☐ 3× wk for _____ wks
☐ 2× month for _____ months
☐ 1× month for _____ months

Specific Instructions/Precautions:

Treatment Type

☐ Manual Therapy _____
☐ Hot/Cold Packs _____
☐ Self-Care/Exercises _____
☐ Other _____

Treatment Goals

☐ Decrease Pain
☐ Decrease Inflammation
☐ Decrease Muscle Tension/Spasms
☐ Decrease Compensatory Patterns
☐ Increase Mobility
☐ Increase Strength
☐ Restore Function
☐ Restore Posture
☐ Patient Education
☐ All of the Above
☐ Other _____

_____

_____

_____

_____

C. Referring Health Care Provider (HCP)

Contact Information
HCP Name _____
Address _____
City _____ State ____ Zip _____
Phone _____
Fax _____
Email _____

Reporting—I will send an initial report after
the first visit and a progress report after
every 6–8 sessions. Please check how you
would like to receive this information:
☐ Fax ☐ Mail ☐ Email
☐ Send Copies of Chart Notes with each report

HCP Signature: _____ Date _____

Revised and reprinted with permission, Adler ◆ Giersch, PS

260

HEALTH REPORT-F

Patient Name _____ Date _____

Date of Injury _____ ID#/DOB _____

A. Draw today's symptoms on the figures.

1. Identify CURRENT symptomatic areas in your body by marking letters on the figures below. Use the letters provided in the key to identify the symptoms you are feeling today.
2. Circle the area around each letter, representing the size and shape of each symptom location.

Key
P = pain or tenderness
S = joint or muscle stiffness
N = numbness or tingling

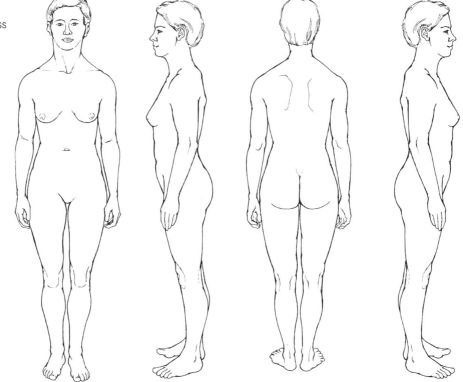

B. Identify the intensity of your symptoms.

1. Pain Scale: Mark a line on the scale to show the amount of pain you are experiencing today.

No Pain |———————————————————————————————| Unbearable Pain

2. Activities Scale: Mark a line on the scale to show the limitations you are experiencing today in your daily activities.

Can Do Anything I Want |———————————————————————————| Cannot Do Anything

C. Comments

_____

_____

_____

_____

Signature _____ Date _____

HEALTH REPORT-M

Patient Name _____ Date _____

Date of Injury _____ ID#/DOB _____

A. Draw today's symptoms on the figures.

1. Identify CURRENT symptomatic areas in your body by marking letters on the figures below. Use the letters provided in the key to identify the symptoms you are feeling today.
2. Circle the area around each letter, representing the size and shape of each symptom location.

Key

P = pain or tenderness
S = joint or muscle stiffness
N = numbness or tingling

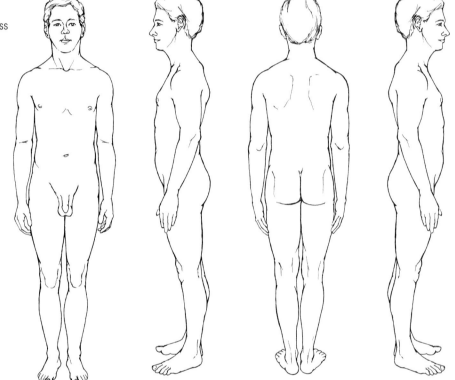

B. Identify the intensity of your symptoms.

1. Pain Scale: Mark a line on the scale to show the amount of pain you are experiencing today.

No Pain ┣━━━━━━━━━━━━━━━━━━━━━━━━━━━━━━━┫ Unbearable Pain

2. Activities Scale: Mark a line on the scale to show the limitations you are experiencing today in your daily activities.

Can Do Anything I Want ┣━━━━━━━━━━━━━━━━━━━━━━━━━━┫ Cannot Do Anything

C. Comments

_____

_____

_____

_____

Signature _____ Date _____

Manual Therapist

HEALTH REPORT

Patient Name _____ Date _____

Date of Injury _____ ID#/DOB _____

A. Draw today's symptoms on the figures.

1. Identify CURRENT symptomatic areas in your body by marking letters on the figures below. Use the letters provided in the key to identify the symptoms you are feeling today.
2. Circle the area around each letter, representing the size and shape of each symptom location.

Key
P = pain or tenderness
S = joint or muscle stiffness
N = numbness or tingling

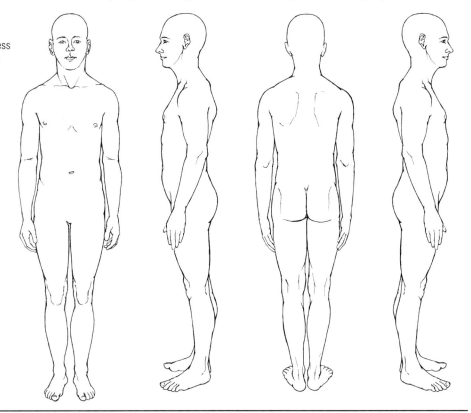

B. Identify the intensity of your symptoms.

1. Pain Scale: Mark a line on the scale to show the amount of pain you are experiencing today.

   No Pain |————————————————————————————| Unbearable Pain

2. Activities Scale: Mark a line on the scale to show the limitations you are experiencing today in your daily activities.

   Can Do Anything I Want |————————————————————————| Cannot Do Anything

C. Comments

_____
_____
_____
_____

Signature _____ Date _____

263

NECK PAIN & DISABILITY INDEX

Patient Name _____ Date _____

Date of Injury _____ ID#/DOB _____

This questionnaire has been designed to give the health care provider information as to how your neck pain has affected your ability to manage everyday life. Please answer every section and mark in each section only the **ONE** box which applies to you. We realize you may consider that two of the statements in any one section relate to you, but please just mark the box which most closely describes your problem today.

Section 1 - Pain Intensity
☐ I have no pain at the moment.
☐ The pain is very mild at the moment.
☐ The pain is moderate at the moment.
☐ The pain is fairly severe at the moment.
☐ The pain is very severe at the moment.
☐ The pain is the worst imaginable at the moment.

Section 2 - Personal Care
(washing, dressing, etc.)
☐ I can look after myself normally without causing pain.
☐ I can look after myself normally but it causes extra pain.
☐ It is painful to look after myself and I am slow and careful.
☐ I need some help but manage most of my personal care.
☐ I need help every day in most aspects of self care.
☐ I do not get dressed, I wash myself with difficulty and I stay in bed.

Section 3 - Lifting
☐ I can lift heavy weights without extra pain.
☐ I can lift heavy weights but it causes extra pain.
☐ Pain prevents me from lifting heavy weights off the floor, but I can manage if they are conveniently positioned, e.g. on a table.
☐ Pain prevents me from lifting heavy weights, but I can manage light to medium weights if they are conveniently positioned.
☐ I can lift very light weights.
☐ I cannot lift or carry anything at all.

Section 4 - Reading
☐ I can read as much as I want to with no pain in my neck.
☐ I can read as much as I want to with slight pain in my neck.
☐ I can read as much as I want to with moderate pain in my neck.
☐ I can't read as much as I want to because of moderate pain in my neck.
☐ I can hardly read at all because of severe pain in my neck.
☐ I cannot read at all.

Section 5 - Headaches
☐ I have no headaches at all.
☐ I have slight headaches which come infrequently.
☐ I have moderate headaches which come infrequently.
☐ I have moderate headaches which come frequently.
☐ I have severe headaches which come frequently.
☐ I have headaches almost all of the time.

Section 6 - Concentration
☐ I can concentrate fully when I want to with no difficulty.
☐ I can concentrate fully when I want to with slight difficulty.
☐ I have a fair degree of difficulty in concentrating when I want to.
☐ I have a lot of difficulty concentrating when I want to.
☐ I have a great deal of difficulty in concentrating when I want to.
☐ I cannot concentrate at all.

Section 7 - Work
☐ I can do as much work as I want to.
☐ I can do my usual work but no more.
☐ I can do most of my usual work but no more.
☐ I cannot do my usual work.
☐ I can hardly do any work at all.
☐ I can't do any work at all.

Section 8 - Driving
☐ I can drive my car without any neck pain.
☐ I can drive my car as long as I want with slight pain in my neck.
☐ I can drive my car as long as I want with moderate pain in my neck.
☐ I can't drive my car as long as I want because of moderate pain in my neck.
☐ I can hardly drive at all because of severe pain in my neck.
☐ I can't drive my car at all.

Section 9 - Sleeping
☐ I have no trouble sleeping.
☐ My sleep is slightly disturbed (less than 1 hour sleepless).
☐ My sleep is mildly disturbed (1–2 hours sleepless).
☐ My sleep is moderately disturbed (2–3 hours sleepless).
☐ My sleep is greatly disturbed (3–5 hours sleepless).
☐ My sleep is completely disturbed (5–7 hours sleepless).

Section 10 - Recreation
☐ I am able to engage in all my recreational activities with no neck pain at all.
☐ I am able to engage in all my recreational activities with some pain in my neck.
☐ I am able to engage in most, but not all of my usual recreational activities because of pain in my neck.
☐ I am able to engage in a few of my usual recreation activities because of pain in my neck.
☐ I can hardly do any recreational activities because of pain in my neck.
☐ I can't do recreational activities at all.

Signature _____ Date _____

LOW BACK PAIN & DISABILITY INDEX

Patient Name _____ Date _____

Date of Injury _____ ID#/DOB _____

This questionnaire has been designed to give the health care provider information about how your back pain has affected your ability to manage everyday life. Please answer every section and mark in each section only the **ONE** box which applies to you. We realize you may consider that two statements in any one section relate to you, but please just mark the box which most closely describes your problem today.

Section 1 - Pain Intensity
☐ The pain comes and goes and is mild.
☐ The pain is mild and does not vary much.
☐ The pain comes and goes and is moderate.
☐ The pain is moderate and does not vary much.
☐ The pain comes and goes and is severe.
☐ The pain is severe and does not vary much.

Section 2 - Personal Care
☐ I can look after myself normally without causing pain.
☐ I can look after myself normally but it causes extra pain.
☐ It is painful to look after myself and I am slow and careful.
☐ I need some help but manage most of my personal care.
☐ I need help every day in most aspects of self care.
☐ I do not get dressed, I wash myself with difficulty, and I stay in bed.

Section 3 - Lifting
☐ I can lift heavy weights without extra pain.
☐ I can lift heavy weights but it causes extra pain.
☐ Pain prevents me from lifting heavy weights off the floor, but I can manage if they are conveniently positioned, e.g. on a table.
☐ Pain prevents me from lifting heavy weights, but I can manage light to medium weights if they are conveniently positioned.
☐ I can lift very light weights.
☐ I cannot lift or carry anything at all.

Section 4 - Walking
☐ I have no pain on walking.
☐ I have some pain on walking but it does not increase with distance.
☐ I cannot walk more than 1 mile without increasing pain.
☐ I cannot walk more than 1/2 mile without increasing pain.
☐ I cannot walk more than 1/4 mile without increasing pain.
☐ I cannot walk at all without increasing pain.

Section 5 - Sitting
☐ I can sit in any chair as long as I like.
☐ I can only sit in my favorite chair as long as I like.
☐ Pain prevents me from sitting more than 1 hour.
☐ Pain prevents me from sitting more than 1/2 hour.
☐ Pain prevents me from sitting more than 10 minutes.
☐ I avoid sitting because it increases my pain straight away.

Section 6 - Standing
☐ I can stand as long as I want without pain.
☐ I have some pain on standing but it does not increase with time.
☐ I cannot stand for longer than 1 hour without increasing pain.
☐ I cannot stand for longer than 1/2 hour without increasing pain.
☐ I cannot stand for longer than 10 minutes without increasing pain.
☐ I avoid standing because it increases the pain straight away.

Section 7 - Sleeping
☐ I have no trouble sleeping.
☐ My sleep is slightly disturbed (less than 1 hour sleepless).
☐ My sleep is mildly disturbed (1–2 hours sleepless).
☐ My sleep is moderately disturbed (2–3 hours sleepless).
☐ My sleep is greatly disturbed (3–5 hours sleepless).
☐ My sleep is completely disturbed (5–7 hours sleepless).

Section 8 - Social Life
☐ My social life is normal and gives me no pain.
☐ My social life is normal but increases the degree of pain.
☐ Pain has no significant effect on my social life apart from limiting my more energetic interests, e.g. dancing, etc.
☐ Pain has restricted my social life and I do not go out very often.
☐ Pain has restricted my social life to my home.
☐ I hardly have any social life because of the pain.

Section 9 - Traveling
☐ I get no pain while traveling.
☐ I get some pain while traveling but none of my usual forms of travel make it any worse.
☐ I get extra pain while traveling but it does not compel me to seek alternate forms of travel.
☐ I get extra pain while traveling which compels me to seek alternative forms of travel.
☐ Pain restricts all forms of travel.
☐ Pain prevents all forms of travel except that done lying down.

Section 10 - Changing Degree of Pain
☐ My pain is rapidly getting better.
☐ My pain fluctuates but overall is definitely getting better.
☐ My pain seems to be getting better but improvement is slow at present.
☐ My pain is neither getting better nor getting worse.
☐ My pain is gradually worsening.
☐ My pain is rapidly worsening.

Signature _____ Date _____

FUNCTIONAL RATING INDEX

Name _____ ID#/DOB _____ Date _____

In order to properly assess your condition, we must understand how much your _____
have affected your ability to manage everyday activities. For each item below, please circle the
number which most closely describes your condition right now.

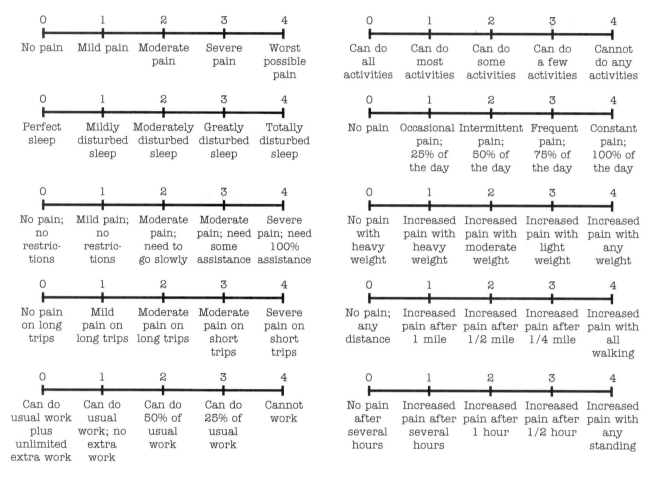

0	1	2	3	4
No pain	Mild pain	Moderate pain	Severe pain	Worst possible pain

0	1	2	3	4
Can do all activities	Can do most activities	Can do some activities	Can do a few activities	Cannot do any activities

0	1	2	3	4
Perfect sleep	Mildly disturbed sleep	Moderately disturbed sleep	Greatly disturbed sleep	Totally disturbed sleep

0	1	2	3	4
No pain	Occasional pain; 25% of the day	Intermittent pain; 50% of the day	Frequent pain; 75% of the day	Constant pain; 100% of the day

0	1	2	3	4
No pain; no restrictions	Mild pain; no restrictions	Moderate pain; need to go slowly	Moderate pain; need some assistance	Severe pain; need 100% assistance

0	1	2	3	4
No pain with heavy weight	Increased pain with heavy weight	Increased pain with moderate weight	Increased pain with light weight	Increased pain with any weight

0	1	2	3	4
No pain on long trips	Mild pain on long trips	Moderate pain on long trips	Moderate pain on short trips	Severe pain on short trips

0	1	2	3	4
No pain; any distance	Increased pain after 1 mile	Increased pain after 1/2 mile	Increased pain after 1/4 mile	Increased pain with all walking

0	1	2	3	4
Can do usual work plus unlimited extra work	Can do usual work; no extra work	Can do 50% of usual work	Can do 25% of usual work	Cannot work

0	1	2	3	4
No pain after several hours	Increased pain after several hours	Increased pain after 1 hour	Increased pain after 1/2 hour	Increased pain with any standing

Dear _____ :

Thank you for referring _____ to my office. Your patient and I were unable to connect for the following reason(s):

_____ The patient did not schedule an appointment.

_____ The patient did not attend the scheduled appointment.

_____ I am not scheduling new patients at this time. I anticipate my schedule to open back up again _____.

_____ I am unable to benefit the patient for the following reason(s):

_____

_____

_____

_____

Thank you for the referral. I hope to work with you again in the future.

Yours in health,

Manual Therapist _____ **SOAP CHART-F**

Patient Name _____ Date _____

Date of Injury _____ ID#/DOB _____ Meds _____

S Focus/Health Concerns: Prioritize

    Symptoms: Location/Intensity/Frequency/Duration/Onset

    Activities of Daily Living: Aggravating/Relieving

O Findings: Visual/Palpable/Test Results

    Techniques/Modalities: Locations/Duration

    Response to Treatment (see Δ)

A Goals: Long-term/Short-term

    Functional Outcomes

P Future Treatment/Frequency

    Homework/Self-care

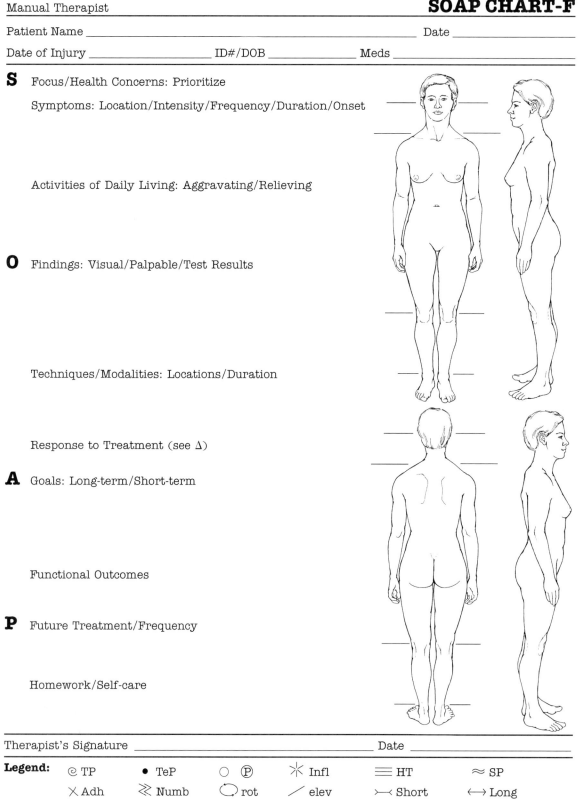

Therapist's Signature _____ Date _____

Legend:

℮ TP	• TeP	○ Ⓟ	⁂ Infl	≡ HT	≈ SP
✕ Adh	≳ Numb	↻ rot	╱ elev	⊱ Short	↔ Long

Manual Therapist _____ **SOAP CHART-M**

Patient Name _____ Date _____

Date of Injury _____ ID#/DOB _____ Meds _____

S Focus/Health Concerns: Prioritize

 Symptoms: Location/Intensity/Frequency/Duration/Onset

 Activities of Daily Living: Aggravating/Relieving

O Findings: Visual/Palpable/Test Results

 Techniques/Modalities: Locations/Duration

 Response to Treatment (see Δ)

A Goals: Long-term/Short-term

 Functional Outcomes

P Future Treatment/Frequency

 Homework/Self-care

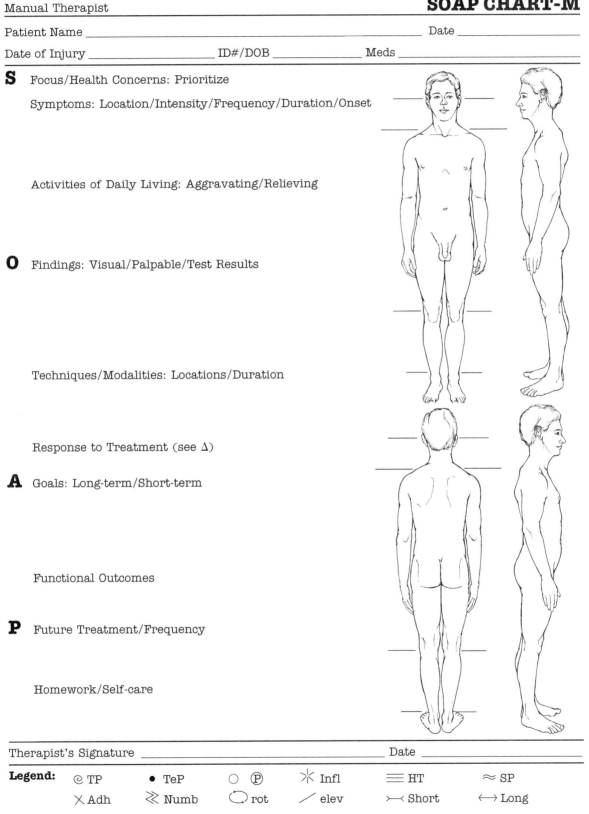

Therapist's Signature _____ Date _____

Legend: ℰ TP   • TeP   ○ Ⓟ   ✳ Infl   ☰ HT   ≈ SP

           ✕ Adh   ≷ Numb   ◯ rot   ╱ elev   ⊃< Short   ↔ Long

Manual Therapist **SOAP CHART**

Patient Name _____ Date _____

Date of Injury _____ ID#/DOB _____ Meds _____

S Focus/Health Concerns: Prioritize

Symptoms: Location/Intensity/Frequency/Duration/Onset

Activities of Daily Living: Aggravating/Relieving

O Findings: Visual/Palpable/Test Results

Techniques/Modalities: Locations/Duration

Response to Treatment (see Δ)

A Goals: Long-term/Short-term

Functional Outcomes

P Future Treatment/Frequency

Homework/Self-care

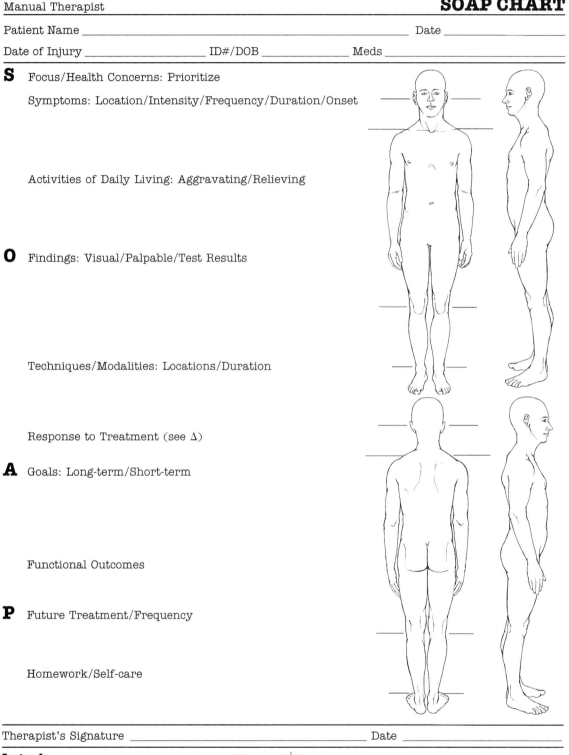

Therapist's Signature _____ Date _____

Legend:
| ℮ TP | ● TeP | ○ Ⓟ | ⁑ Infl | ≡ HT | ≈ SP |
| ✕ Adh | ≋ Numb | ↻ rot | ╱ elev | ⤙ Short | ↔ Long |

Manual Therapist _____   **SOAP CHART-F**

Patient Name _____   Date _____

Date of Injury _____ ID#/DOB _____ Meds _____

S

O

A

P

Therapist's Signature _____   Date _____

S

O

A

P

Therapist's Signature _____   Date _____

Legend: ℮ TP   ● TeP   ○ ⓟ   ⋇ Infl   ≡ HT   ≈ SP
        ⤫ Adh   ≋ Numb   ◯ rot   ╱ elev   ⤙ Short   ⟷ Long

271

Manual Therapist _____ **SOAP CHART-M**

Patient Name _____ Date _____

Date of Injury _____ ID#/DOB _____ Meds _____

S

O

A

P

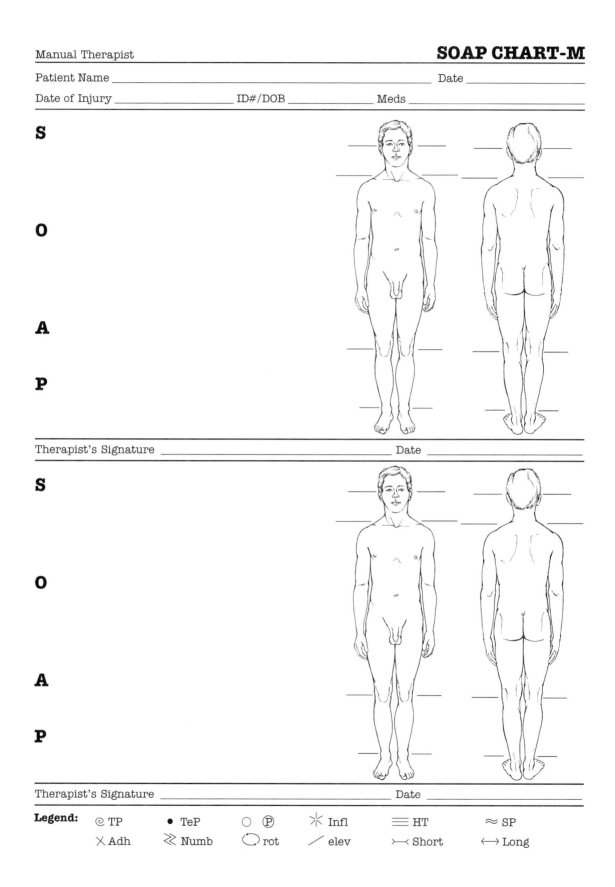

Therapist's Signature _____ Date _____

S

O

A

P

Therapist's Signature _____ Date _____

Legend: ℮ TP   • TeP   ○ Ⓟ   ✳ Infl   ≡ HT   ≈ SP

✕ Adh   ≋ Numb   ◯ rot   ╱ elev   ⤙ Short   ⟷ Long

Patient Name _____ Date _____

Date of Injury _____ ID#/DOB _____ Meds _____

S

O

A

P

Therapist's Signature _____ Date _____

S

O

A

P

Therapist's Signature _____ Date _____

Legend: ℮ TP   ● TeP   ○ Ⓟ   ✳ Infl   ☰ HT   ≈ SP

✕ Adh   ≋ Numb   ⟳ rot   ╱ elev   ⟞ Short   ⟷ Long

WELLNESS CHART—F

Name _____ ID#/DOB _____ Meds _____

Tx: _____   Tx: _____

C: _____   C: _____
_____   _____

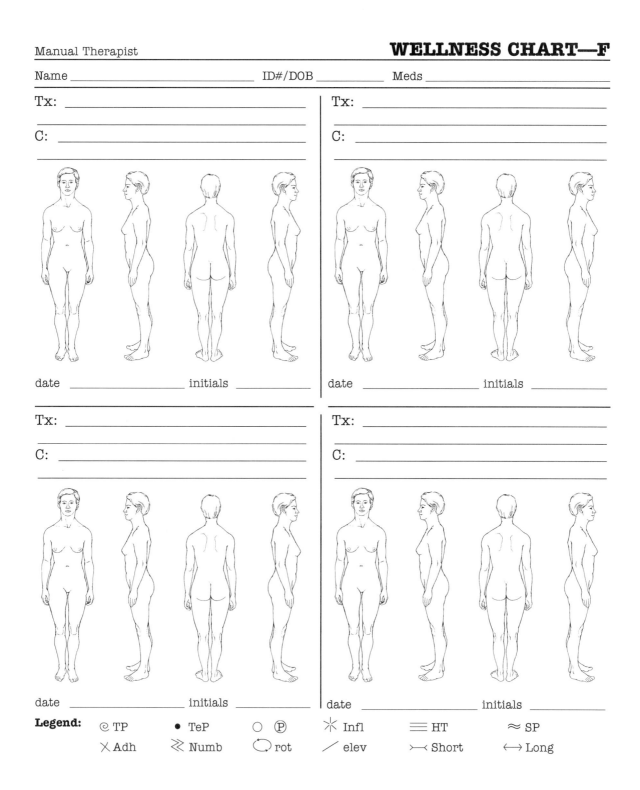

date _____ initials _____   date _____ initials _____

Tx: _____   Tx: _____

C: _____   C: _____
_____   _____

date _____ initials _____   date _____ initials _____

Legend:

℃ TP	• TeP	○ Ⓟ	⁎ Infl	≡ HT	≈ SP
✕ Adh	≋ Numb	↺ rot	╱ elev	↦ Short	↔ Long

WELLNESS CHART—M

Name _____ ID#/DOB _____ Meds _____

Tx: _____

C: _____
_____

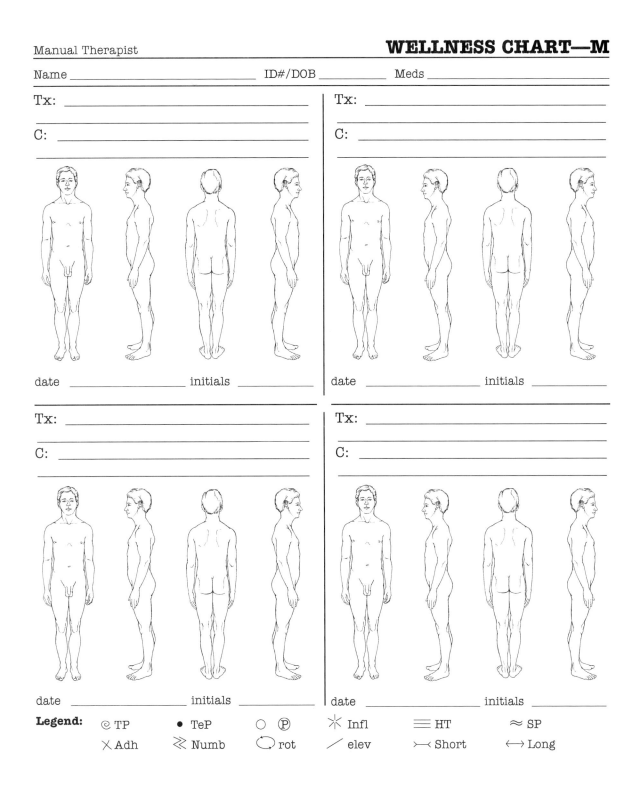

date _____ initials _____

Tx: _____

C: _____
_____

date _____ initials _____

Tx: _____
_____

C: _____
_____

date _____ initials _____

Tx: _____
_____

C: _____
_____

date _____ initials _____

Legend: ℮ TP   • TeP   ○ ⓟ   ✳ Infl   ☰ HT   ≈ SP
             ✕ Adh   ≋ Numb   ⟲ rot   ╱ elev   ⊱ Short   ↔ Long

Manual Therapist

Name _____ ID#/DOB _____ Meds _____

Tx: _____   Tx: _____

C: _____   C: _____

_____   _____

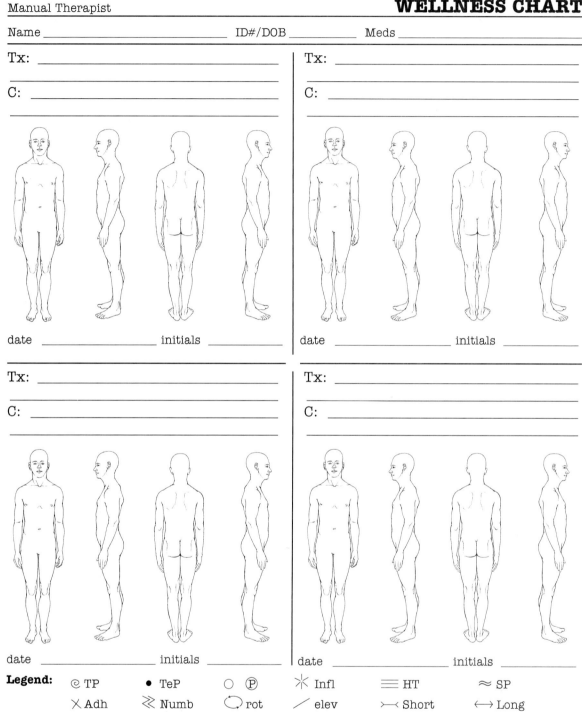

date _____ initials _____   date _____ initials _____

Tx: _____   Tx: _____

C: _____   C: _____

_____   _____

date _____ initials _____   date _____ initials _____

Legend: ℮ TP   ● TeP   ○ Ⓟ   ✳ Infl   ≡ HT   ≈ SP

✕ Adh   ≋ Numb   ↺ rot   ╱ elev   ⊷ Short   ↔ Long

WELLNESS CHART—SEATED

Name _____ ID#/DOB _____ Meds _____

Tx: _____

C: _____

Tx: _____

C: _____

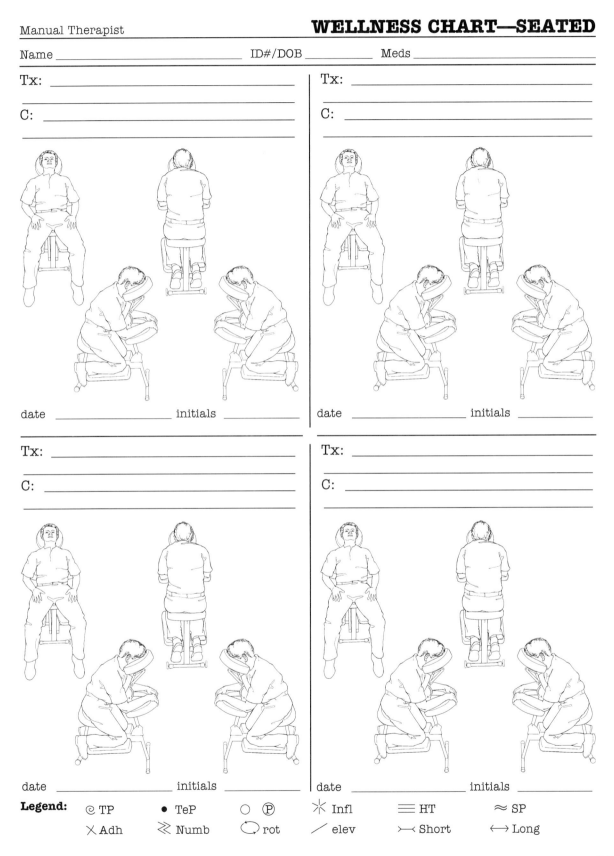

date _____ initials _____

Tx: _____

C: _____

date _____ initials _____

Tx: _____

C: _____

date _____ initials _____

date _____ initials _____

Legend:

℮ TP	● TeP	○ Ⓟ	✳ Infl	☰ HT	≈ SP
✕ Adh	≋ Numb	↺ rot	╱ elev	⊶ Short	⟷ Long

277

WELLNESS CHART—SPORTS

Manual Therapist _____ Date _____

Event _____ Location _____

Ask each athlete the following: (Note individual responses below—concerns only.)

1. Are you currently experiencing any of the following?
   - pain, tenderness, stiffness
   - swelling
   - numbness, tingling
   - dizziness
   - cold, clammy skin
   - shaking

2. How soon do you compete? / When did you finish competing?

3. Have you warmed up? / Cooled down?

4. Have you consumed water since the event?

Athlete's Name _____ Athlete's initials: _____

Hx: (note concerns) _____

Tx: (check all that apply) _____ Pre-event _____ Post-event _____ Refer-first aid/med

C: _____ Initials: _____

Athlete's Name _____ Athlete's initials: _____

Hx: (note concerns) _____

Tx: (check all that apply) _____ Pre-event _____ Post-event _____ Refer-first aid/med

C: _____ Initials: _____

Athlete's Name _____ Athlete's initials: _____

Hx: (note concerns) _____

Tx: (check all that apply) _____ Pre-event _____ Post-event _____ Refer-first aid/med

C: _____ Initials: _____

Athlete's Name _____ Athlete's initials: _____

Hx: (note concerns) _____

Tx: (check all that apply) _____ Pre-event _____ Post-event _____ Refer-first aid/med

C: _____ Initials: _____

Athlete's Name _____ Athlete's initials: _____

Hx: (note concerns) _____

Tx: (check all that apply) _____ Pre-event _____ Post-event _____ Refer-first aid/med

C: _____ Initials: _____

Athlete's Name _____ Athlete's initials: _____

Hx: (note concerns) _____

Tx: (check all that apply) _____ Pre-event _____ Post-event _____ Refer-first aid/med

C: _____ Initials: _____

Manual Therapist _____ **RANGE OF MOTION**

Patient Name _____ Date _____

Date of Injury _____ ID#/DOB _____

PRE-TEST 1 Initials _____ Date _____

Position of patient: prone, sidelying, sitting, standing, supine, other: _____

Type of test: active, active assisted, passive, resistive, other: _____

Joint: C-spine, T-spine, L-spine, hip, knee, ankle, shoulder, elbow, wrist, other: _____

Action	Quantify ↓ or ↑		Rate Pain		Rate Quality	
	Ⓡ	Ⓛ	Ⓡ	Ⓛ	Ⓡ	Ⓛ

PRE-TEST 2 Initials _____ Date _____

Position of patient: prone, sidelying, sitting, standing, supine, other: _____

Type of test: active, active assisted, passive, resistive, other: _____

Joint: C-spine, T-spine, L-spine, hip, knee, ankle, shoulder, elbow, wrist, other: _____

Action	Quantify ↓ or ↑		Rate Pain		Rate Quality	
	Ⓡ	Ⓛ	Ⓡ	Ⓛ	Ⓡ	Ⓛ

PRE-TEST 3 Initials _____ Date _____

Position of patient: prone, sidelying, sitting, standing, supine, other: _____

Type of test: active, active assisted, passive, resistive, other: _____

Joint: C-spine, T-spine, L-spine, hip, knee, ankle, shoulder, elbow, wrist, other: _____

Action	Quantify ↓ or ↑		Rate Pain		Rate Quality	
	Ⓡ	Ⓛ	Ⓡ	Ⓛ	Ⓡ	Ⓛ

POST-TEST 1 Initials _____ Date _____

Position of patient: prone, sidelying, sitting, standing, supine, other: _____

Type of test: active, active assisted, passive, resistive, other: _____

Joint: C-spine, T-spine, L-spine, hip, knee, ankle, shoulder, elbow, wrist, other: _____

Action	Quantify ↓ or ↑		Rate Pain		Rate Quality	
	Ⓡ	Ⓛ	Ⓡ	Ⓛ	Ⓡ	Ⓛ

POST-TEST 2 Initials _____ Date _____

Position of patient: prone, sidelying, sitting, standing, supine, other: _____

Type of test: active, active assisted, passive, resistive, other: _____

Joint: C-spine, T-spine, L-spine, hip, knee, ankle, shoulder, elbow, wrist, other: _____

Action	Quantify ↓ or ↑		Rate Pain		Rate Quality	
	Ⓡ	Ⓛ	Ⓡ	Ⓛ	Ⓡ	Ⓛ

POST-TEST 3 Initials _____ Date _____

Position of patient: prone, sidelying, sitting, standing, supine, other: _____

Type of test: active, active assisted, passive, resistive, other: _____

Joint: C-spine, T-spine, L-spine, hip, knee, ankle, shoulder, elbow, wrist, other: _____

Action	Quantify ↓ or ↑		Rate Pain		Rate Quality	
	Ⓡ	Ⓛ	Ⓡ	Ⓛ	Ⓡ	Ⓛ

Directions for charting Range of Motion Results: For each test, fill in the form blanks as follows:
ACTION—Identify the action tested: abd, add, DF, ever, ext, ext rot, flex, int rot, inv, lat flex, PF, pro, SB, and Sup
QUANTIFY—Quantify the available range of motion: ↓ (hypomobility), ↑ (hypermobility); L, M, S; 0–10; N, G, F, P (Normal, Good, Fair, Poor).
PAIN—Identify if Pain is present with movement: If present, rate pain. If absent: Ø.
QUALITY—Identify and Rate the quality of movement: sm, seg, Sp, rig (smooth, segmented, spastic, rigid)

PATIENT'S RELEASE OF HEALTH CARE INFORMATION

Patient's Name _____

Social Security Number _____ Date of Birth _____

I hereby instruct my providers to provide full and complete information to _____
_____ and to accept this authorization form and release the protected information
requested without requiring any additional authorizations. I specifically waive any "minimally
necessary" limitations of HIPAA.

Health Care Provider/Facility _____
is hereby authorized to release health care information, including intake forms, chart notes,
reports, correspondence, billing statements, and other written information to my attorneys,
employees, and designated agents of my attorneys, to wit:

Attorney's Name _____ Phone _____
Address _____
City _____ State _____ Zip _____

This request and authorization applies to:
____ Health care information relating to the following treatment, condition, or dates of
treatment: _____
____ All health care information:
____ Other: _____

How the Information will be used: Said information shall be used for any and all purposes for
_____ to pursue payment of care expenses and in providing legal
services to me in conjunction with my case. Following said disclosure the information may no
longer be subject to HIPAA protection, as it may be subject to re-disclosure that is unprotected
absent specific laws protecting specific sensitive information.

Revocation of Prior Authorization: All medical authorizations by the patient or patient's
authorized representatives given before the date of this release for any reason whatsoever are
hereby revoked.

Unlawful Disclosure Prohibited: State and Federal prohibits any health care provider from
releasing any health care information about a patient to another person without the consent of the
patient. You are requested to disclose no such information to any insurance adjuster or any other
person without written authority from me which is printed on the letterhead of my attorny.

Effect of Photocopy: A photocopy of this release shall have the same force and effect as a signed
original.

Authorization expires 90 days from date of signature. Thereafter, no authorization exists unless
an updated release is provided by: _____

I understand that I have the right to revoke this release for any information not yet provided to
_____ by providing notice of revocation in writing to the above named
care provider. I also understand that I have the right to refuse to authorize disclosure at all.

_____   _____
Signature of Patient or Patient's Authorized Representative   Date

Authorization to Use and Disclose Health Care Information

Name _____ ID#/DOB _____ Date _____

I: _____, authorize my manual therapist: _____,
to disclose my health care information with the following health care providers and/or insurance companies:

Name(s): _____

Address: _____

The following information may be disclosed (check all that apply):

☐ All health care information in my medical chart.

☐ Only health care information relating to the following injury, illness, or treatment: _____

_____

☐ Only health care information for the following dates or time periods: _____

_____

☐ Including information regarding HIV, STD, mental health, drug or alcohol abuse.

I give my authorization to release health care information for the following purposes (check all that apply):

☐ To share information with my health care team in an attempt to coordinate care

☐ To obtain payment of care expenses I have incurred for my treatments.

☐ To take part in research

☐ Other: _____

This authorization expires on:

Date: _____ (no longer than 90 days from the date signed)

Event: _____

I understand that I may refuse to sign this authorization.

I may also revoke this authorization at any time by writing a letter to my manual therapist.

I understand that once my health care information is disclosed, the recipient may redisclose the information and it may no longer be protected HIPAA or state privacy laws.

I also understand my obtaining care can not be conditioned on my signing this release.

Signature _____ Date _____

INSURANCE STATUS— PERSONAL INJURY

Patient Name _____ Date _____

Date of Injury _____ ID#/DOB _____

A. Reporting to Attorney
Which information would you like to receive monthly and how do you prefer to receive information:
- ☐ copies of billing
- ☐ monthly statements
- ☐ SOAP charts
- ☐ Progress reports

- ☐ fax
- ☐ mail
- ☐ email
- ☐ upon request

B. Primary Insurance Coverage   Effective dates: from _____ to _____
Please provide the following information regarding your client's/my patient's insurance status:

Insured _____
Insurance ID# _____
Insurance Carrier _____
Billing Address _____
City _____ State _____ Zip _____
Adjuster _____
Phone _____ Fax _____
PIP policy amount $ _____
Dates of coverage _____
PIP available $ _____
Med Pay policy amount $ _____
Dates of coverage _____
Med Pay available $ _____

C. Secondary Insurance Coverage   ☐ N/A   ☐ Effective date: _____

Insured _____
Insurance ID# _____
Insurance Carrier _____
Billing Address _____
City _____ State _____ Zip _____
Adjuster _____
Phone _____ Fax _____
PIP policy amount $ _____
Dates of coverage _____
PIP available $ _____
Med Pay policy amount $ _____
Dates of coverage _____
Med Pay available $ _____
If secondary coverage is through the patients' private health insurance, is manual therapy a covered benefit: ☐ Yes   ☐ No   ☐ Don't Know

D. Third Party Insurance Coverage   ☐ N/A   ☐ Effective date: _____

Insured _____
Insurance ID# _____
Insurance Carrier _____
Billing Address _____
City _____ State _____ Zip _____
Adjuster _____
Phone _____ Fax _____
Liability policy amount $ _____
Dates of coverage _____
Liability available $ _____
Uninsured/underinsured Motorist (UIM)$ _____
Policy Amount $ _____
UIM available $ _____

CONTRACTUAL GUARANTEE OF PAYMENT FOR MEDICAL SERVICES

I hereby authorize and direct you, my attorney, to pay directly to my health care provider(s), _____, the total dollar amount owing for health care services, including applicable interest charges, provided for injuries arising from the motor vehicle accident on _____. I hereby authorize my attorney and the involved insurance companies to withhold sums from any settlement, judgment, or verdict as may be necessary to adequately protect my health care provider(s) and their office. I hereby further consent to a lien being filed on my case by said health care provider(s) and their office against any and all proceeds of my settlement, judgment, or verdict which may be paid to you, my attorney, or myself as the result of the injuries for which I have been treated.

I agree never to rescind this document and that any attempt at recession will not be honored by my attorney. I hereby instruct that in the event another attorney is substituted in this matter, the new attorney shall honor this Contractual Guarantee of Payment for Health Care Services as inherent in the settlement and enforceable upon the case as if it were executed by him/her.

I fully understand that I am directly and fully responsible to said health care provider(s) or their office for all health care bills submitted by them for services rendered to me. Further, this agreement is made solely for said health care providers' additional protection and in consideration of their forbearance on payment. I also understand that such payment is not contingent on any settlement, judgment, or verdict by which I may eventually recover damages.

I specifically request my attorney to acknowledge this letter by signing below and returning it to the office of said health care provider(s). I have been advised that if my attorney does not wish to cooperate in protecting the health care providers' interest, the health care provider(s) will not await payment, but will require me to make payments on a current basis.

Date _____ Patient's Signature _____

Patient's Social Security Number or Driver's License Number _____

The undersigned, being attorney of record for the above patient, does hereby agree to observe all the terms of the above, and agrees to withhold such sums from any settlement, judgment, or verdict as may be necessary to adequately protect said health care provider(s) named above.

Date _____ Attorney's Signature _____

Please date, sign, and return one original to   _____

_____

_____

_____

_____

THANK YOU.

Provider _____ **INSURANCE VERIFICATION**

Patient Name _____ Date _____

Date of Injury _____ ID#/DOB _____

Verify and Authorize Patient Benefits

Company Name _____

Phone _____ Fax _____

Provider Service Rep _ _____

Date/time called _____

Check all verified:
- ☐ Physical medicine/rehab benfit
- ☐ I can provide services
- ☐ Covered services (from worksheet):

_____

Check all authorized:
- ☐ Number of visits _____
- ☐ Dates of coverage _____

Authorization # _____

Billing procedures:
- ☐ HCFA 1500 ☐ electronic ☐ other

Send with each bill:
- ☐ Prescription/referral ☐ Reports
- ☐ SOAPS ☐ License/certification

What is the expected turnaround time on
claim reimbursement? _____

_____

Comments _____

Re-Authorize

Provider Service Rep _____

Date/time called _____

Check all authorized:
- ☐ Number of visits _____
- ☐ Dates of coverage _____

Authorization # _____

Total # of visits to date _____

Total $ spent to date _____

Comments _____

Re-Authorize

Provider Service Rep _____

Date/time called _____

Check all authorized:
- ☐ Number of visits _____
- ☐ Dates of coverage _____

Authorization # _____

Total # of visits to date _____

Total $ spent to date _____

Comments _____

Referring Health Care Provider Info

Name _____

Phone _____ Fax _____

Prescription received? ☐ Yes ☐ No

Dates of coverage _____

# of visits _____

Diagnosis (ICD-9 codes) _____

_____

Comments _____

Renewal

Date _____
Progress report sent? ☐ Yes ☐ No
Prescription received? ☐ Yes ☐ No

Dates of coverage _____

# of visits _____

ICD-9 codes _____

Comments _____

Renewal

Date _____
Progress report sent? ☐ Yes ☐ No
Prescription received? ☐ Yes ☐ No

Dates of coverage _____

# of visits _____

ICD-9 codes _____

Comments _____

Attorney Information (if applicable)

Name _____

Phone _____ Fax _____

Guarantee of Payment contract signed?
☐ Yes ☐ No

Date requested _____ Received _____

Medical Lien filed? ☐ Yes ☐ No

Date _____ Expires _____
Renewed _____ Expires _____
Renewed _____ Expires _____

Requests for patient files:

Date requested _____ Date sent _____
Authorization received? ☐ Yes ☐ No
Exclusive? ☐ Yes ☐ No Expires _____

Date requested _____ Date sent _____
Authorization received? ☐ Yes ☐ No
Exclusive? ☐ Yes ☐ No Expires _____

Provider _____ **VERIFICATION WORKSHEET**

Patient Name _____ Date _____

Date of Injury _____ ID#/DOB _____

Verify and Authorize Physical Medicine and Rehabilitation Services
(Common modality codes and procedure codes for manual therapists.)

Authorized?	Code #	Description	Restrictions	Max Rate
☐ Yes ☐ No	95831	Muscle testing, ROM, manual, with report		
☐ Yes ☐ No	97010	Hot or cold packs		
☐ Yes ☐ No	97012	Mechanical traction		
☐ Yes ☐ No	97039	Unlisted modality, Specify:		
☐ Yes ☐ No	97110	Therapeutic exercise		
☐ Yes ☐ No	97112	Neuromuscular reeducation		
☐ Yes ☐ No	97113	Aquatic therapy		
☐ Yes ☐ No	97116	Gait training		
☐ Yes ☐ No	97124	Massage therapy		
☐ Yes ☐ No	97139	Unlisted therapeutic procedure, Specify:		
☐ Yes ☐ No	97140	Manual therapy: eg, mobilization/manip., MLD, MFR, manual traction		
☐ Yes ☐ No	97050	Therapeutic procedure(s), group (2 or more)		
☐ Yes ☐ No	99056	Home/Hospital visit		
☐ Yes ☐ No	99075	Medical testimony		
☐ Yes ☐ No		Other:		
☐ Yes ☐ No		Other:		
☐ Yes ☐ No		Other:		
☐ Yes ☐ No		Other:		
☐ Yes ☐ No		Other:		
☐ Yes ☐ No		Other:		
☐ Yes ☐ No		Other:		

See CPT codebook for detailed descriptions of modalities and procedures listed above and for additional modalities and therapeutic procedures not listed on worksheet.

PAYMENT LOG

Name _____ Date _____

Date of Injury_____ ID#/DOB _____

Billing Date: _____ Total Billed: $ _____

Patient Paid: $ _____ Insurance Paid: $ _____ Total Paid: $ _____

If Total Paid does NOT equal Total Billed, complete below for each date of service (from lines 1-6, Section 24 of HCFA 1500)

Line 1, Initial Billing

Treatment Date: _____ Bill Date: _____

Charges: ____ Adjustments: ____ Amount Billed: _____

Due from patient: _____ Due from Insurance: _____

Patient Paid: _____ Insurance paid: _____

Line 1, Rebilling

Rebill Date: _____ Rebilled to: _____

Outstanding: _____ Interest: _____ Amount Billed: _____

Rebill Date: _____ Rebilled to: _____

Outstanding: _____ Interest: _____ Amount Billed: _____

Rebill Date: _____ Rebilled to: _____

Outstanding: _____ Interest: _____ Amount Billed: _____

Line 2, Initial Billing

Treatment Date: _____ Bill Date: _____

Charges: ____ Adjustments: ____ Amount Billed: _____

Due from patient: _____ Due from Insurance: _____

Patient Paid: _____ Insurance paid: _____

Line 2, Rebilling

Rebill Date: _____ Rebilled to: _____

Outstanding: _____ Interest: _____ Amount Billed: _____

Rebill Date: _____ Rebilled to: _____

Outstanding: _____ Interest: _____ Amount Billed: _____

Rebill Date: _____ Rebilled to: _____

Outstanding: _____ Interest: _____ Amount Billed: _____

Line 3, Initial Billing

Treatment Date: _____ Bill Date: _____

Charges: ____ Adjustments: ____ Amount Billed: _____

Due from patient: _____ Due from Insurance: _____

Patient Paid: _____ Insurance paid: _____

Line 3, Rebilling

Rebill Date: _____ Rebilled to: _____

Outstanding: _____ Interest: _____ Amount Billed: _____

Rebill Date: _____ Rebilled to: _____

Outstanding: _____ Interest: _____ Amount Billed: _____

Rebill Date: _____ Rebilled to: _____

Outstanding: _____ Interest: _____ Amount Billed: _____

Line 4, Initial Billing

Treatment Date: _____ Bill Date: _____

Charges: ____ Adjustments: ____ Amount Billed: _____

Due from patient: _____ Due from Insurance: _____

Patient Paid: _____ Insurance paid: _____

Line 4, Rebilling

Rebill Date: _____ Rebilled to: _____

Outstanding: _____ Interest: _____ Amount Billed: _____

Rebill Date: _____ Rebilled to: _____

Outstanding: _____ Interest: _____ Amount Billed: _____

Rebill Date: _____ Rebilled to: _____

Outstanding: _____ Interest: _____ Amount Billed: _____

Line 5, Initial Billing

Treatment Date: _____ Bill Date: _____

Charges: ____ Adjustments: ____ Amount Billed: _____

Due from patient: _____ Due from Insurance: _____

Patient Paid: _____ Insurance paid: _____

Line 5, Rebilling

Rebill Date: _____ Rebilled to: _____

Outstanding: _____ Interest: _____ Amount Billed: _____

Rebill Date: _____ Rebilled to: _____

Outstanding: _____ Interest: _____ Amount Billed: _____

Rebill Date: _____ Rebilled to: _____

Outstanding: _____ Interest: _____ Amount Billed: _____

Line 6, Initial Billing

Treatment Date: _____ Bill Date: _____

Charges: ____ Adjustments: ____ Amount Billed: _____

Due from patient: _____ Due from Insurance: _____

Patient Paid: _____ Insurance paid: _____

Line 6, Rebilling

Rebill Date: _____ Rebilled to: _____

Outstanding: _____ Interest: _____ Amount Billed: _____

Rebill Date: _____ Rebilled to: _____

Outstanding: _____ Interest: _____ Amount Billed: _____

Rebill Date: _____ Rebilled to: _____

Outstanding: _____ Interest: _____ Amount Billed: _____

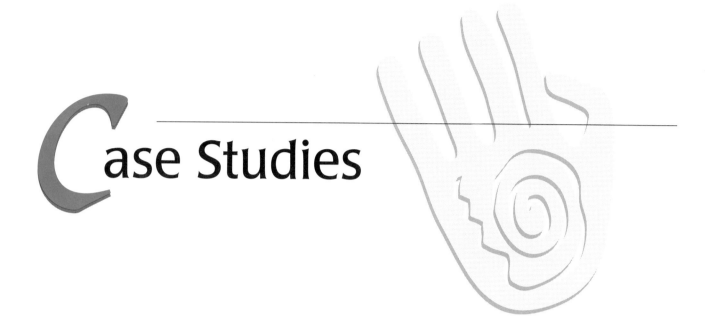

Case Studies

Personal Injury

Flow Charts: Use of intake forms, progress summaries, treatment notes, attorney forms and billing forms as needed for personal injury cases, workers' compensation, and wellness care.

Case Study: Darnel Washington, a 64-year-old retired male, sustained mild sprain-strain injuries typical of a motor vehicle collision, with moderate complications—the collision triggered onset of previously dormant degenerative scoliosis. Mr. Washington was a passenger in a 1982 Honda Accord and was rear-ended by a 1991 Ford F250 truck. Mr. Washington was turned to the left talking with his nephew, the driver. They were driving to a hockey game, traffic was heavy, and road conditions were icy. He was wearing a seatbelt with a shoulder harness. They were slowing down to stop for a yellow light; the truck behind them was speeding up to go through the light. No ambulance was called to the scene. All involved drove away from the scene after assisting the police in filing a report. Mr. Washington and his nephew attended the remainder of the hockey game.

Initially, Mr. Washington felt fine, just a little stiff and sore. After a few weeks, his back pain worsened and headaches became more frequent. He scheduled an appointment with his physician who diagnosed the degenerative scoliosis and referred him to a massage therapist. Mr. Washington's massage therapist used manual lymphatic drainage, CranioSacral therapy, and Feldenkrais as his primary treatment techniques for addressing the whiplash condition and the scoliosis.

John Olson, the massage therapist, was experiencing difficulty determining who to bill for the treatment sessions. He referred Mr. Washington to a personal injury attorney. Ms. Storro, the attorney retained to represent Mr. Washington, discovered that the driver, Mr. Washington's nephew, had PIP insurance, which was the appropriate insurance to bill for the first year of treatment.

This flow chart demonstrates the forms that are recommended for use with patients involved in personal injury cases: who completes the form, how often the form is used, and any additional comments for using the form.

Personal Injury INTAKE FORMS	Who	Frequency	Comments
Fees and Policies	Patient	Initial visit	Update as needed
Health Information	Patient	Initial visit	Update annually
Health Info—Wellness	—		
Injury Information, part 1	Patient	Initial visit	Per incident
Injury Information, part 2	Patient	Initial visit	Per incident
Billing Information	Patient	Initial visit	If you provide billing services
Prescription	HCP	As needed	A progress report should precede each renewal
PROGRESS SUMMARIES			
Health Report	Patient	Monthly	Patient reports current status
Pain Questionnaires	Patient	Monthly	Daily or weekly, if used as a pain journal
Initial Report w/o Tx	MT	As needed	If patient does not receive tx
Initial Report w/ Tx	MT	Initial visit	Summarizes tx and proposes tx plan

Progress Report	MT	Monthly	Practitioner reports to HCP
Narrative Report	MT	1x	If requested by patient's attorney

TREATMENT NOTES

Initial SOAP	MT	Initial visit	Summarizes all findings; sets goals, plan
Subsequent SOAP	MT	Each visit	(excluding initial, progress, and discharge sessions) brief, focused
Progress SOAP	MT	monthly	Summarizes all findings; updates goals, plan
Discharge SOAP	MT	Final visit	Summarizes all findings; ongoing care plan
Wellness	—		
Range of Motion	MT	As needed	

ATTORNEY FORMS

Release of Health Care Information	Attorney	As needed	Must have on file before releasing any PHI
Guarantee of Payment	MT, Patient, Attorney		If end-of-settlement case
Insurance Status–Personal Injury	Attorney	As needed	If insurance status is unknown/unclear

BILLING FORMS

Insurance Verification	MT	As needed	With renewal of prescribed services
HCFA 1500 Billing Form	MT	Each visit	May bill for multiple sessions per HCFA form after initial billing if total amount is under $250 and sessions fall within the same month
Payment Log	MT	As needed	If payments do not match bills

HANDS HEAL

John Olson, LMP, GCFP
345 Moon River Rd. Ste. 6
Minnehaha, MN   55987
TEL   612 555 9889

FEES AND POLICIES

A. Fee Schedule

Fees for services are as follows:

- CranioSacral/Lymph Drainage $100 per hour
  (97140)   ($25 per 15 minute units)
- Feldenkrais $100 per hour
  (97112)   ($25 per 15 minute unit)
- Hot and Cold Packs $15 per session
  (97101)   ($15 per session)
- Therapeutic Massage $80 Per Hour
  (97124)   ($20 per 15 minute unit)

B. Payment Policies

Cash or Check

- A 10% discount is available when payment is made at the time services are provided.
- Pre-payment discounts: 6 sessions for the price of 5.

Billing

I will bill your insurance company directly under the following conditions:

Private Health: verbal verification of coverage
Worker's Compensation: verbal verification of coverage

Auto Accident

- PIP: verbal verification of coverage
- Second Party Coverage: written verification of coverage
- Third Party Coverage: health care lien will be filed and/or letter of guarantee signed by the patient's attorney

All insurance accounts not paid in full within 90 days from date of service will be charged interest. Interest rates are 12% annually and are charged at 1% monthly. Interest is calculated on the principal amount; interest is not compounded.

C. Office Policies

Cancellations

Cancellations must be made 24 hours in advance of the scheduled appointment time. If cancellations are not made within 24 hours, payment in full is required. This charge will be waived if a replacement can be found for your appointment time. Your insurance company will not be charged for your missed appointment; you will be responsible for payment out-of-pocket.

Right of Refusal

I reserve the right to refuse service to anyone. This includes but is not limited to anyone who requests treatment or services that are outside my scope of practice. I will exercise this right if anyone arrives for treatment under the influence of alcohol or recreational drugs; I reserve the right to charge for the session time, whether or not services were rendered, if I so choose.

Patient Agreement

I have read the policies stated above and agree to abide by them.

Signature ___Darnel G. Washington_____   Date ___2-6-04_____

John Olson, LMP, GCFP

345 Moon River Rd. Ste. 6
Minnehaha, MN   55987
TEL   612 555 9889

HANDS HEAL

HEALTH INFORMATION

Patient Name __Darnel G. Washington__   Date __2-6-04__

Date of Injury __1-6-04__   ID#/DOB __123-45-6789/4-22-37__

A. Patient Information

Address __1209 Lake Winnetonka Dr.__

City __Minnehaha__   State __MN__ Zip __55987__

Phone: Home __(612) 555-1515__

   Work __N/A__   Cell __555-5511__

Employer __IBM__

Work Address __N/A__

Occupation __retired__

Emergency Contact __Shalonda-wife__

Phone: Home __same__

   Work __N/A__   Cell __555-5511__

Primary Health Care Provider

Name __Sage Redtree, MD__

Address __87 Old Trail Pkwy__

City/State/Zip __Minnehaha MN 55987__

Phone: __555-0009__   Fax __555-9000__

I give my massage therapist permission to
consult with my health care providers
regarding my health and treatment.

Comments _____

Initials __DGW__   Date __2-6-02__

B. Current Health Information

List Health Concerns Check all that apply

Primary __back pain__
☐ mild ☒ moderate ☐ disabling
☒ constant ☐ intermittant
☒ symptoms ↑ w/activity   ☐ ↓ w/activity
☒ getting worse ☐ getting better ☐ no change
treatment received __pain pills, back brace__

Secondary __headaches__
☐ mild ☒ moderate ☐ disabling
☐ constant ☒ intermittant
☒ symptoms ↑ w/activity   ☐ ↓ w/activity
☒ getting worse ☐ getting better ☐ no change
treatment received __pain pills__

Additional __neck stiff__
☒ mild ☐ moderate ☐ disabling
☒ constant ☐ intermittant
☒ symptoms ↑ w/activity   ☐ ↓ w/activity
☐ getting worse ☒ getting better ☐ no change
treatment received __stretching__

List Daily Activities Limited by Condition

Work __N/A__

Home/Family __gardening, vacuuming__

Sleep/Self-care __sleep, exercise__

Social/Recreational __play w/ grandchildren,__
__dancing, bowling, bridge group__

List Self-Care Routines

How do you reduce stress? __watch sports,__
__garden__
Pain? __heat, back brace, meds__

List current medications (include pain relievers
and herbal remedies) _____
__hydrocodone 500 mg every 4 hrs__

Have you ever received massage therapy
before? __no__   Frequency? _____

What are your goals for receiving massage
therapy? __get around easier, less pain__

C. Health History

List and Explain. Include dates and treatment
received.
Surgeries __appendicitis 1949 removed,__
__torn meniseus Ⓛ knee 1980 arthoscopy__

Injuries __bowling injury Ⓡ knee 1979__
__no treatment until surgery 1980__

Major Illnesses __scoliosis 1949__
__Milwaukee brace, exercise, pain meds__

Check All Current and Previous Conditions Please Explain

General

current	past		comments
☒	☐	headaches	_____
☒	☒	pain	_scoliosis_
☒	☐	sleep disturbances	
		can't get comfortable	
☐	☒	fatigue	_scoliosis_
☐	☐	infections	_____
☐	☐	fever	_____
☐	☐	sinus	_____
☐	☐	other	_____

Skin Conditions

current	past		comments
☐	☐	rashes	_____
☐	☐	athlete's foot, warts	_____
☐	☐	other	_____

Muscles and Joints

current	past		comments
☐	☐	rheumatoid arthritis	
☒	☐	osteoarthritis	_____
☐	☐	osteoporosis	_____
☒	☒	scoliosis	_____
☐	☐	broken bones	_____
☐	☐	spinal problems	_____
☐	☐	disk problems	_____
☐	☐	lupus	_____
☐	☐	TMJ, jaw pain	_____
☐	☐	spasms, cramps	
☐	☐	sprains, strains	
☐	☐	tendonitis, bursitis	
☐	☐	stiff or painful joints	_____
☐	☒	weak or sore muscles	
		scoliosis	
☐	☐	neck, shoulder, arm pain	
☒	☒	low back, hip, leg pain	
		MVA, scoliosis	
☐	☐	other	_____

Nervous System

current	past		comments
☐	☐	head injuries, concussions	
☐	☐	dizziness, ringing in ears	
☐	☐	loss of memory, confusion	
☐	☐	numbness, tingling	
☐	☐	sciatica, shooting pain	
☐	☐	chronic pain	_____
☐	☐	depression	_____
☐	☐	other	_____

Respiratory, Cardiovascular

current	past		comments
☐	☐	heart disease	_____
☐	☐	blood clots	_____
☐	☐	stroke	_____
☐	☐	lymphadema	_____
☐	☐	high, low blood pressure	
☐	☐	irregular heart beat	
☐	☐	poor circulation	_____
☐	☐	swollen ankles	_____
☐	☐	varicose veins	_____
☐	☐	chest pain, shortness of breath	_____
☐	☐	asthma	_____

Allergies

current	past		comments
☐	☐	scents, oils, lotions	_____
☐	☐	detergents	_____
☐	☐	other	_____

Digestive/Elimination System

current	past		comments
☐	☐	bowel problems	_____
☐	☐	gas, bloating	_____
☐	☐	bladder/kidney/prostrate	
☐	☐	abdominal pain	_____
☐	☐	other	_____

Endocrine System

current	past		comments
☐	☐	thyroid	_____
☐	☐	diabetes	_____

Reproductive System

current	past		comments
☐	☐	pregnancy	_____
☐	☐	painful, emotional menses	
☐	☐	fibrotic cysts	_____

Cancer/Tumors

current	past		comments
☐	☐	benign	_____
☐	☐	malignant	_____

Habits

current	past		comments
☐	☒	tobacco	_quit chew 30 yrs ago_
☐	☐	alcohol	_____
☐	☐	drugs	_____
☒	☐	coffee, soda	_1-2 cups/day_

Contract for Care

I promise to participate fully as a member of my health care team. I will make sound choices regarding my treatment plan based on the information provided by my manual therapist and other members of my health care team, and my experience of those suggestions. I agree to participate in the self care program we select. I promise to inform my practitioner any time I feel my well-being is threatened or compromised. I expect my manual therapist to provide safe and effective treatment.

Consent for Care

It is my choice to receive manual therapy, and I give my consent to receive treatment. I have reported all health conditions that I am aware of and will inform my practitioner of any changes in my health.

Signature _Darnel G. Washington_   Date _2-6-04_

293

John Olson, LMP, GCFP
345 Moon River Rd. Ste. 6
Minnehaha, MN 55987
Tel 612 555 9889

INJURY INFORMATION

Patient Name __Darnel G. Washington__   Date __2-6-04__

Date of Injury __1-6-04__   Insurance ID# __123-45-6789__

A. General Injury Information

1. How did the accident occur?
   [X] Auto   ☐ On-the-Job   ☐ Other _____

2. Was a police report filed?   [X] Yes   ☐ No
   Was a work incident report filed?
   ☐ Yes   [X] No

3. Describe your injury and how it occurred:
   My nephew was driving. We were slowing down for a yellow light and a truck hit us from behind

4. Describe how you felt during and immediately after the injury:
   fine

   Later that same day: soreness and stiff neck and back after sitting at hockey game, headache
   The next day: headache - pounding, stiff and sore neck and back

   The next week: headache worse, neck stiffness better but back pain worse
   The next month: headache and back pain

   Describe any bruises, cuts, or abrasions as a result of the injury:
   0

5. Are your symptoms ☐ getting better
   [X] getting worse   ☐ no change
   What makes them better? _____
   nothing yet

   Worse? sitting, lifting grandkids, pushing them in swing, bending over in garden

6. Did you return to work on the day of the injury? ☐ Yes   ☐ No
   Have you lost time from work since the injury? ☐ Yes   ☐ No

7. What are your work responsibilities?
   N/A
   Which work activities are affected by this injury? _____

   Have your work responsibilities changed as a result of this injury?   ☐ Yes   ☐ No
   Explain _____
   What other daily activities are affected by this injury? _____

8. Did you go to the emergency room?
   ☐ Yes   [X] No
   Were you hospitalized?   ☐ Yes   [X] No
   List the health care providers who have treated you for this injury, the type of treatment provided, and their diagnosis.
   Dr. Redtree—pain pills, back support, stretching exercises, says I have mild whiplash and a reoccurance of scolios

9. Have you ever had this type of injury before? [X] Yes   ☐ No
   Explain I've had scoliosis most of my life.

   Did you have any physical complaints before the injury? ☐ Yes   [X] No
   Explain My scoliosis wasn't bothering me at all
   Do you have any illnesses or previous injuries that may have been affected by this injury? [X] Yes   ☐ No
   Explain just the scoliosis

Signature __Darnel G. Washington__   Date __2-6-01__

HANDS HEAL

John Olson, LMP, GCFP
345 Moon River Rd. Ste. 6
Minnehaha, MN   55987
Tᴇʟ   612 555 9889

B. Motor Vehicle Accident Information

1. Did the police arrive at the accident?
   ☒ Yes   ☐ No

2. How was your vehicle hit?
   ☒ Rear end   ☐ Head on   ☐ Side swipe
   OR Did your vehicle hit another vehicle/object?
   ☐ Rear end   ☐ Head on   ☐ Side swipe
   If you were hit from behind, was your vehicle pushed forward upon impact?
   ☒ Yes   ☐ No   If yes, how much?
   about 50 feet
   Did your vehicle hit anything else after the initial impact?   ☐ Yes   ☐ No
   Explain _____
   _____
   _____
   _____

3. Were you at a stop or moving at the time of impact?   ☐ Stopped   ☒ Moving
   If you were stopped, was your foot on the brake?   ☐ Yes   ☐ No
   If you were moving, were you:
   ☐ Increasing speed
   ☒ Decreasing speed
   ☐ Traveling at a steady speed
   Was the other vehicle moving at the time of impact?   ☒ Yes   ☐ No
   If yes, was it: ☒ Increasing speed
   ☐ Decreasing speed   ☐ Traveling at a steady speed

4. Where were you seated in the vehicle?
   passenger side-front seat
   _____

5. Which way was your head facing upon impact?
   facing nephew-driver, we were talking
   _____

6. Were you aware of the approaching vehicle or did the impact catch you by surprise?
   ☐ Aware   ☒ Surprise

7. Did you lose consciousness?
   ☐ Yes   ☒ No

8. Were you wearing a seat belt?   ☐ No
   ☐ Lap belt   ☐ Shoulder harness   ☒ Both

9. Is your vehicle equipped with an airbag?
   ☐ Yes ☒ No
   Did it activate?   ☐ Yes   ☐ No

10. Is the top of your head rest:
    ☐ Above your head   ☒ Below your head
    Does your head touch the head rest?
    ☐ Yes   ☒ No
    If no, how far in front of the head rest is your head?
    a few inches

11. What were the road conditions?
    ☐ Wet   ☐ Dry   ☒ Icy   ☐ Oily

12. What type of vehicle were you in? (make, model, year)
    '82 Honda Accord
    What type of vehicle hit you? (make, model, year)
    '91 Ford F250 Truck

13. Did any part of your body come into contact with the vehicle?   ☐ Yes   ☒ No
    Explain _____
    _____
    _____
    Did any parts of the vehicle break?
    ☒ Yes   ☐ No
    Explain _fender damage_____
    _____
    _____

14. Check all of the following symptoms that you have experienced since the accident:
    ☐ Loss of memory _____
    ☐ Loss of balance_____
    ☒ Visual disturbances _eye strain_____
    ☐ Hearing difficulties _____
    ☒ Difficulty breathing _tight & painful_
    ☒ Sleep disturbances _pain keeps me up_

15. Anything else you want to tell me about the accident or how you feel?
    _____
    _____
    _____

Patient Signature _Darnel G. Washington_____   Date _2-6-04_____

295

HANDS HEAL

John Olson, LMP, GCFP
345 Moon River Rd. Ste. 6
Minnehaha, MN   55987
Tel   612 555 9889

BILLING INFORMATION

Patient Name _Darnel G. Washington_   Date _02-16-04_

Date of Injury _01-06-04_   ID#/DOB _123-45-6789_

Billing Policy

Our office is set up to receive direct payment from insurance companies. For the best chance of reimbursement from your insurance carrier, <u>we ask that you</u>:

• Contact your insurance company to determine your manual therapy coverage and provider stipulations. Coverage depends on your insurance company and the specific plan you have chosen. We have provided a list of questions for you to ask your insurance representative or attorney that will help determine your eligibility for our billing service.

• You will need a current prescription for manual therapy from a primary health care provider, such as a physician or a chiropractor in order to submit your claim. Referrals are current for 90 days unless otherwise specified.

    It is important that you understand your insurance policies in order for you to budget for your manual therapy services. You are personally responsible for all charges incurred in our office. We expect payment in full until your insurance coverage has been verified.

    We realize that the completion of this form is an added burden to you as a consumer, and we thank you very much for your assistance. This completed form will provide both you and our billing department with important information regarding your manual therapy insurance benefits, and enable us to process your claim in a timely fashion.

Patient Information

Is patient's condition related to:

☒ auto collsion—In what state? _MN_
☐ other accident _____
☐ employment ☐ illness

Patient status: ☒ male ☐ female
☐ single ☒ married/partnered ☐ other

Patient relationship to insured
☐ self ☐ spouse/partner ☐ child ☒ other

Insured's Information (if other than patient)

Name _James Washington_
Address _33 W. Holden Court_
City _Minnehaha_   State _MN_ Zip _55987_
Phone: _612-555-7654_
Date of birth _5-31-60_
Sex: ☒ Male ☐ Female
Employer's Name or School Name _____
Maad Printing and Design

Insurance Information

Insurance plan name or program name: _Farmington States_

Member ID#: _989-76-6789_   Group #: _____

Customer service phone #: _612-555-7887_   Date and time you called: _2-15-04   2:15 pm_

Name of customer service representative: _Clifford Glens_

Insurance claim address: _PO Box 3778 O'Claire_   State: _MN_   Zip: _55978_

Does the plan include a Physical Medicine and Rehabilitation benefit? ☒ Yes ☐ No

Who may provide the services? ☒ Massage Therapist ☐ Physical Therapist ☐ Other

Is pre-authorization required? ☐ Yes ☒ No   Who can authorize the services? _N/A_

Is a prescription required? ☒ Yes ☐ No   Is a referral required? ☐ Yes ☒ No

Who may refer? ☒ MD ☒ DC ☐ ND ☐ PT ☐ Other _____

How often does the referral need to be updated to ensure continuous coverage? _____

Is there a Preferred Provider list for Manual Therapists? ☐ Yes ☒ No

Is _____ on the list? ☐ Yes ☐ No

HANDS HEAL

John Olson, LMP, GCFP

345 Moon River Rd. Ste. 6
Minnehaha, MN   55987
TEL   612 555 9889

BILLING INFORMATION page 2

If this is a Workers' Compensation Claim, please fill out the following information:

Who is the attending HCP? _____ Phone: _____

Claim number: _____ Date eligibility began: _____

Number of visits authorized: _____ Number of visits remaining: _____

Dates of coverage: _____ Date claim closed: _____

If this is a Personal Injury Claim, please fill out the following information:

PIP policy amount: _30 K___ Dates of coverage: _1-6-04 to 05_ PIP available: ___30 K___

MedPay amount: __10 K___ Dates of coverage: _1-6-04 to 05_ MedPay available: _10 K_

Liability amount: _____ Dates of coverage: _____ Liability available: _____

Uninsured/Underinsured (UMI) policy amount: _____ UMI available: _____

Has the PIP application been received? ☒ Yes ☐ No

Has an attorney been consulted? ☒ Yes ☐ No   Retained? ☒ Yes ☐ No

Name/Firm _B. Charma Storro, JD_____

Address ___5 Hive Lane_____ City _Minnehaha_____ State _MN__ Zip _55987_

Phone ___612-555-2337_____ Fax _612-555-7332_____

If this is a Private Health Insurance Claim, please fill out the following information:
(Or, if your Personal Injury claim defaults to secondary coverage, fill this out)

Maximum allowable benefit for Physical Medicine/Rehabilitation: _____

In network: $_____ # visits _____ Remaining $_____ # visits _____

Deductible: $_____ Satisifed to date: $_____ Co-Pay: $_____

Out-of-network: $_____ # visits _____ Remaining $_____ # visits _____

Deductible: $_____ Satisifed to date: $_____ Co-Insurance: $_____

Are these limits just for manual therapy? ☐ Yes ☐ No

If no, what other types of treatment do they include? _____
(i.e., chiropractic, physical therapy, occupational therapy, naturopathy, etc.)

Assignment of Benefits

My signature below authorizes and directs payment of medical benefits for services billed to my health care provider: _John Olson_____

Release of Medical Records

My signature below authorizes the release of my medical records including intake forms, chart notes, reports, and billing statements to my attorneys, health care providers, and insurance case managers, for the purpose of processing my claims. (I will inform my practitioner immediately upon signing any exclusive Release of Medical Records with my attorney.)

Financial Responsibility

It is my responsibility to pay for all services provided. In the event that my insurance company denies payment or makes a partial payment, I agree to be and remain responsible for the balance. It is also my understanding and agreement that if you have contracted with my insurance company at a discount rate and the agreed-upon fee has been satisfied, the balance owed on those specific visits will be waived.

Signature _Darnel G. Washington_____ Date _2-16-04_____

John Olson, LMP, GCFP

345 Moon River Rd. Ste. 6
Minnehaha, MN   55987
TEL   612 555 9889

PRESCRIPTION

Patient Name __Darnel G. Washington__   Date __2-30-04__

Date of Injury __1-6-04__   ID#/DOB __123-45-6789__

A. Diagnosis

(Include ICD-9 codes that specifically
address Manual Therapy Treatment)

Scoliosis   754.2

Spasm   728.85

Neck Pain   723.1

Thoracic Pain   724.1

Condition is related to

X Auto Accident
☐ Work Injury
☐ Illness
X Other: __concomittant scoliosis recurrance__

B. Medically Necessary Treatment: Implement Plan as Prescribed Below

Application (Primary & Secondary)

☐ Head __whiplash__
☐ Neck __whiplash__
☐ Chest __scoliosis__
☐ Shoulders __2°—as needed__
☐ Abdomen __2°—as needed__
☐ Back __scoliosis__
☐ Lowback/Hips __whiplash__
☐ Upper extremities __2°—as needed__
☐ Lower extremities __2°—as needed__
X All of the above _____
☐ Other: _____

Frequency & Duration

X 1× wk for __6__ wks
☐ 2× wk for _____ wks
☐ 3× wk for _____ wks
☐ 2× month for _____ months
☐ 1× month for _____ months

Specific Instructions/Precautions:
__as needed__

Treatment Type

X Manual Therapy _____
X Hot/Cold Packs _____
X Self-Care/Exercises _____
☐ Other _____

Treatment Goals

☐ Decrease Pain
☐ Decrease Inflammation
☐ Decrease Muscle Tension/Spasms
☐ Decrease Compensatory Patterns
☐ Increase Mobility
☐ Increase Strength
☐ Restore Function
☐ Restore Posture
☐ Patient Education
X All of the Above
☐ Other _____

C. Referring Health Care Provider (HCP)

Contact Information
HCP Name __Sage Redtree MD__
Address __87 Old Trail PKWY__
City __Minnehaha__   State __MN__ Zip __55987__
Phone __555-0009__
Fax __555-9000__
Email _____

Reporting—I will send an initial report after
the first visit and a progress report after
every 6–8 sessions. Please check how you
would like to receive this information:
X Fax ☐ Mail ☐ Email
X Send Copies of Chart Notes with each report

HCP Signature: __Sage Redtree MD__   Date __2-30-04__

Revised and reprinted with permission, Adler ♦ Giersch, PS

298

John Olson, LMP, GCFP

345 Moon River Rd. Ste. 6
Minnehaha, MN   55987
Tel   612 555 9889

HEALTH REPORT

Patient Name _Darnel G. Washington_   Date _2-6-04_

Date of Injury _1-6-04_   ID#/DOB _123-45-6789/4-22-37_

A. Draw today's symptoms on the figures.

1. Identify CURRENT symptomatic areas in your body by marking letters on the figures below.
   Use the letters provided in the key to identify the symptoms you are feeling today.
2. Circle the area around each letter, representing the size and shape of each symptom location.

Key
P = pain or tenderness
S = joint or muscle stiffness
N = numbness or tingling

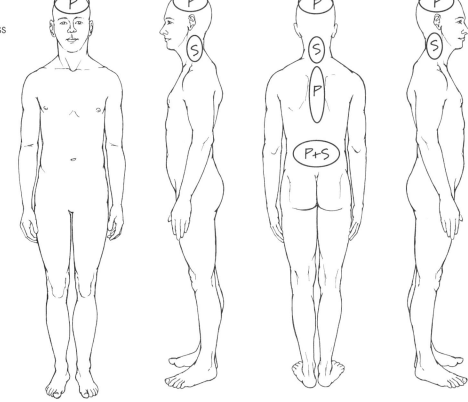

B. Identify the intensity of your symptoms.

1. Pain Scale: Mark a line on the scale to show the amount of pain you are experiencing today.

   No Pain ├────────────────┼────────────────┤ Unbearable Pain   (5.5)

2. Activities Scale: Mark a line on the scale to show the limitations you are experiencing today   (5.5)
   in your daily activities.

   Can Do Anything I Want ├────────────────┼────────────────┤ Cannot Do Anything

C. Comments

_____

_____

_____

_____

Signature _Darnel G. Washington_   Date _2-6-04_

299

LOW BACK PAIN & DISABILITY INDEX

Provider Name _John Olson LMT GCFP_

Patient Name _Darnel G. Washington_   Date _2-6-04_

Date of Injury _1-6-04_   ID#/DOB _123-45-6789_

This questionnaire has been designed to give the health care provider information about how your back pain has affected your ability to manage everyday life. Please answer every section and mark in each section only the **ONE** box which applies to you. We realize you may consider that two statements in any one section relate to you, but please just mark the box which most closely describes your problem today.

Section 1 - Pain Intensity
- ☐ The pain comes and goes and is mild.
- ☐ The pain is mild and does not vary much.
- ☐ The pain comes and goes and is moderate.
- 3 ☒ The pain is moderate and does not vary much.
- ☐ The pain comes and goes and is severe.
- ☐ The pain is severe and does not vary much.

Section 2 - Personal Care
- ☐ I can look after myself normally without causing pain.
- ☐ I can look after myself normally but it causes extra pain.
- 2 ☒ It is painful to look after myself and I am slow and careful.
- ☐ I need some help but manage most of my personal care.
- ☐ I need help every day in most aspects of self care.
- ☐ I do not get dressed, I wash myself with difficulty, and I stay in bed.

Section 3 - Lifting
- ☐ I can lift heavy weights without extra pain.
- ☐ I can lift heavy weights but it causes extra pain.
- ☐ Pain prevents me from lifting heavy weights off the floor, but I can manage if they are conveniently positioned, e.g. on a table.
- 3 ☒ Pain prevents me from lifting heavy weights, but I can manage light to medium weights if they are conveniently positioned.
- ☐ I can lift very light weights.
- ☐ I cannot lift or carry anything at all.

Section 4 - Walking
- ☐ I have no pain on walking.
- ☐ I have some pain on walking but it does not increase with distance.
- 2 ☒ I cannot walk more than 1 mile without increasing pain.
- ☐ I cannot walk more than 1/2 mile without increasing pain.
- ☐ I cannot walk more than 1/4 mile without increasing pain.
- ☐ I cannot walk at all without increasing pain.

Section 5 - Sitting
- ☐ I can sit in any chair as long as I like.
- ☐ I can only sit in my favorite chair as long as I like.
- ☐ Pain prevents me from sitting more than 1 hour.
- 3 ☒ Pain prevents me from sitting more than 1/2 hour.
- ☐ Pain prevents me from sitting more than 10 minutes.
- ☐ I avoid sitting because it increases my pain straight away.

Section 6 - Standing
- ☐ I can stand as long as I want without pain.
- ☐ I have some pain on standing but it does not increase with time.
- 2 ☒ I cannot stand for longer than 1 hour without increasing pain.
- ☐ I cannot stand for longer than 1/2 hour without increasing pain.
- ☐ I cannot stand for longer than 10 minutes without increasing pain.
- ☐ I avoid standing because it increases the pain straight away.

Section 7 - Sleeping
- ☐ I have no trouble sleeping.
- ☐ My sleep is slightly disturbed (less than 1 hour sleepless).
- ☐ My sleep is mildly disturbed (1–2 hours sleepless).
- 3 ☒ My sleep is moderately disturbed (2–3 hours sleepless).
- ☐ My sleep is greatly disturbed (3–5 hours sleepless).
- ☐ My sleep is completely disturbed (5–7 hours sleepless).

Section 8 - Social Life
- ☐ My social life is normal and gives me no pain.
- ☐ My social life is normal but increases the degree of pain.
- 2 ☒ Pain has no significant effect on my social life apart from limiting my more energetic interests, e.g. dancing, etc.
- ☐ Pain has restricted my social life and I do not go out very often.
- ☐ Pain has restricted my social life to my home.
- ☐ I hardly have any social life because of the pain.

Section 9 - Traveling
- ☐ I get no pain while traveling.
- ☐ I get some pain while traveling but none of my usual forms of travel make it any worse.
- 2 ☒ I get extra pain while traveling but it does not compel me to seek alternate forms of travel.
- ☐ I get extra pain while traveling which compels me to seek alternative forms of travel.
- ☐ Pain restricts all forms of travel.
- ☐ Pain prevents all forms of travel except that done lying down.

Section 10 - Changing Degree of Pain
- ☐ My pain is rapidly getting better.
- ☐ My pain fluctuates but overall is definitely getting better.
- 4 ☐ My pain seems to be getting better but improvement is slow at present.
- ☐ My pain is neither getting better nor getting worse.
- ☒ My pain is gradually worsening.
- ☐ My pain is rapidly worsening.

$$\frac{26}{52\%} \times 2$$

Signature _Darnel G. Washington_   Date _2-6-04_

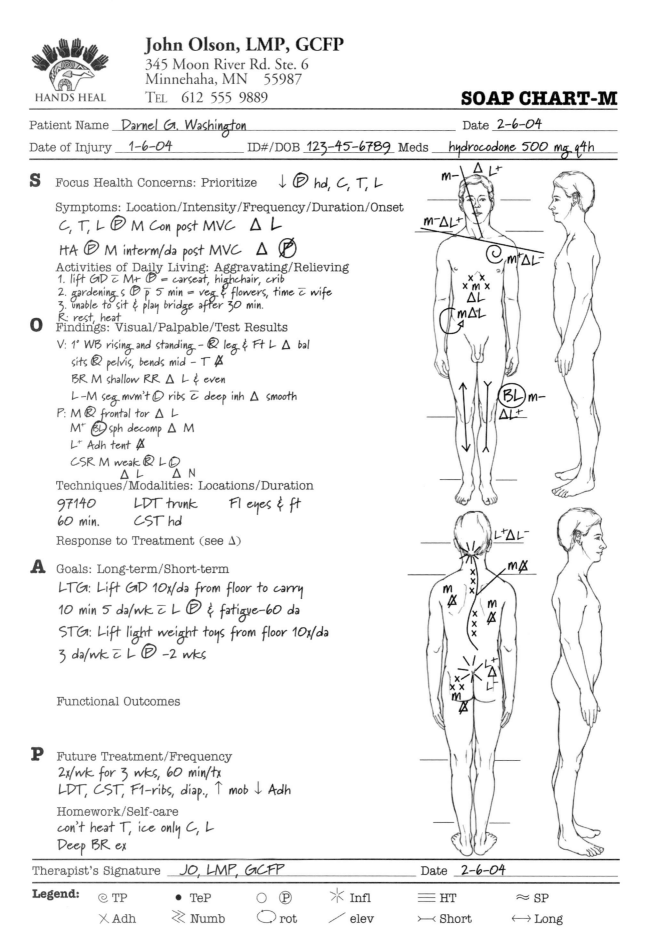

John Olson, LMP, GCFP
345 Moon River Rd. Ste. 6
Minnehaha, MN   55987
TEL   612 555 9889

HANDS HEAL

SOAP CHART-M

Patient Name _Darnel G. Washington_   Date _2-6-04_

Date of Injury _1-6-04_   ID#/DOB _123-45-6789_ Meds _hydrocodone 500 mg q4h_

S Focus Health Concerns: Prioritize   ↓ Ⓟ hd, C, T, L

Symptoms: Location/Intensity/Frequency/Duration/Onset

C, T, L Ⓟ M Con post MVC Δ L

HA Ⓟ M interm/da post MVC Δ Ⓟ

Activities of Daily Living: Aggravating/Relieving
1. lift GD c̄ M+ Ⓟ = carseat, highchair, crib
2. gardening s Ⓟ p̄ 5 min = veg & flowers, time c̄ wife
3. unable to sit & play bridge after 30 min.
R: rest, heat

O Findings: Visual/Palpable/Test Results

V: 1° WB rising and standing - Ⓡ leg & Ft L Δ bal

sits Ⓡ pelvis, bends mid - T ⍉

BR M shallow RR Δ L & even

L-M seg mvm't Ⓛ ribs c̄ deep inh Δ smooth

P: M Ⓡ frontal tor Δ L

M⁺ ⒝Ⓛ sph decomp Δ M

L⁺ Adh tent ⍉

CSR M weak Ⓡ L Ⓛ
    Δ L   Δ N

Techniques/Modalities: Locations/Duration

97140   LDT trunk   Fl eyes & ft
60 min.   CST hd

Response to Treatment (see Δ)

A Goals: Long-term/Short-term

LTG: Lift GD 10x/da from floor to carry

10 min 5 da/wk c̄ L Ⓟ & fatigue-60 da

STG: Lift light weight toys from floor 10x/da

3 da/wk c̄ L Ⓟ -2 wks

Functional Outcomes

P Future Treatment/Frequency
2x/wk for 3 wks, 60 min/tx
LDT, CST, F1-ribs, diap., ↑ mob ↓ Adh

Homework/Self-care
con't heat T, ice only C, L
Deep BR ex

Therapist's Signature _JO, LMP, GCFP_   Date _2-6-04_

Legend: ⓒ TP   • TeP   ○ Ⓟ   ✳ Infl   ≡ HT   ≈ SP

✕ Adh   ≋ Numb   ⬭ rot   ╱ elev   ⤝ Short   ⟷ Long

301

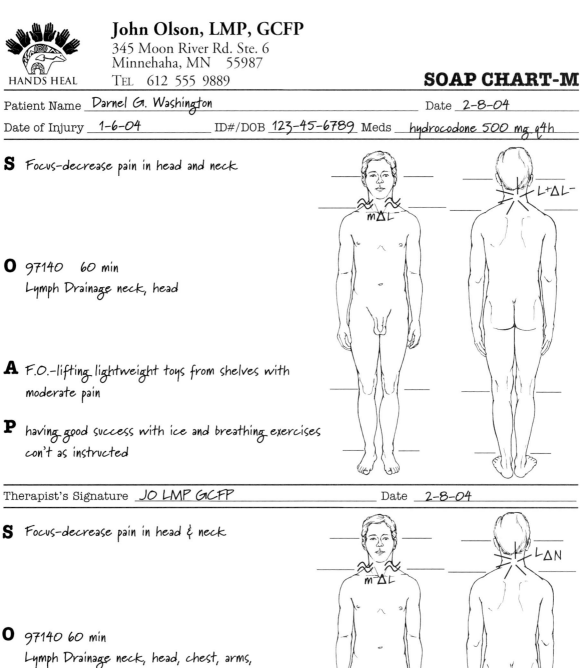

John Olson, LMP, GCFP
345 Moon River Rd. Ste. 6
Minnehaha, MN   55987
TEL   612 555 9889

HANDS HEAL

SOAP CHART-M

Patient Name   _Darnel G. Washington_   Date _2-8-04_

Date of Injury _1-6-04_   ID#/DOB _123-45-6789_ Meds   _hydrocodone 500 mg q4h_

S Focus-decrease pain in head and neck

O 97140   60 min
Lymph Drainage neck, head

A F.O.-lifting lightweight toys from shelves with
moderate pain

P having good success with ice and breathing exercises
con't as instructed

Therapist's Signature   _JO LMP GCFP_   Date   _2-8-04_

S Focus-decrease pain in head & neck

O 97140 60 min
Lymph Drainage neck, head, chest, arms,
all passive cervical ranges of motion limited-mild
minus-with mild pain at end ranges Δ N
with L⁻ pain
A con't

P con't

Therapist's Signature   _JO LMP GCFP_   Date   _2-11-04_

Legend:
| ℰ TP | ● TeP | ○ ℗ | ✳ Infl | ≡ HT | ≈ SP |
| ✕ Adh | ≋ Numb | ↻ rot | ╱ elev | ⊱ Short | ↔ Long |

302

John Olson, LMP, GCFP

345 Moon River Rd. Ste. 6
Minnehaha, MN   55987
T℮ʟ   612 555 9889

HANDS HEAL

Dr. Sage Redtree
87 Old Trail Parkway
Minnehaha, MN 55987

Client: Darnel G. Washington
DOI: 1-6-04
Insurance ID #: 123-45-6789

3-8-04

Dear Dr. Redtree:

Thank you for the referral of Mr. Washington. We have had six treatments in the last 30 days. In this time he has reached his initial short-term goal of being able to lift lightweight toys from the floor up to a high shelf at least 10 times a day, three days a week—on the days that he takes care of his granddaughter—with no more than mild pain in his back. We have also resolved the inflammation in his neck and reduced his headaches to mild and infrequent.

Mr. Washington has yet to accomplish his long-term goal of lifting his granddaughter at least 10 times a day and carrying her at least 10 minutes twice a day during the three days a week he cares for her. To support him in accomplishing this goal, I would like to continue to see Mr. Washington twice per week for one hour sessions of Manual Lymphatic Drainage, CranioSacral Therapy, and Feldenkrais. My goals are to reduce the scar tissue and muscle spasms in his neck and back and improve the mobility of his ribs, neck, and shoulders. Mr. Washington will continue to use alternating heat and ice packs on his neck and back as per the handouts and instructions I have provided, and he is diligent about doing the breathing exercises as instructed.

Please let me know by fax if this treatment plan is acceptable to you.

I am aware that Mr. Washington has a history of scoliosis, and I have asked him to schedule an appointment with you for an evaluation of that condition. I am concerned that it may interfere with his progress.

Sincerely,
John Olson, LMP, GCFP

John Olson, LMP, GCFP
345 Moon River Rd. Ste. 6
Minnehaha, MN   55987
TEL   612 555 9889

HANDS HEAL

SOAP CHART—M

Patient Name _Darnel G. Washington_   Date _2-11-05_

Date of Injury _1-6-04_   ID#/DOB _123-45-6789_ Meds _Ø_

S   Focus for Today   ↓ stiff back

Symptoms: Location/Intensity/Frequency/Duration/Onset

Stiff T L cons, 4 da-bridge marathon 2-7—05
Δ WNL

Activities of Daily Living: Aggravating/Relieving

A: carrying GD ↑ 10 min, sit or garden ↑ 2 hrs = ↑ ℗ M
R: ex, stretch, rest

O   Findings: Visual/Palpable/Test Results

M weak c̄ sit Δ L
mvm't T vs hip
rib mob M ↓   BR L ↓ Δ N
Δ L

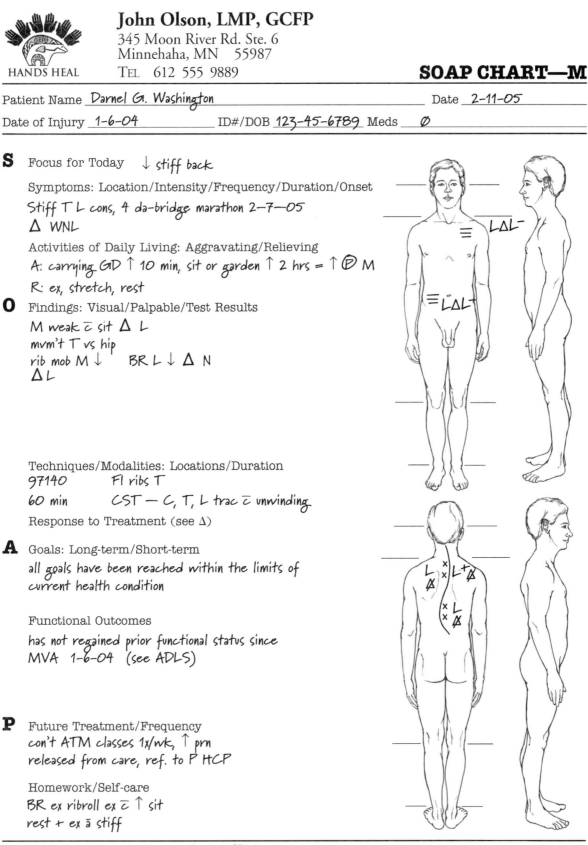

Techniques/Modalities: Locations/Duration
97140   Fl ribs T
60 min   CST — C, T, L trac c̄ unwinding

Response to Treatment (see Δ)

A   Goals: Long-term/Short-term

all goals have been reached within the limits of
current health condition

Functional Outcomes

has not regained prior functional status since
MVA 1-6-04   (see ADLS)

P   Future Treatment/Frequency
con't ATM classes 1x/wk, ↑ prn
released from care, ref. to P HCP

Homework/Self-care
BR ex ribroll ex c̄ ↑ sit
rest + ex ā stiff

Therapist's Signature _JO LMP, GCFP_   Date _2-11-05_

Legend:

℮ TP	• TeP	○ ℗	⋇ Infl	≡ HT	≈ SP
✕ Adh	≳ Numb	⟲ rot	∕ elev	⊱ Short	⟷ Long

HANDS HEAL

John Olson, LMP, GCFP

345 Moon River Rd. Ste. 6
Minnehaha, MN   55987

Tel   612 555 9889   •   Fax   612 555 9887   •   Email   olsen@email.com

January 20, 2005

Patient: Darnel G. Washington

DOI: 1-6-04

Claim Number: 123-45-6789

Date of Exam: 1-20-05

Mr. Washington was first seen in my office on 2-6-04 for manual therapy treatment to injuries sustained in a motor vehicle accident on 1-6-04. He was referred by Dr. Sage Redtree, MD, with an initial diagnosis of spinal sprain-strain in the neck, mid-back and low back areas, and headaches. Within 2 months of the accident, Dr. Redtree diagnosed Mr. Washington with a flare-up of scoliosis with accelerated spinal degeneration.

Mr. Washington stated: he was a passenger in a Honda Accord and was rear-ended by a Ford F250 pick-up truck. The Honda was stopping for a yellow light, and the Ford was speeding up to go through the intersection. It was a cold and snowy January afternoon and the roads were slick. The car was pushed across the intersection but did not come in contact with any other vehicles or objects. Mr. Washington was turned to his left in his seat to chat with the driver at the time of impact. His head was thrown from side to side.

Initial Subjective Data:

On 2-6-04, Mr. Washington complained of mild neck pain and stiffness, moderate mid-back pain and stiffness, mild low back stiffness, and a moderate headache. The symptoms were constant since the evening of the accident, and increased in severity with all attempts to to lift his granddaughter, garden with his wife, or sit for over 30 minutes playing bridge with the club he presides over.

Initial Objective Findings:

I palpated moderate muscle spasms in the right sternocleidomastoid and scalene muscles, left trapezius and rhomboids, and right quadratus lumborum. Trigger points were elicited with light digital pressure in the paraspinal muscles, intercostals, and diaphragm. Muscle tension was mild to moderate throughout the spinal postural muscles. Cervical range of motion was moderately limited with active flexion and extension, and passive lateral flexion bilateraly. Inflammation was palpable in the cervical and thoracic regions: redness, heat, swelling, and loss of function; pain and inflammation seemed to be preventing full range of motion. Mr. Washington's posture showed a moderate left shoulder elevation with internal rotation, mild right hip elevation, mild "hump" or kyphosis in the mid-back, mild curvature of the thoracic spine, and a mild forward head position. He was weight-bearing moderately more on the right, his leg swing mildly closed on the right and arm swing moderately closed on the left when I observed his gait.

Initial Functional Goals:

Mr. Washington is the primary caregiver for his granddaughter during the day. Because of her age, he needed to pick her up to put her into the high chair at meals, and into the car seat, and to put her to bed at nap time. At the beginning of treatment, he was unable to lift or carry her because of pain and stiffness. His initial goal was to be able to lift her 10 times a day with mild pain and fatigue.

After the scoliosis flared up, his activity level dropped considerably. Simple activities such as getting dressed and driving a car became too painful without assistance or frequent rest periods. His goal was to wash himself, dress himself, and walk around the block every day.

A year later, he was able to accomplish his initial goal.

Current Subjective Data:

Mr. Washington has infrequent and mild episodes of pain and stiffness with mild activity, which increase to moderate episodes of pain and stiffness lasting for several hours if he exceeds the following: 5 minutes of carrying his granddaughter, 1 hour of gardening, and 2 hours of sitting.

Current Objective Data:

Mr. Washington's kyphosis and spinal curvature are more pronounced than they were initially. The muscles around the scoliosis are constantly and moderately tight. His muscles in the mid-back area spasm only with activities in excess of the limitations described above, the rest of the spasms have resolved. The trigger points have resolved except around the scoliosis, the headaches are gone, and his cervical range of motion is normal. His gait is excellent and his posture is compromised only by the scoliosis.

Treatment:

Initially, I used full body lymphatic drainage techniques to reduce the swelling and pain, increase mobility, and strengthen the immune system. Soon I began incorporating movement re-education techniques to find ways that allowed Mr. Washington to move and perform daily activities, such as sitting, standing, and lifting, with more comfort and ease. Initially, the treatment frequency was weekly, increasing to bi-weekly with the exacerbation of scoliosis. After one year of treatment, the frequency returned to weekly, then bimonthly as progress permitted. There was one gap in treatment, due to an extended vacation, during which time Mr. Washington increased his self-care activities.

Progress Summary:

Within six sessions, the neck pain and stiffness, headaches, and low back stiffness were infrequent and mild. Unfortunately, the mid-back pain and stiffness worsened for several months and were debilitating. After several months, the treatments slowly and steadily diminished the pain and increased Mr. Washington's ability to return to a modified level of activity, but it was more than a year before Mr. Washington's scoliosis stabilized and he could return to his normal activities.

Mr. Washington is able to lift his granddaughter as needed, but can carry her for only 5 minutes at a time. He is able to garden for up to 1 hour, and can sit at a bridge table for 2 hours, after which time the pain kicks in.

Patient Status:

Mr. Washington participates in a daily stretching and strengthening routine, and comes in monthly for group movement classes to maintain his daily activity level. We have attempted to discontinue his treatments and rely solely on his self-care routine; however, after 45–50 days without treatment, his ability to function is compromised and his pain increases to moderate and frequent.

In summary, Mr. Washington responded positively to treatments and adapted to a higher level of self-care responsibilities. Please call if you have questions.

Yours in health,

John Olson, LMP, GCFP

306

PATIENT'S RELEASE OF HEALTH CARE INFORMATION

Patient's Name _Darnel G. Washington_

Social Security Number _123-45-6789_ Date of Birth _4-22-37_

I hereby instruct my providers to provide full and complete information to _B. Charma Storro, JD_ and to accept this authorization form and release the protected information requested without requiring any additional authorizations. I specifically waive any "minimally necessary" limitations of HIPAA.

Health Care Provider/Facility _John Olson, LMP, GCFP_

is hereby authorized to release health care information, including intake forms, chart notes, reports, correspondence, billing statements, and other written information to my attorneys, employees, and designated agents of my attorneys, to wit:

Attorney's Name _B. Charma Storro, JD_ Phone _(612) 555-2337_

Address _5 Hive Lane_

City _Minnehaha_ State _MN_ Zip _55987_

This request and authorization applies to:

_✓_ Health care information relating to the following treatment, condition, or dates of treatment: _MVC 1-6-04_

____ All health care information:

____ Other: _____

How the Information will be used: Said information shall be used for any and all purposes for _B. Charma Storro, JD_ to pursue payment of care expenses and in providing legal services to me in conjunction with my case. Following said disclosure the information may no longer be subject to HIPAA protection, as it may be subject to re-disclosure that is unprotected absent specific laws protecting specific sensitive information.

Revocation of Prior Authorization: All medical authorizations by the patient or patient's authorized representatives given before the date of this release for any reason whatsoever are hereby revoked.

Unlawful Disclosure Prohibited: State and Federal prohibits any health care provider from releasing any health care information about a patient to another person without the consent of the patient. You are requested to disclose no such information to any insurance adjuster or any other person without written authority from me which is printed on the letterhead of my attorny.

Effect of Photocopy: A photocopy of this release shall have the same force and effect as a signed original.

Authorization expires 90 days from date of signature. Thereafter, no authorization exists unless an updated release is provided by: _B. Charma Storro, JD_

I understand that I have the right to revoke this release for any information not yet provided to _B. Charma Storro, JD_ by providing notice of revocation in writing to the above named care provider. I also understand that I have the right to refuse to authorize disclosure at all.

Darnel G. Washington _2-15-05_

Signature of Patient or Patient's Authorized Representative Date

John Olson, LMP, GCFP

345 Moon River Rd. Ste. 6
Minnehaha, MN   55987
Tel   612 555 9889

HANDS HEAL

INSURANCE STATUS—
PERSONAL INJURY

Patient Name _Darnel G. Washington_ Date _2-15-04_

Date of Injury _1-6-04_ ID#/DOB _123-45-6789_

A. Reporting to Attorney

Which information would you like to receive monthly and how do you prefer to receive information:

☒ copies of billing ☐ fax
☐ monthly statements ☒ mail
☒ SOAP charts ☐ email
☒ Progress reports ☒ upon request

B. Primary Insurance Coverage   Effective dates: from _1-6-04_ to _1-6-05_

Please provide the following information regarding your client's/my patient's insurance status:
Insured _James Washington_
Insurance ID# _989-76-6789_
Insurance Carrier _Farmington States_
Billing Address _PO Box 5778_
City _O'Claire_ State _MN_ Zip _55978_
Adjuster _Clifford Glens_
Phone _612-555-7887_ Fax _612-555-8778_
PIP policy amount $ _30,000_
Dates of coverage _____
PIP available $ _28,000_
Med Pay policy amount $ _10,000_
Dates of coverage _1-6-04 to 1-6-05_
Med Pay available $ _10,000_

C. Secondary Insurance Coverage   ☐ N/A   ☒ Effective date: _1-6-05_

Insured _Darnel G. Washington_
Insurance ID# _123-45-6789_
Insurance Carrier _Allied_
Billing Address _PO Box 2988_
City _Omaha_ State _NE_ Zip _68144_
Adjuster _Jarma Jones_
Phone _402-555-1991_ Fax _402-555-9119_
PIP policy amount $ _N/A Private Health Plan_
Dates of coverage _____
PIP available $ _____
Med Pay policy amount $ _____
Dates of coverage _____
Med Pay available $ _____
If secondary coverage is through the patients' private health insurance, is manual therapy a
covered benefit: ☐ Yes   ☐ No   ☒ Don't Know

D. Third Party Insurance Coverage   ☐ N/A   ☐ Effective date: _____

Insured _Peter O'Malley_
Insurance ID# _987-63-4321_
Insurance Carrier _Safe Hands_
Billing Address _PO Box 4321_
City _St. Petersburg_ State _MD_ Zip _10111_
Adjuster _David Davies_
Phone _512-555-7733_ Fax _512-555-7337_
Liability policy amount $ _100,000_
Dates of coverage _1-6-04 to 1-6-07_
Liability available $ _100,000_
Uninsured/underinsured Motorist (UIM)$ _____
Policy Amount $ _____
UIM available $ _____

308

CONTRACTUAL GUARANTEE OF PAYMENT FOR MEDICAL SERVICES

I hereby authorize and direct you, my attorney, to pay directly to my health care provider(s), ___John Olson___, the total dollar amount owing for health care services, including applicable interest charges, provided for injuries arising from the motor vehicle accident on ___1-6-04___. I hereby authorize my attorney and the involved insurance companies to withhold sums from any settlement, judgment, or verdict as may be necessary to adequately protect my health care provider(s) and their office. I hereby further consent to a lien being filed on my case by said health care provider(s) and their office against any and all proceeds of my settlement, judgment, or verdict which may be paid to you, my attorney, or myself as the result of the injuries for which I have been treated.

I agree never to rescind this document and that any attempt at recession will not be honored by my attorney. I hereby instruct that in the event another attorney is substituted in this matter, the new attorney shall honor this Contractual Guarantee of Payment for Health Care Services as inherent in the settlement and enforceable upon the case as if it were executed by him/her.

I fully understand that I am directly and fully responsible to said health care provider(s) or their office for all health care bills submitted by them for services rendered to me. Further, this agreement is made solely for said health care providers' additional protection and in consideration of their forbearance on payment. I also understand that such payment is not contingent on any settlement, judgment, or verdict by which I may eventually recover damages.

I specifically request my attorney to acknowledge this letter by signing below and returning it to the office of said health care provider(s). I have been advised that if my attorney does not wish to cooperate in protecting the health care providers' interest, the health care provider(s) will not await payment, but will require me to make payments on a current basis.

Date ___1-3-05___ Patient's Signature ___Darnel G. Washington___

Patient's Social Security Number or Driver's License Number ___123-45-6789___

The undersigned, being attorney of record for the above patient, does hereby agree to observe all the terms of the above, and agrees to withhold such sums from any settlement, judgment, or verdict as may be necessary to adequately protect said health care provider(s) named above.

Date ___1-6-05___ Attorney's Signature ___B. Charma Storro, JD___

Please date, sign, and return one original to   ___John Olson, LMP, GCFP___

                                                                    ___345 Moon River Rd. Ste. 6___

                                                                    ___Minnehaha, MN 55987___

                                                                    ___(612) 555-9889___

                                                                     ___fax (612) 555-8998___

THANK YOU.

Revised and reprinted with permission, Adler ♦ Giersch, PS

John Olson, LMP, GCFP
345 Moon River Rd. Ste. 6
Minnehaha, MN   55987
Tel   612 555 9889

INSURANCE VERIFICATION

HANDS HEAL

Patient Name _Darnel G. Washington_   Date _2-17-04_

Date of Injury _1-6-04_   ID#/DOB _123-45-6789_

Verify and Authorize Patient Benefits

Company Name _Farmington States_

Phone _612-555-7887_ Fax _555-8778_

Provider Service Rep _Clifford Glens_

Date/time called _2-17-04   11 am_

Check all verified:
- ☒ Physical medicine/rehab benfit
- ☒ I can provide services
- ☒ Covered services (from worksheet):
  _97140, 97010, 97110_

Check all authorized:
- ☐ Number of visits _N/A_
- ☐ Dates of coverage _____
Authorization # _____

Billing procedures:
- ☒ HCFA 1500 ☐ electronic ☐ other

Send with each bill:
- ☒ Prescription/referral ☐ Reports
- ☐ SOAPS ☐ License/certification

What is the expected turnaround time on claim reimbursement? _30 da_

Comments _____

Re-Authorize

Provider Service Rep _____

Date/time called _____

Check all authorized:
- ☐ Number of visits _____
- ☐ Dates of coverage _____
Authorization # _____

Total # of visits to date _____

Total $ spent to date _____

Comments _____

Re-Authorize

Provider Service Rep _____

Date/time called _____

Check all authorized:
- ☐ Number of visits _____
- ☐ Dates of coverage _____
Authorization # _____

Total # of visits to date _____

Total $ spent to date _____

Comments _____

Referring Health Care Provider Info

Name _Sage Redtree MD_

Phone _612-555-0009_ Fax _612-555-9000_

Prescription received? ☒ Yes ☐ No

Dates of coverage _2-6-04 to 3-6-04_

# of visits _6_

Diagnosis (ICD-9 codes) _723.1_
_728.85, 724.1, 784.0_

Comments _____

Renewal

Date _____
Progress report sent? ☐ Yes ☐ No
Prescription received? ☐ Yes ☐ No

Dates of coverage _____

# of visits _____

ICD-9 codes _____

Comments _____

Renewal

Date _____
Progress report sent? ☐ Yes ☐ No
Prescription received? ☐ Yes ☐ No

Dates of coverage _____

# of visits _____

ICD-9 codes _____

Comments _____

Attorney Information (if applicable)

Name _B. Charma Storro_

Phone _612-555-2337_ Fax _612-555-7332_

Guarantee of Payment contract signed?
☒ Yes ☐ No

Date requested _1-3-05_ Received _1-6-05_

Medical Lien filed? ☐ Yes ☒ No

Date _____ Expires _____
Renewed _____ Expires _____
Renewed _____ Expires _____

Requests for patient files:

Date requested _2-15-05_ Date sent _2-20-05_
Authorization received? ☒ Yes ☐ No
Exclusive? ☒ Yes ☐ No Expires _5-15-05_

Date requested _____ Date sent _____
Authorization received? ☐ Yes ☐ No
Exclusive? ☐ Yes ☐ No Expires _____

310

John Olson, LMP, GCFP
345 Moon River Rd. Ste. 6
Minnehaha, MN   55987
TEL   612 555 9889

HANDS HEAL

VERIFICATION WORKSHEET

Patient Name _Darnel G. Washington_   Date _2-17-04_

Date of Injury _1-6-04_   ID#/DOB _123-45-6789_

Verify and Authorize Physical Medicine and Rehabilitation Services
(Common modality codes and procedure codes for manual therapists.)

Authorized?	Code #	Description	Restrictions	Max Rate
☐ Yes ☐ No	95831	Muscle testing, ROM, manual, with report		
☒ Yes ☐ No	97010	Hot or cold packs	must be supervised	N/A
☐ Yes ☐ No	97012	Mechanical traction		
☐ Yes ☐ No	97039	Unlisted modality, Specify:		
☒ Yes ☐ No	97110	Therapeutic exercise	N/A	N/A
☐ Yes ☐ No	97112	Neuromuscular reeducation		
☐ Yes ☐ No	97113	Aquatic therapy		
☐ Yes ☐ No	97116	Gait training		
☐ Yes ☐ No	97124	Massage therapy		
☐ Yes ☐ No	97139	Unlisted therapeutic procedure, Specify:		
☒ Yes ☐ No	97140	Manual therapy: eg, mobilization/manip., MLD, MFR, manual traction	4 unit limit	N/A
☐ Yes ☐ No	97050	Therapeutic procedure(s), group (2 or more)		
☐ Yes ☐ No	99056	Home/Hospital visit		
☐ Yes ☐ No	99075	Medical testimony		
☐ Yes ☐ No		Other:		
☐ Yes ☐ No		Other:		
☐ Yes ☐ No		Other:		
☐ Yes ☐ No		Other:		
☐ Yes ☐ No		Other:		
☐ Yes ☐ No		Other:		
☐ Yes ☐ No		Other:		

See CPT codebook for detailed descriptions of modalities and procedures listed above and for additional modalities and therapeutic procedures not listed on worksheet.

HEALTH INSURANCE CLAIM FORM

	PICA								PICA

1. MEDICARE ☐ (Medicare #) **MEDICAID** ☐ (Medicaid #) **CHAMPUS** ☐ (Sponsor's SSN) **CHAMPVA** ☐ (VA File #) **GROUP HEALTH PLAN** ☐ (SSN or ID) **FECA BLK LUNG** ☐ (SSN) **OTHER** ☐ (ID)

1a. INSURED'S I.D. NUMBER (FOR PROGRAM IN ITEM 1)

2. PATIENT'S NAME (Last Name, First Name, Middle Initial)
Washington Darnel G.

3. PATIENT'S BIRTH DATE MM 04 DD 22 YY 37 **SEX** M ☒ F ☐

4. INSURED'S NAME (Last Name, First Name, Middle Initial)
Washington James

5. PATIENT'S ADDRESS (No., Street)
1209 Lake Minnetonka Dr

6. PATIENT RELATIONSHIP TO INSURED
Self ☐ Spouse ☐ Child ☐ Other ☒

7. INSURED'S ADDRESS (No., Street)
32 W. Holden Court

CITY Minnehaha **STATE** MN

8. PATIENT STATUS
Single ☐ Married ☒ Other ☐
Employed ☐ Full-Time Student ☐ Part-Time Student ☐

CITY Minnehaha **STATE** MN

ZIP CODE 55987 **TELEPHONE** (Include Area Code) (612) 555-1515

ZIP CODE 55987 **TELEPHONE** (INCLUDE AREA CODE) (612) 555-1515

9. OTHER INSURED'S NAME (Last Name, First Name, Middle Initial)
Washington Darnel G.

10. IS PATIENT'S CONDITION RELATED TO:

11. INSURED'S POLICY GROUP OR FECA NUMBER

a. OTHER INSURED'S POLICY OR GROUP NUMBER
Allied

a. EMPLOYMENT? (CURRENT OR PREVIOUS) YES ☐ NO ☒

a. INSURED'S DATE OF BIRTH MM 05 DD 31 YY 60 **SEX** M ☒ F ☐

b. OTHER INSURED'S DATE OF BIRTH MM DD YY **SEX** M ☐ F ☐

b. AUTO ACCIDENT? YES ☒ NO ☐ **PLACE (State)** MN

b. EMPLOYER'S NAME OR SCHOOL NAME
Maad Printing & Design

c. EMPLOYER'S NAME OR SCHOOL NAME

c. OTHER ACCIDENT? YES ☐ NO ☒

c. INSURANCE PLAN NAME OR PROGRAM NAME
Farmington States

d. INSURANCE PLAN NAME OR PROGRAM NAME
P56789-0

10d. RESERVED FOR LOCAL USE

d. IS THERE ANOTHER HEALTH BENEFIT PLAN?
YES ☒ NO ☐ *If yes, return to and complete item 9 a-d.*

READ BACK OF FORM BEFORE COMPLETING & SIGNING THIS FORM.
12. PATIENT'S OR AUTHORIZED PERSON'S SIGNATURE I authorize the release of any medical or other information necessary to process this claim. I also request payment of government benefits either to myself or to the party who accepts assignment below.
SIGNED signature on file DATE 2-6-04

13. INSURED'S OR AUTHORIZED PERSON'S SIGNATURE I authorize payment of medical benefits to the undersigned physician or supplier for services described below.
SIGNED signature on file

14. DATE OF CURRENT: MM 01 DD 06 YY 04 ◄ ILLNESS (First symptom) OR INJURY (Accident) OR PREGNANCY(LMP)

15. IF PATIENT HAS HAD SAME OR SIMILAR ILLNESS. GIVE FIRST DATE MM DD YY

16. DATES PATIENT UNABLE TO WORK IN CURRENT OCCUPATION FROM MM DD YY TO MM DD YY

17. NAME OF REFERRING PHYSICIAN OR OTHER SOURCE
Sage Redtree, MD

17a. I.D. NUMBER OF REFERRING PHYSICIAN

18. HOSPITALIZATION DATES RELATED TO CURRENT SERVICES FROM MM DD YY TO MM DD YY

19. RESERVED FOR LOCAL USE

20. OUTSIDE LAB? YES ☐ NO ☐ **$ CHARGES**

21. DIAGNOSIS OR NATURE OF ILLNESS OR INJURY. (RELATE ITEMS 1,2,3 OR 4 TO ITEM 24E BY LINE)
1. 728.85
2. 723.1
3. 724.1
4. 784.0

22. MEDICAID RESUBMISSION CODE **ORIGINAL REF. NO.**

23. PRIOR AUTHORIZATION NUMBER

24. A. DATE(S) OF SERVICE From / To						B. Place of Service	C. Type of Service	D. PROCEDURES, SERVICES, OR SUPPLIES (Explain Unusual Circumstances) CPT/HCPCS	MODIFIER	E. DIAGNOSIS CODE	F. $ CHARGES	G. DAYS OR UNITS	H. EPSDT Family Plan	I. EMG	J. COB	K. RESERVED FOR LOCAL USE
MM	DD	YY	MM	DD	YY											
02	06	04				3	9	97140		1,2,3,4	$100 00	4				
02	06	04				3	9	97140		1,2,3,4	$100 00	4				

25. FEDERAL TAX I.D. NUMBER 567-89-1234 SSN ☒ EIN ☐

26. PATIENT'S ACCOUNT NO.

27. ACCEPT ASSIGNMENT? (For govt. claims, see back) YES ☐ NO ☐

28. TOTAL CHARGE $ 160 00

29. AMOUNT PAID $ 0

30. BALANCE DUE $ 160 00

31. SIGNATURE OF PHYSICIAN OR SUPPLIER INCLUDING DEGREES OR CREDENTIALS (I certify that the statements on the reverse apply to this bill and are made a part thereof.)
John Olson LMP, GCFB 2-8-04
SIGNED DATE

32. NAME AND ADDRESS OF FACILITY WHERE SERVICES WERE RENDERED (If other than home or office)

33. PHYSICIAN'S, SUPPLIER'S BILLING NAME, ADDRESS, ZIP CODE & PHONE #
John Olson, LMP, GCFP
345 Moon River Rd. Ste. 6
Minnehaha, MN 55987
PIN# (612) 555-9889 GRP#

FORM HCFA-1500 (12-90)
NORTHWEST BUSINESS FORMS (206) 728-8181

PLEASE PRINT OR TYPE

FORM OWCP-1500   FORM RRB-1500   APPROVED OMB-0938-0008
(APPROVED BY AMA COUNCIL ON MEDICAL SERVICE 8/88)

Workers' Compensation

Case Study: Zamora Hostetter, a 24-year-old woman, suffers from a severe shoulder injury. She cannot use her right arm at all due to a complete acromioclavicular separation. She slipped on a banana peel while carrying a 25-pound bag of rice at work. The bag of rice fell on top of her, magnifying the impact of the humerus into the AC joint and increasing the severity of the injury. She has concommitant symptoms: headache, neck stiffness, and back pain. She was taken to the emergency room and released the same day. She went to see her chiropractor the next day and was referred to Helena LaLuna for structural integration therapy.

Ms. Hostetter is a very motivated, young, healthy woman who is eager to get back to her active lifestyle. She has clear goals for her chiropractic care and her manual therapy and is familiar with stretching and strengthening routines. She is used to riding her bike everywhere and does not have a car, so she is having to take the bus to and from her appointments. This has not stopped her from being on time to every appointment. However, she is having difficulty adhering to the firm instructions from the chiropractor—no strengthening exercises for the first three weeks. The manual therapist is reinforcing the instructions, and Ms. Hostetter is healing quickly.

This flow chart demonstrates the forms that are recommended for use with patients involved in workers' compensation cases: who completes the form, how often the form is used, and any additional comments for using the form.

Workers' Compensation INTAKE FORMS	Who	Frequency	Comments
Fees and Policies	Patient	Initial visit	Update as needed
Health Information	Patient	Initial visit	Update annually
Health Info—Wellness	—		
Injury Information, Part 1	Patient	Initial visit	Per incident
Injury Information, Part 2	—		
Billing Information	Patient	Initial visit	If you provide billing services
Prescription	HCP	As needed	A progress report should precede each renewal
PROGRESS SUMMARIES			
Health Report	Patient	Monthly	Patient reports current status
Pain Questionnaires	Patient	Monthly	Daily or weekly, if used as a pain journal
Initial Report w/o Tx	MT	As needed	If patient does not receive tx
Initial Report w/ Tx	MT	Initial visit	Summarizes tx and proposes tx plan
Progress Report	MT	Monthly	Practitioner reports to HCP
Narrative Report	—		
TREATMENT NOTES			
Initial SOAP	MT	Initial visit	Summarizes all findings; sets goals, plan
Subsequent SOAP	MT	Each visit	(excluding initial, progress, and discharge sessions) brief, focused
Progress SOAP	MT	Monthly	Summarizes all findings; updates goals, plan

Discharge SOAP	MT	Final visit	Summarizes all findings; ongoing care plan
Wellness Chart	—		
Range of Motion	MT	As needed	Minimal ROM assessment necessary each subsequent note, extensive ROM for initial and progress notes

ATTORNEY FORMS

Release of Health Care Information	Attorney	As needed	must have on file before releasing any PHI
Guarantee of Payment	MT, Patient, Attorney		If end-of-settlement case
Insurance Status—Personal Injury	Attorney	As needed	If insurance status is unknown/unclear

BILLING FORMS

Insurance Verification	MT	As needed	With renewal of prescribed services
HCFA 1500 billing form	MT	Each visit	May bill for multiple sessions per HCFA form after initial billing if total amount is under $250 and sessions fall within the same month
Payment Log	MT	As needed	If payments do not match bills

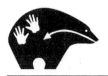

Helena LaLuna, CR
123 Sun Moon and Stars Drive
Capitol Hill, WA   98119
TEL   206 555 4446

A. My Fees for Services Are as Follows:

Structural Integration	$100 per hour
(CTP code #97140)	($25 per 15 minute Unit)

B. Payment for Services Are as Follows:

Cash, Check, or Credit Card (Mastercard, Visa, or American Express):
- A 15% discount when payment is made at the time of service.
- Monthly accounts may be pre-arranged, payment in full required monthly.

I will bill your insurance company directly under the following conditions:

- Private Health Insurance: No
- Worker's Compensation: Yes—verbal authorization OK, active claims only, HCP prescription required

- Auto Accident:
  - PIP: Yes—written authorization required or Insurance Status–Personal Injury from Attorney verifying insurance status, HCP prescription required
  - Second Party Coverage: Yes—if PIP, see above
  - Third Party Coverage: Yes—Guarantee of Payment contract required, helath care lien required, HCP perscription required

All insurance accounts not paid in full within 90 days from date of service will be charged interest. Interest rates are 12% annually and are charged at 1% monthly. Interest is calculated on the principal amount; interest is not compounded.

C. Office Policies

Cancellations

Cancellations must be made 24 hours in advance of the scheduled appointment time. If cancellations are not made within 24 hours, payment in full is required. This charge will be waived if a replacement can be found for your appointment time. Your insurance company will not be charged for your missed appointment; you will be responsible for payment out-of-pocket.

Right of Refusal

I reserve the right to refuse service to anyone. This includes but is not limited to anyone who requests treatment or services that are outside my scope of practice. I will exercise this right if anyone arrives for treatment under the influence of alcohol or recreational drugs; I reserve the right to charge for the session time, whether or not services were rendered, if I so choose.

Patient Agreement

I have read the policies stated above and agree to abide by them.

Signature   *Zamora Hostetter*   Date   *4-4-04*

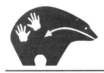

Helena LaLuna, CR
123 Sun Moon and Stars Drive
Capitol Hill, WA   98119
TEL   206 555 4446

HEALTH INFORMATION

Patient Name _Zamora Hostetter_   Date _4-4-04_

Date of Injury _3-31-04_   ID#/DOB _C98-7654321 / 5-22-80_

A. Patient Information

Address _63 18th Ave W_

City _Capitol Hill_   State _WA_ Zip _98119_

Phone: Home _(206) 555-1221_

  Work _555-2112_   Cell _555-1122_

Employer _Howling Moon Cafe_

Work Address _1421 37th Ave NW 98122_

Occupation _chef_

Emergency Contact _Mary Lou Hostetter_

Phone: Home _(206) 555-0909_

  Work _555-9090_ Cell _555-9900_

Primary Health Care Provider

Name _Manda Rae Yuricich, DC_

Address _4041 Bell Town Wy Ste. 200_

City/State/Zip _Capitol Hill, WA 98119_

Phone: _555-3535_   Fax _555-4646_

I give my massage therapist permission to consult with my health care providers regarding my health and treatment.

Comments _re: work inj only_

Initials _ZH_   Date _4-4-04_

B. Current Health Information

List Health Concerns Check all that apply

Primary _shoulder pain_
☐ mild ☐ moderate ☒ disabling
☒ constant ☐ intermittant
☒ symptoms ↑ w/activity   ☐ ↓ w/activity
☐ getting worse ☐ getting better ☒ no change
treatment received _ER—x-ray, sling_

Secondary _back pain_
☐ mild ☒ moderate ☐ disabling
☒ constant ☐ intermittant
☒ symptoms ↑ w/activity   ☐ ↓ w/activity
☐ getting worse ☒ getting better ☐ no change
treatment received _ER DC—adjust_

Additional _neck pain & headaches_
☒ mild ☐ moderate ☐ disabling
☐ constant ☒ intermittant
☒ symptoms ↑ w/activity   ☐ ↓ w/activity
☐ getting worse ☒ getting better ☐ no change
treatment received _ER, DC_

List Daily Activities Limited by Condition

Work _standing, lifting, cooking, chopping food_

Home/Family _cooking, cleaning, yardwork_

Sleep/Self-care _restless sleep, can't pull shirts on, tie shoes, button_

Social/Recreational _biking, roller hockey, dancing_

List Self-Care Routines

How do you reduce stress? _____
sports, being outdoors
Pain? _arnica, ice packs, visualization_

List current medications (include pain relievers and herbal remedies) _____
arnica, calcium, vitamins

Have you ever received massage therapy before? _No_   Frequency? _____

What are your goals for receiving massage therapy? _get back to work and sports_

C. Health History

List and Explain. Include dates and treatment received.

Surgeries _____ _None_

Injuries _broken arm Ⓡ, fell out of tree house in 1987, in case for 8 weeks_

Major Illnesses _____ _None_

316

Check All Current and Previous Conditions Please Explain

General

current	past		comments
☒	☐	headaches	
☒	☐	pain	_SH, back, neck_
☒	☐	sleep disturbances	
			pain wakes me up
☐	☐	fatigue	
☐	☐	infections	
☐	☐	fever	
☐	☐	sinus	
☐	☐	other	

Skin Conditions

current	past		comments
☐	☐	rashes	
☐	☐	athlete's foot, warts	
☐	☐	other	

Muscles and Joints

current	past		comments
☐	☐	rheumatoid arthritis	
☐	☐	osteoarthritis	
☐	☐	osteoporosis	
☐	☐	scoliosis	
☐	☒	broken bones	Ⓡ _arm_
☒	☐	spinal problems	
			neck and back
☐	☐	disk problems	
☐	☐	lupus	
☐	☐	TMJ, jaw pain	
☐	☐	spasms, cramps	
☐	☐	sprains, strains	
☐	☐	tendonitis, bursitis	
☒	☐	stiff or painful joints	_SH_
☐	☐	weak or sore muscles	
☒	☐	neck, shoulder, arm pain	
☒	☐	low back, hip, leg pain	
☐	☐	other	

Nervous System

current	past		comments
☐	☐	head injuries, concussions	
☐	☐	dizziness, ringing in ears	
☐	☐	loss of memory, confusion	
☐	☐	numbness, tingling	
☐	☐	sciatica, shooting pain	
☐	☐	chronic pain	
☐	☐	depression	
☐	☐	other	

Respiratory, Cardiovascular

current	past		comments
☐	☐	heart disease	
☐	☐	blood clots	
☐	☐	stroke	
☐	☐	lymphadema	
☐	☐	high, low blood pressure	
☐	☐	irregular heart beat	
☐	☐	poor circulation	
☐	☐	swollen ankles	
☐	☐	varicose veins	
☐	☐	chest pain, shortness of breath	
☐	☐	asthma	

Allergies

current	past		comments
☐	☐	scents, oils, lotions	
☐	☐	detergents	
☐	☐	other	

Digestive/Elimination System

current	past		comments
☐	☐	bowel problems	
☐	☐	gas, bloating	
☐	☐	bladder/kidney/prostrate	
☐	☐	abdominal pain	
☐	☐	other	

Endocrine System

current	past		comments
☐	☐	thyroid	
☐	☐	diabetes	

Reproductive System

current	past		comments
☐	☐	pregnancy	
☐	☐	painful, emotional menses	
☐	☐	fibrotic cysts	

Cancer/Tumors

current	past		comments
☐	☐	benign	
☐	☐	malignant	

Habits

current	past		comments
☐	☒	tobacco	_quit 1998_
☒	☐	alcohol	_mild use_
☐	☐	drugs	
☐	☐	coffee, soda	

Contract for Care

I promise to participate fully as a member of my health care team. I will make sound choices regarding my treatment plan based on the information provided by my manual therapist and other members of my health care team, and my experience of those suggestions. I agree to participate in the self care program we select. I promise to inform my practitioner any time I feel my well-being is threatened or compromised. I expect my manual therapist to provide safe and effective treatment.

Consent for Care

It is my choice to receive manual therapy, and I give my consent to receive treatment. I have reported all health conditions that I am aware of and will inform my practitioner of any changes in my health.

Signature _Zamora Hostetter_   Date _4-4-04_

Helena LaLuna, CR
123 Sun Moon and Stars Drive
Capitol Hill, WA 98119
Tel 206 555 4446

INJURY INFORMATION

Patient Name _Zamora Hostetter_   Date _4-4-04_

Date of Injury _3-31-04_   ID#/DOB _C98-7654321_

A. General Injury Information

1. How did the accident occur?
   ☐ Auto   ☐ On-the-Job   ☐ Other _____

2. Was a police report filed?   ☐ Yes   ☐ No
   Was a work incident report filed?
   ☒ Yes   ☐ No

3. Describe your injury and how it occurred:
   slipped on banana peel, carrying 25 lb. bag of
   rice over left shoulder, fell backwards
   onto right arm, then right hip, head
   bounced on tile floor, rice landed on top of
   _me._

4. Describe how you felt during and
   immediately after the injury:
   shoulder "popped"-immediate pain, head
   throbbing
   Later that same day: _backache_

   The next day: _neck stiff, back stiff, can't_
   use right arm at all

   The next week: _N/A_

   The next month: _N/A_

   Describe any bruises, cuts, or abrasions
   as a result of the injury:
   bruise on right hip

5. Are your symptoms ☒ getting better
   ☐ getting worse   ☒ no change _-shoulder_
   What makes them better? _only_
   ice, arnica, visualization ex., chiropractor

   Worse? _everything using my arm, sleep_

6. Did you return to work on the day of the
   injury? ☐ Yes   ☒ No
   Have you lost time from work since the
   injury? ☒ Yes   ☒ No

7. What are your work responsibilities?
   cooking, prep, stocking supplies

   Which work activities are affected by this
   injury? _everything_

   Have your work responsibilities changed as
   a result of this injury?   ☒ Yes   ☐ No
   Explain _____
   What other daily activities are affected by
   this injury? _everything using my right arm_

8. Did you go to the emergency room?
   ☒ Yes   ☐ No
   Were you hospitalized?   ☐ Yes   ☒ No
   List the health care providers who have
   treated you for this injury, the type of
   treatment provided, and their diagnosis.
   ER-separated shoulder-sling
   DC-whiplash, spinal subluxations, muscle
   spasms-adjust, ice

9. Have you ever had this type of injury
   before? ☐ Yes   ☒ No
   Explain _____

   Did you have any physical complaints
   before the injury? ☐ Yes   ☒ No
   Explain _____

   Do you have any illnesses or previous
   injuries that may have been affected by
   this injury? ☐ Yes   ☒ No
   Explain _____

Signature _Zamora Hostetter_   Date _4-4-04_

HANDS HEAL

John Olson, LMP, GCFP
345 Moon River Rd. Ste. 6
Minnehaha, MN   55987
Tel   612 555 9889

BILLING INFORMATION

Patient Name _Zamora Hostetter_ Date _4-3-04_

Date of Injury _3-31-04_ ID#/DOB _C98-7654321 / 5-22-80_

Billing Policy

Our office is set up to receive direct payment from insurance companies. For the best chance of reimbursement from your insurance carrier, <u>we ask that you</u>:

• Contact your insurance company to determine your manual therapy coverage and provider stipulations. Coverage depends on your insurance company and the specific plan you have chosen. We have provided a list of questions for you to ask your insurance representative or attorney that will help determine your eligibility for our billing service.

• You will need a current prescription for manual therapy from a primary health care provider, such as a physician or a chiropractor in order to submit your claim. Referrals are current for 90 days unless otherwise specified.

It is important that you understand your insurance policies in order for you to budget for your manual therapy services. You are personally responsible for all charges incurred in our office. We expect payment in full until your insurance coverage has been verified.

We realize that the completion of this form is an added burden to you as a consumer, and we thank you very much for your assistance. This completed form will provide both you and our billing department with important information regarding your manual therapy insurance benefits, and enable us to process your claim in a timely fashion.

Patient Information

Is patient's condition related to:

☐ auto collsion—In what state? _____
☐ other accident _____
☒ employment ☐ illness

Patient status: ☐ male ☒ female
☒ single ☐ married/partnered ☐ other

Patient relationship to insured
☒ self ☐ spouse/partner ☐ child ☐ other

Insured's Information (if other than patient)

Name _N/A_

Address _____

City _____ State ____ Zip _____

Phone: _____

Date of birth _____

Sex: ☐ Male ☐ Female

Employer's Name or School Name _____

Insurance Information

Insurance plan name or program name: _WA Dept. of L & I_

Member ID#: _C98-7654321_ Group #: _____

Customer service phone #: _360-555-6655_ Date and time you called: _4-3-04_

Name of customer service representative: _Megan Yaskell_

Insurance claim address: _PO Box 323, Olympia_ State: _WA_ Zip: _98055_

Does the plan include a Physical Medicine and Rehabilitation benefit? ☒ Yes ☐ No

Who may provide the services? ☒ Massage Therapist ☐ Physical Therapist ☐ Other

Is pre-authorization required? ☒ Yes ☐ No   Who can authorize the services? _L & I_

Is a prescription required? ☒ Yes ☐ No   Is a referral required? ☐ Yes ☒ No

Who may refer? ☐ MD ☒ DC ☐ ND ☐ PT ☐ Other _____

How often does the referral need to be updated to ensure continuous coverage? _30 da_

Is there a Preferred Provider list for Manual Therapists? ☒ Yes ☐ No

Is _Helena LaLuna_ on the list? ☒ Yes ☐ No

319

HANDS HEAL

John Olson, LMP, GCFP
345 Moon River Rd. Ste. 6
Minnehaha, MN   55987
Tel   612 555 9889

BILLING INFORMATION page 2

If this is a Workers' Compensation Claim, please fill out the following information:

Who is the attending HCP? _Manda Rae Yuricich_   Phone: _(206)555-3535_

Claim number: _C98-7654321_   Date eligibility began: _3-31-04_

Number of visits authorized: _6_   Number of visits remaining: _6_

Dates of coverage: _3-31-04 to 4-30-04_   Date claim closed: _____

If this is a Personal Injury Claim, please fill out the following information:

PIP policy amount: _____   Dates of coverage: _____   PIP available: _____

MedPay amount: _____   Dates of coverage: _____   MedPay available: _____

Liability amount: _____   Dates of coverage: _____   Liability available: _____

Uninsured/Underinsured (UMI) policy amount: _____   UMI available: _____

Has the PIP application been received?   ☐ Yes   ☐ No

Has an attorney been consulted?   ☐ Yes   ☐ No   Retained?   ☐ Yes   ☐ No

Name/Firm _____

Address _____   City _____   State _____   Zip _____

Phone _____   Fax _____

If this is a Private Health Insurance Claim, please fill out the following information:
(Or, if your Personal Injury claim defaults to secondary coverage, fill this out)

Maximum allowable benefit for Physical Medicine/Rehabilitation: _____

In network: $_____   # visits _____   Remaining $_____   # visits _____

Deductible: $_____   Satisfied to date: $_____   Co-Pay: $_____

Out-of-network: $_____   # visits _____   Remaining $_____   # visits _____

Deductible: $_____   Satisfied to date: $_____   Co-Insurance: $_____

Are these limits just for manual therapy?   ☐ Yes   ☐ No

If no, what other types of treatment do they include? _____
(i.e., chiropractic, physical therapy, occupational therapy, naturopathy, etc.)

Assignment of Benefits

My signature below authorizes and directs payment of medical benefits for services billed to my health care provider: _Helena LaLuna_

Release of Medical Records

My signature below authorizes the release of my medical records including intake forms, chart notes, reports, and billing statements to my attorneys, health care providers, and insurance case managers, for the purpose of processing my claims. (I will inform my practitioner immediately upon signing any exclusive Release of Medical Records with my attorney.)

Financial Responsibility

It is my responsibility to pay for all services provided. In the event that my insurance company denies payment or makes a partial payment, I agree to be and remain responsible for the balance. It is also my understanding and agreement that if you have contracted with my insurance company at a discount rate and the agreed-upon fee has been satisfied, the balance owed on those specific visits will be waived.

Signature   _Zamorra Hostetter_   Date   _4-3-04_

320

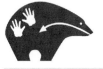

Helena LaLuna, CR
123 Sun Moon and Stars Drive
Capitol Hill, WA   98119
TEL   206 555 4446

PRESCRIPTION

Patient Name _Zamora Hostetter_   Date _4-1-04_

Date of Injury _3-31-04_   ID#/DOB _C98-7654321_

A. Diagnosis

(Include ICD-9 codes that specifically
address Manual Therapy Treatment)

Lowback Ⓟ 724.2

Neck Ⓟ 723.1

Shoulder sp/st 840.9, Headache 784.0

Spasm 728.85

Condition is related to

☐ Auto Accident
☒ Work Injury
☐ Illness
☐ Other: _____

B. Medically Necessary Treatment: Implement Plan as Prescribed Below

Application (Primary & Secondary)

☐ Head _____
☐ Neck _____
☐ Chest _____
☐ Shoulders _separated Ⓡ SH_
☐ Abdomen _____
☐ Back _____
☐ Lowback/Hips _____
☐ Upper extremities _as related to sh injury_
☐ Lower extremities _a related to LB injury_
☐ All of the above _____
☐ Other: _____

Frequency & Duration

☐ 1× wk for _____ wks
☒ 2× wk for _5_ wks
☐ 3× wk for _____ wks
☐ 2× month for _____ months
☐ 1× month for _____ months

Treatment Type

☒ Manual Therapy _____
☒ Hot/Cold Packs _____
☒ Self-Care/Exercises _____
☐ Other _____

Treatment Goals

☐ Decrease Pain
☐ Decrease Inflammation
☐ Decrease Muscle Tension/Spasms
☐ Decrease Compensatory Patterns
☐ Increase Mobility
☐ Increase Strength
☐ Restore Function
☐ Restore Posture
☐ Patient Education
☒ All of the Above
☐ Other _____

Specific Instructions/Precautions:

Techniques at your discretion

No strengthening for first 3 wks

C. Referring Health Care Provider (HCP)

Contact Information
HCP Name _Manda Rae Yuricich DC_
Address _4041 Bell Town Wy Ste 200_
City _Capitol Hill_   State _WA_ Zip _98119_
Phone _206) 555-3535_
Fax _(206) 555-4646_
Email _____

Reporting—I will send an initial report after
the first visit and a progress report after
every 6–8 sessions. Please check how you
would like to receive this information:

☒ Fax ☐ Mail ☐ Email
☐ Send Copies of Chart Notes with each report

HCP Signature: _Manda Rae Yuricich, DC_   Date _4-1-04_

Revised and reprinted with permission, Adler ♦ Giersch, PS

321

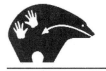

Helena LaLuna, CR
123 Sun Moon and Stars Drive
Capitol Hill, WA   98119
Tel   206 555 4446

HEALTH REPORT-F

Patient Name _Zamora Hostetter_   Date _4-4-04_

Date of Injury _3-31-04_   ID#/DOB _C98-7654321 / 5-22-80_

A. Draw today's symptoms on the figures.

1. Identify CURRENT symptomatic areas in your body by marking letters on the figures below. Use the letters provided in the key to identify the symptoms you are feeling today.
2. Circle the area around each letter, representing the size and shape of each symptom location.

Key
P = pain or tenderness
S = joint or muscle stiffness
N = numbness or tingling

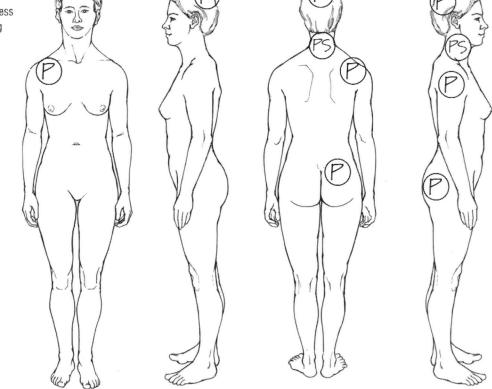

B. Identify the intensity of your symptoms.

1. Pain Scale: Mark a line on the scale to show the amount of pain you are experiencing today.

No Pain ├──────────────────────┼──────────────────┤ Unbearable Pain   (6.5)

2. Activities Scale: Mark a line on the scale to show the limitations you are experiencing today in your daily activities.   (8.5)

Can Do Anything I Want ├──────────────────────────┼────────┤ Cannot Do Anything

C. Comments

_____

_____

_____

_____

Signature _Zamora Hostetter_   Date _4-4-04_

Helena LaLuna, CR

123 Sun Moon and Stars Drive
Capitol Hill, WA   98119
TEL   206 555 4446

® shoulder   (revised Vernon-Mior)
NECK PAIN & DISABILITY INDEX

Patient Name _Zamora Hostetter_   Date _4-4-04_

Date of Injury _3-31-04_   ID#/DOB _C98-7654321_

This questionnaire has been designed to give the health care provider information as to how your neck pain has affected your ability to manage everyday life. Please answer every section and mark in each section only the **ONE** box which applies to you. We realize you may consider that two of the statements in any one section relate to you, but please just mark the box which most closely describes your problem today.

3 Section 1 - Pain Intensity
- ☐ I have no pain at the moment.
- ☐ The pain is very mild at the moment.
- ☐ The pain is moderate at the moment.
- ☒ The pain is fairly severe at the moment.
- ☐ The pain is very severe at the moment.
- ☐ The pain is the worst imaginable at the moment.

3 Section 2 - Personal Care
(washing, dressing, etc.)
- ☐ I can look after myself normally without causing pain.
- ☐ I can look after myself normally but it causes extra pain.
- ☐ It is painful to look after myself and I am slow and careful.
- ☒ I need some help but manage most of my personal care.
- ☐ I need help every day in most aspects of self care.
- ☐ I do not get dressed, I wash myself with difficulty and I stay in bed.

5 Section 3 - Lifting
- ☐ I can lift heavy weights without extra pain.
- ☐ I can lift heavy weights but it causes extra pain.
- ☐ Pain prevents me from lifting heavy weights off the floor, but I can manage if they are conveniently positioned, e.g. on a table.
- ☐ Pain prevents me from lifting heavy weights, but I can manage light to medium weights if they are conveniently positioned.
- ☐ I can lift very light weights.
- ☒ I cannot lift or carry anything at all.

1 Section 4 - Reading
- ☐ I can read as much as I want to with no pain in my neck.
- ☒ I can read as much as I want to with slight pain in my neck.
- ☐ I can read as much as I want to with moderate pain in my neck.
- ☐ I can't read as much as I want to because of moderate pain in my neck.
- ☐ I can hardly read at all because of severe pain in my neck.
- ☐ I cannot read at all.

3 Section 5 - Headaches
- ☐ I have no headaches at all.
- ☐ I have slight headaches which come infrequently.
- ☐ I have moderate headaches which come infrequently.
- ☒ I have moderate headaches which come frequently.
- ☐ I have severe headaches which come frequently.
- ☐ I have headaches almost all of the time.

1 Section 6 - Concentration
- ☐ I can concentrate fully when I want to with no difficulty.
- ☒ I can concentrate fully when I want to with slight difficulty.
- ☐ I have a fair degree of difficulty in concentrating when I want to.
- ☐ I have a lot of difficulty concentrating when I want to.
- ☐ I have a great deal of difficulty in concentrating when I want to.
- ☐ I cannot concentrate at all.

5 Section 7 - Work
- ☐ I can do as much work as I want to.
- ☐ I can do my usual work but no more.
- ☐ I can do most of my usual work but no more.
- ☐ I cannot do my usual work.
- ☐ I can hardly do any work at all.
- ☒ I can't do any work at all.

1 Section 8 - Driving
- ☐ I can drive my car without any neck pain.
- ☒ I can drive my car as long as I want with slight pain in my neck.
- ☐ I can drive my car as long as I want with moderate pain in my neck.
- ☐ I can't drive my car as long as I want because of moderate pain in my neck.
- ☐ I can hardly drive at all because of severe pain in my neck.
- ☐ I can't drive my car at all.

4 Section 9 - Sleeping
- ☐ I have no trouble sleeping.
- ☐ My sleep is slightly disturbed (less than 1 hour sleepless).
- ☐ My sleep is mildly disturbed (1–2 hours sleepless).
- ☐ My sleep is moderately disturbed (2–3 hours sleepless).
- ☒ My sleep is greatly disturbed (3–5 hours sleepless).
- ☐ My sleep is completely disturbed (5–7 hours sleepless).

30 × 2 = 60%

4 Section 10 - Recreation
- ☐ I am able to engage in all my recreational activities with no neck pain at all.
- ☐ I am able to engage in all my recreational activities with some pain in my neck.
- ☐ I am able to engage in most, but not all of my usual recreational activities because of pain in my neck.
- ☐ I am able to engage in a few of my usual recreation activities because of pain in my neck.
- ☒ I can hardly do any recreational activities because of pain in my neck.
- ☐ I can't do recreational activities at all.

Signature _Zamora Hostetter_   Date _4-4-04_

Helena LaLuna, CR
123 Sun Moon and Stars Drive
Capitol Hill, WA   98119
Tel   206 555 4446

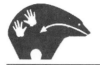

SOAP CHART-F

Patient Name _Zamora Hostetter_   Date _4-4-04_

Date of Injury _3-31-04_   ID#/DOB _C98-7654321_ Meds _arnica every 2 hrs_

S Focus/Health Concerns: Prioritize ↓ Ⓟ & ↑ ROM SH, neck, LB
Dx: Sep SH, SI jt sublux., whiplash
Symptoms: Location/Intensity/Frequency/Duration/Onset

Ⓡ SH/ Ⓟ/ S-/ cons / fall 3-31-04   Δ M
LB/ Ⓟ/ M / cons/ fall 3-31-04   Δ M-
Neck / Ⓟ/ L / interm / daily / fall   Δ N

Activities of Daily Living: Aggravating/Relieving

Unable to stand more than 10 min.

Unable to lift anything c̄ Ⓡ SH/arm

Unable to work, play hockey, bike

O Findings: Visual/Palpable/Test Results

See figures

Techniques/Modalities: Locations/Duration

97140 FB MFR 60 min — _gentle_

Response to Treatment (see Δ)

A Goals: Long-term/Short-term
LTG—stand for 1/2 hr cooking 3 da/wk
5 wks   < M Ⓟ & fatigue
STG—stand for 20 min. slicing kiwis and decorating cake
2 wks   c̄ M Ⓟ & fatigue

Functional Outcomes

P Future Treatment/Frequency
2x/wk for 5 wks, 60 min each
10 session rolfing protocol
focus on ↓ Ⓟ ↑ROM Ⓡ SH & Ⓡ SI jt
Homework/Self-care
ice pack wrapped in towel 8-10 min SH & hip
SH ex: wall climb 3-5x/da as shown

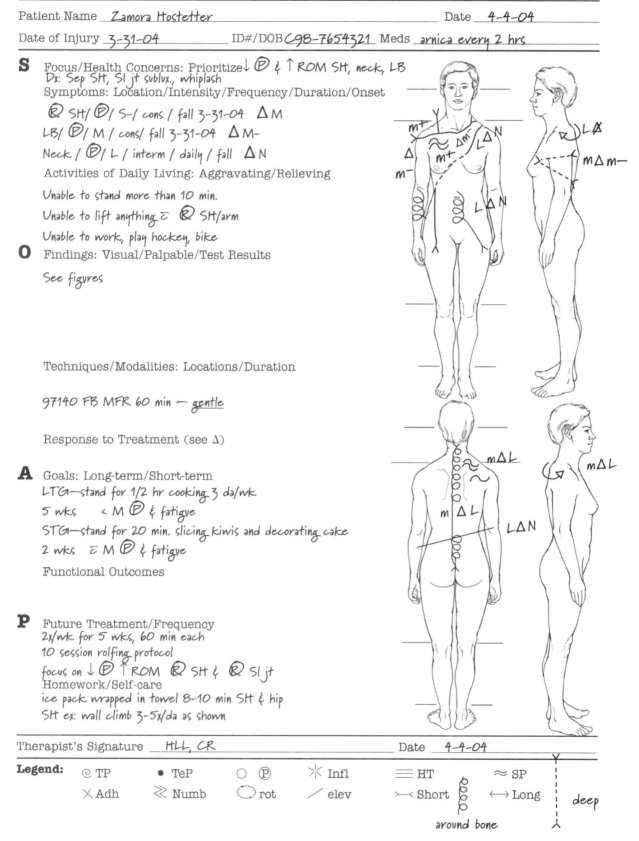

Therapist's Signature _HLL, CR_   Date _4-4-04_

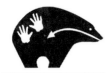

Helena LaLuna, CR

123 Sun Moon and Stars Drive
Capitol Hill, WA   98119
TEL   206 555 4446   •   FAX   206 555 4447   •   EMAIL   laluna@email.com

Manda Rae Yuricich, DC   4-6-04

4041 Bell Town Way, Ste. 200

Capitol Hill, WA 98119

Thank you, Dr. Yuricich, for referring Ms. Hostetter to my office. Our first appointment was on
April 4, 2001. The results of the sessions are as follows:

Functional goals: Ms. Hostetter would like to return to work as a chef as soon as possible. To
facilitate that, our initial goal is to have her cooking for 30 minutes per day, 3 days per week,
with moderate pain and fatigue within 30 days. Currently, she is unable to cook due to severe
pain and muscle spasms in her neck, shoulders and back.

Together, we will resolve those findings and accomplish those goals with the following
treatment plan: myofascial release for 10 sessions, addressing her shoulder, neck, back and
sacral soft tissue injuries, ice packs to reduce the inflammation, and homework exercises to
facilitate self-care.

I will report back to you by May 5. Please contact me if you have questions, comments, or
feedback.

Yours in health,

Helena LaLuna, CR

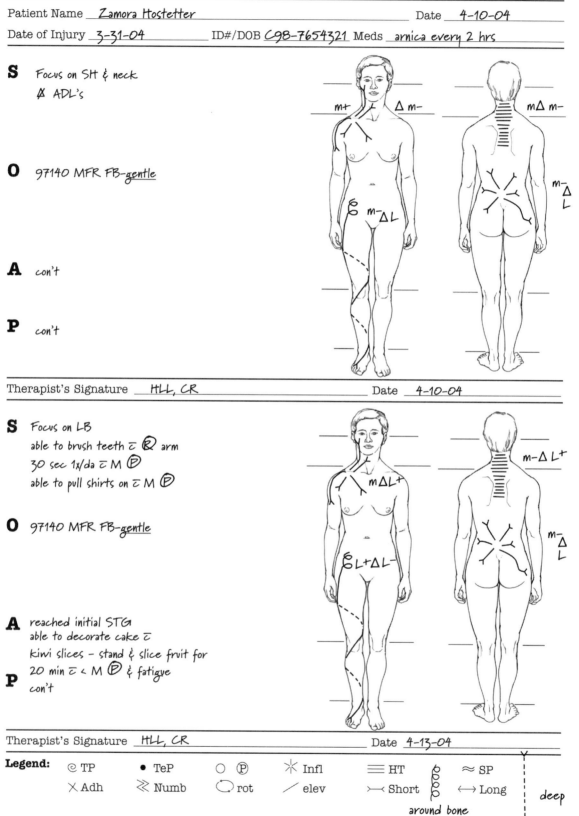

Helena LaLuna, CR
123 Sun Moon and Stars Drive
Capitol Hill, WA   98119
TEL   206 555 4446

SOAP CHART-F

Patient Name __Zamora Hostetter__   Date __4-10-04__

Date of Injury __3-31-04__   ID#/DOB __C98-7654321__ Meds __arnica every 2 hrs__

S   Focus on SH & neck
    ∆ ADL's

O   97140 MFR FB-_gentle_

A   con't

P   con't

m+   ∆ m-   m∆ m-

m-∆ L   m-∆ L

Therapist's Signature ___HLL, CR___   Date ___4-10-04___

S   Focus on LB
    able to brush teeth c̄ Ⓡ arm
    30 sec 1x/da c̄ M Ⓟ
    able to pull shirts on c̄ M Ⓟ

O   97140 MFR FB-_gentle_

A   reached initial STG
    able to decorate cake c̄
    kiwi slices - stand & slice fruit for
    20 min c̄ < M Ⓟ & fatigue
P   con't

m∆L+   m-∆ L+

L+∆L-   m-∆ L

Therapist's Signature __HLL, CR__   Date __4-13-04__

Legend: ℮ TP   • TeP   ○ Ⓟ   ✳ Infl   ≡ HT   ঙ ≈ SP
          ✕ Adh   ≫ Numb   ↻ rot   ∕ elev   ⊱ Short   ঙ ↔ Long   Ⲩ deep
                                                   around bone

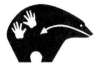

Helena LaLuna, CR
123 Sun Moon and Stars Drive
Capitol Hill, WA   98119
TEL   206 555 4446

SOAP CHART-F

Patient Name _Zamora Hostetter_   Date _5-11-04_

Date of Injury _3-31-04_   ID#/DOB _C98-7654321_ Meds _arnica every 2 hrs_

S   Focus/Health Concerns: Prioritize ↓ Ⓟ & ↑ ROM SH & LB

Symptoms: Location/Intensity/Frequency/Duration/Onset

Ⓡ SH/ Ⓟ/ M / freq / daily / fall ΔL

LB/ Ⓟ/ M / freq / daily / fall ΔL

No HA Ⓟ for 10 days

Activities of Daily Living: Aggravating/Relieving

able to dress, wash hair c̄ M Ⓟ

Unable to work but cooking @ home for

30 min c̄ M Ⓟ, unable to play hockey or bike

O   Findings: Visual/Palpable/Test Results

See figures

Techniques/Modalities: Locations/Duration

97140 MFR FB 60 min — mod press.

Response to Treatment (see Δ)

A   Goals: Long-term/Short-term
LTG—cook for 90 min + 3 hrs prep
4 wks   3 da/wk c̄ L Ⓟ & M fatigue
STG—cook for 60 min + 1¹/₂ hrs prep
2 wks   3 da/wk c̄ M Ⓟ & fatigue

Functional Outcomes
Now able to cook for 30 min 3 da/wk lifting up to
25 lbs c̄ M Ⓟ & fatigue

P   Future Treatment/Frequency
1x wk/4 wks ↓ Ⓟ & ↑ ROM ↑ strength
rolfing protocol – Adv series

Homework/Self-care
begin aerobic ex 30 min/da 4/7
see PT for strength training
con't ice prn

Therapist's Signature _HLL, CR_   Date _5-11-04_

Legend: ℰ TP   • TeP   ○ Ⓟ   ⋇ Infl   ≡ HT   ≈ SP

              ✕ Adh   ≋ Numb   ⌒ rot   ╱ elev   ⤙ Short   ↔ Long

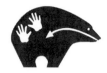

Helena LaLuna, CR
123 Sun Moon and Stars Drive
Capitol Hill, WA   98119
TEL   206 555 4446   •   FAX   206 555 4447   •   EMAIL   laluna@email.com

4041 Bell Town Way, Ste. 200   5-12-04

Capitol Hill, WA 98119

Patient: Zamora Hostetter

DOI: 3-31-04

Claim #: C98-7654321

Dear Dr. Yuricich:

Thank you for referring Ms. Hostetter to my office for manual therapy. After 10 sessions of myofascial release, Ms. Hostetter has achieved her initial goal. She is able to stand and cook for 30 minutes, while repeatedly lifting and extending up to 25 pounds over a stove and tossing food, 3 days a week, with moderate pain and fatigue.

To facilitate Ms. Hostetter's to return to work, ongoing care is requested. We must extend her cooking time to 90 minutes, 3 days a week, and include 3 hours of additional time at work preparing food. However, Ms. Hostetter is able to sit down at work and take frequent breaks during her preparation time. With 3 additional sessions of myofascial release, we should be able to reach the new goal of cooking for 90 minutes, while repeatedly lifting and extending up to 25 pounds over a stove and tossing food, 3 days a week, with mild pain and moderate fatigue. Ms. Hostetter will attend session weekly for 3 weeks, receive additional self-care instructions including alternating hot and cold pack applications, and participate in home exercises and to stretch and strengthen injured areas during this time.

Please inform me of your decision to continue Ms. Hostetter's manual therapy. I look forward to working with you in the future.

Yours in health,

Helena LaLuna, CR

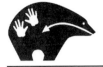

Helena LaLuna, CR
123 Sun Moon and Stars Drive
Capitol Hill, WA   98119
TEL   206 555 4446

RANGE OF MOTION

Patient Name _Zamora Hostetter_   Date _4-4-04_

Date of Injury _3-31-04_   ID#/DOB _C98-7654321_

PRE-TEST 1 Initials _____ Date _____

Position of patient: prone, sidelying, (sitting)
standing, supine, other: _____

Type of test: (active), active assisted, passive,
resistive, other: _____

Joint: C-spine, T-spine, L-spine, hip, knee,
ankle, (shoulder), elbow, wrist, other: _____

Action	Quantify ↓ or ↑		Rate Pain		Rate Quality	
	(R)	(L)	(R)	(L)	(R)	(L)
flex	S↓	N	S(P)	Ø	/	N
ext	S↓	N	S(P)	Ø	/	N
Abd	S↓	N	S(P)	Ø	/	N
Add	S↓	N	S(P)	Ø	/	N

PRE-TEST 2 Initials _____ Date _____

Position of patient: prone, sidelying, (sitting),
standing, supine, other: _____

Type of test: active, active assisted, (passive),
resistive, other: _____

Joint: C-spine, T-spine, L-spine, hip, knee,
ankle, (shoulder), elbow, wrist, other: _____

Action	Quantify ↓ or ↑		Rate Pain		Rate Quality	
	(R)	(L)	(R)	(L)	(R)	(L)
flex	S↓	N	S(P)	Ø	Mseg	N
ext	M↓	N	M(P)	Ø	Mseg	N
Abd	S↓	N	S(P)	Ø	Mseg	N
Add	M↓	N	M(P)	Ø	Mseg	N

PRE-TEST 3 Initials _____ Date _____

Position of patient: prone, sidelying, sitting,
standing, supine, other: _____

Type of test: active, active assisted, passive,
resistive, other: _____

Joint: C-spine, T-spine, L-spine, hip, knee,
ankle, shoulder, elbow, wrist, other: _____

Action	Quantify ↓ or ↑		Rate Pain		Rate Quality	
	(R)	(L)	(R)	(L)	(R)	(L)

POST-TEST 1 Initials _____ Date _____

Position of patient: prone, sidelying, (sitting),
standing, supine, other: _____

Type of test: (active), active assisted, passive,
resistive, other: _____

Joint: C-spine, T-spine, L-spine, hip, knee,
ankle, (shoulder), elbow, wrist, other: _____

Action	Quantify ↓ or ↑		Rate Pain		Rate Quality	
	(R)	(L)	(R)	(L)	(R)	(L)
flex						
ext						
Abd						
Add						

POST-TEST 2 Initials _____ Date _____

Position of patient: prone, sidelying, (sitting),
standing, supine, other: _____

Type of test: (active), active assisted, passive,
resistive, other: _____

Joint: C-spine, T-spine, L-spine, hip, knee,
ankle, (shoulder), elbow, wrist, other: _____

Action	Quantify ↓ or ↑		Rate Pain		Rate Quality	
	(R)	(L)	(R)	(L)	(R)	(L)
flex						
ext						
Abd						
Add						

POST-TEST 3 Initials _____ Date _____

Position of patient: prone, sidelying, sitting,
standing, supine, other: _____

Type of test: active, active assisted, passive,
resistive, other: _____

Joint: C-spine, T-spine, L-spine, hip, knee,
ankle, shoulder, elbow, wrist, other: _____

Action	Quantify ↓ or ↑		Rate Pain		Rate Quality	
	(R)	(L)	(R)	(L)	(R)	(L)

Directions for charting Range of Motion Results: For each test, fill in the form blanks as follows:
ACTION—Identify the action tested: abd, add, DF, ever, ext, ext rot, flex, int rot, inv, lat flex, PF, pro, SB, and Sup
QUANTIFY—Quantify the available range of motion: ↓ (hypomobility), ↑ (hypermobility); L, M, S; 0–10; N, G, F, P
(Normal, Good, Fair, Poor).
PAIN—Identify if Pain is present with movement: If present, rate pain. If absent: Ø.
QUALITY—Identify and Rate the quality of movement: sm, seg, Sp, rig (smooth, segmented, spastic, rigid)

Helena LaLuna, CR
123 Sun Moon and Stars Drive
Capitol Hill, WA   98119
TEL   206 555 4446

INSURANCE VERIFICATION

Patient Name _Zamora Hostetter_   Date _4-5-04_

Date of Injury _3-31-04_   ID#/DOB _C98-7654321_

Verify and Authorize Patient Benefits

Company Name _L & I_

Phone _(360)555-6655_ Fax _555-5566_

Provider Service Rep _Aziz Amaden_

Date/time called _4-5-04 9:30am_

Check all verified:

☒ Physical medicine/rehab benfit
☒ I can provide services
☒ Covered services (from worksheet):
    97124 bundled

Check all authorized:

☒ Number of visits _12_
☒ Dates of coverage _4-1-04—5-11-04_
Authorization # _A31CLA_

Billing procedures:

☒ HCFA 1500 ☐ electronic ☐ other

Send with each bill:

☐ Prescription/referral ☒ Reports
☒ SOAPS ☐ License/certification

What is the expected turnaround time on
claim reimbursement? _14 da_

Comments _all services allowed_

Re-Authorize

Provider Service Rep _Rosa Perez_

Date/time called _5-13-04_

Check all authorized:

☒ Number of visits _4_
☒ Dates of coverage _5-11-s04—6-11-04_
Authorization # _D42BCG_

Total # of visits to date _____

Total $ spent to date _____

Comments _____

Re-Authorize

Provider Service Rep _____

Date/time called _____

Check all authorized:

☐ Number of visits _____
☐ Dates of coverage _____
Authorization # _____

Total # of visits to date _____

Total $ spent to date _____

Comments _____

Referring Health Care Provider Info

Name _Manda Rae Yuricich, DC_

Phone _(206)555-3535_ Fax _(206)555-4646_

Prescription received? ☒ Yes ☐ No

Dates of coverage _4-4-04 to 5-11-04_

# of visits _10_

Diagnosis (ICD-9 codes) _724.2_
_____ _723.1, 840.9, 728.85, 784.0_

Comments _____

Renewal

Date _5-13-04_

Progress report sent? ☒ Yes ☐ No
Prescription received? ☒ Yes ☐ No

Dates of coverage _5-13-04—6-10-04_

# of visits _4_

ICD-9 codes _same_

Comments _____

Renewal

Date _____

Progress report sent? ☐ Yes ☐ No
Prescription received? ☐ Yes ☐ No

Dates of coverage _____

# of visits _____

ICD-9 codes _____

Comments _____

Attorney Information (if applicable)

Name _____

Phone _____ Fax _____

Guarantee of Payment contract signed?
  ☐ Yes ☐ No

Date requested _____ Received _____

Medical Lien filed? ☐ Yes ☐ No

Date _____ Expires _____
Renewed _____ Expires _____
Renewed _____ Expires _____

Requests for patient files:

Date requested _____ Date sent _____
Authorization received? ☐ Yes ☐ No
Exclusive? ☐ Yes ☐ No Expires _____

Date requested _____ Date sent _____
Authorization received? ☐ Yes ☐ No
Exclusive? ☐ Yes ☐ No Expires _____

330

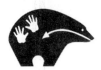

Helena LaLuna, CR
123 Sun Moon and Stars Drive
Capitol Hill, WA   98119
TEL   206 555 4446

VERIFICATION WORKSHEET

Patient Name _Zamora Hostetter_   Date _4-5-04_

Date of Injury _3-31-04_   ID#/DOB   _C98-7654321_

Verify and Authorize Physical Medicine and Rehabilitation Services
(Common modality codes and procedure codes for manual therapists.)

Authorized?	Code #	Description	Restrictions	Max Rate
☐ Yes ☐ No	95831	Muscle testing, ROM, manual, with report		
☐ Yes ☐ No	97010	Hot or cold packs		
☐ Yes ☐ No	97012	Mechanical traction		
☐ Yes ☐ No	97039	Unlisted modality, Specify:		
☐ Yes ☐ No	97110	Therapeutic exercise		
☐ Yes ☐ No	97112	Neuromuscular reeducation		
☐ Yes ☐ No	97113	Aquatic therapy		
☐ Yes ☐ No	97116	Gait training		
☒ Yes ☐ No	97124	Massage therapy	bundled, 4 units	$26/unit
☐ Yes ☐ No	97139	Unlisted therapeutic procedure, Specify:		
☐ Yes ☐ No	97140	Manual therapy: eg, mobilization/manip., MLD, MFR, manual traction		
☐ Yes ☐ No	97050	Therapeutic procedure(s), group (2 or more)		
☐ Yes ☐ No	99056	Home/Hospital visit		
☐ Yes ☐ No	99075	Medical testimony		
☐ Yes ☐ No		Other:		
☐ Yes ☐ No		Other:		
☐ Yes ☐ No		Other:		
☐ Yes ☐ No		Other:		
☐ Yes ☐ No		Other:		
☐ Yes ☐ No		Other:		
☐ Yes ☐ No		Other:		

See CPT codebook for detailed descriptions of modalities and procedures listed above and for additional modalities and therapeutic procedures not listed on worksheet.

CARRIER →

| | PICA | | | | | | | **HEALTH INSURANCE CLAIM FORM** | | PICA | |

1. MEDICARE   MEDICAID   CHAMPUS   CHAMPVA   GROUP HEALTH PLAN   FECA BLK LUNG   OTHER

☐ (Medicare #) ☐ (Medicaid #) ☐ (Sponsor's SSN) ☐ (VA File #) ☐ (SSN or ID) ☐ (SSN) ☒ (ID)

1a. INSURED'S I.D. NUMBER (FOR PROGRAM IN ITEM 1)
C98-7654321

2. PATIENT'S NAME (Last Name, First Name, Middle Initial)
Hostetter Zamora

3. PATIENT'S BIRTH DATE MM DD YY 05 22 80   SEX M ☐ F ☒

4. INSURED'S NAME (Last Name, First Name, Middle Initial)
same

5. PATIENT'S ADDRESS (No., Street)
63 18TH Ave W

6. PATIENT RELATIONSHIP TO INSURED
Self ☒   Spouse ☐   Child ☐   Other ☐

7. INSURED'S ADDRESS (No., Street)

CITY
Capitol Hill   **STATE** WA

8. PATIENT STATUS
Single ☒   Married ☐   Other ☐

Employed ☒   Full-Time Student ☐   Part-Time Student ☐

CITY   **STATE**

ZIP CODE
98119   **TELEPHONE** (Include Area Code)
(206) 555-1221

ZIP CODE   **TELEPHONE** (INCLUDE AREA CODE)
(   )

9. OTHER INSURED'S NAME (Last Name, First Name, Middle Initial)
same

10. IS PATIENT'S CONDITION RELATED TO:

11. INSURED'S POLICY GROUP OR FECA NUMBER

a. OTHER INSURED'S POLICY OR GROUP NUMBER
555-63-1819

a. EMPLOYMENT? (CURRENT OR PREVIOUS)
☒ YES   ☐ NO

a. INSURED'S DATE OF BIRTH MM DD YY   SEX M ☐ F ☐

b. OTHER INSURED'S DATE OF BIRTH MM DD YY   SEX M ☐ F ☐

b. AUTO ACCIDENT?   PLACE (State)
☐ YES   ☒ NO

b. EMPLOYER'S NAME OR SCHOOL NAME
Howling Moon Cafe

c. EMPLOYER'S NAME OR SCHOOL NAME

c. OTHER ACCIDENT?
☐ YES   ☒ NO

c. INSURANCE PLAN NAME OR PROGRAM NAME
WA Dept. L & I

d. INSURANCE PLAN NAME OR PROGRAM NAME
Health Co Selections

10d. RESERVED FOR LOCAL USE

d. IS THERE ANOTHER HEALTH BENEFIT PLAN?
☒ YES   ☐ NO   If yes, return to and complete item 9 a-d.

READ BACK OF FORM BEFORE COMPLETING & SIGNING THIS FORM.
12. PATIENT'S OR AUTHORIZED PERSON'S SIGNATURE I authorize the release of any medical or other information necessary to process this claim. I also request payment of government benefits either to myself or to the party who accepts assignment below.

SIGNED signature on file   DATE 4-4-04

13. INSURED'S OR AUTHORIZED PERSON'S SIGNATURE I authorize payment of medical benefits to the undersigned physician or supplier for services described below.

SIGNED signature on file

14. DATE OF CURRENT: MM DD YY 03 31 01   ◀ ILLNESS (First symptom) OR INJURY (Accident) OR PREGNANCY(LMP)

15. IF PATIENT HAS HAD SAME OR SIMILAR ILLNESS. GIVE FIRST DATE MM DD YY

16. DATES PATIENT UNABLE TO WORK IN CURRENT OCCUPATION FROM MM DD YY TO MM DD YY

17. NAME OF REFERRING PHYSICIAN OR OTHER SOURCE
Manda Rae Yuricich, DC

17a. I.D. NUMBER OF REFERRING PHYSICIAN

18. HOSPITALIZATION DATES RELATED TO CURRENT SERVICES FROM MM DD YY TO MM DD YY

19. RESERVED FOR LOCAL USE

20. OUTSIDE LAB? $ CHARGES
☐ YES   ☐ NO

21. DIAGNOSIS OR NATURE OF ILLNESS OR INJURY. (RELATE ITEMS 1,2,3 OR 4 TO ITEM 24E BY LINE)

1. 724.2   3. 840.9
2. 723.1,784.0   4. 728.85

22. MEDICAID RESUBMISSION CODE   ORIGINAL REF. NO.

23. PRIOR AUTHORIZATION NUMBER

24.	A DATE(S) OF SERVICE						B Place of Service	C Type of Service	D PROCEDURES, SERVICES, OR SUPPLIES (Explain Unusual Circumstances) CPT/HCPCS	MODIFIER	E DIAGNOSIS CODE	F $ CHARGES		G DAYS OR UNITS	H EPSDT Family Plan	I EMG	J COB	K RESERVED FOR LOCAL USE
	From MM DD YY			To MM DD YY														
1	4 4 04						3	9	97124		1,2,3,4	25	—	1				
2	4 4 04						3	9	97124		1,2,3,4	25	—	1				
3	4 4 04						3	9	97124		1,2,3,4	25	—	1				
4	4 4 04						3	9	97124		1,2,3,4	25	—	1				
5																		
6																		

25. FEDERAL TAX I.D. NUMBER SSN EIN
91-1777771   ☐ ☒

26. PATIENT'S ACCOUNT NO.

27. ACCEPT ASSIGNMENT? (For govt. claims, see back)
☐ YES   ☐ NO

28. TOTAL CHARGE $ 100 —

29. AMOUNT PAID $ 0

30. BALANCE DUE $ 100

31. SIGNATURE OF PHYSICIAN OR SUPPLIER INCLUDING DEGREES OR CREDENTIALS (I certify that the statements on the reverse apply to this bill and are made a part thereof.)

Helena LaLuna, CR 4-4-04
SIGNED   DATE

32. NAME AND ADDRESS OF FACILITY WHERE SERVICES WERE RENDERED (If other than home or office)

33. PHYSICIAN'S, SUPPLIER'S BILLING NAME, ADDRESS, ZIP CODE & PHONE #
Helena LaLuna, CR
123 Sun Moon and Stars Dr.
Capitol Hill, WA 98119
PIN# (206) 555-4446   GRP#

FORM HCFA-1500 (12-90)   **PLEASE PRINT OR TYPE**   FORM OWCP-1500   FORM RRB-1500   APPROVED OMB-0938-0008
NORTHWEST BUSINESS FORMS (206) 728-8181   (APPROVED BY AMA COUNCIL ON MEDICAL SERVICE 8/88)

PATIENT AND INSURED INFORMATION / PHYSICIAN OR SUPPLIER INFORMATION

332

Helena LaLuna, CR
123 Sun Moon and Stars Drive
Capitol Hill, WA 98119
TEL 206 555 4446

PAYMENT LOG

Name _Zamora Hostetter_   Date _6-18-04_

Date of Injury _3-31-04_   ID#/DOB _C98-7654321_

Insurance Company _____ Phone _____

Billing Date: _5-18-04_   Total Billed: $ _100_

Patient Paid: $ _0_   Insurance Paid: $ _0_   Total Paid: $ _0_

If Total Paid does NOT equal Total Billed, complete below for each date of service (from lines 1-6, Section 24 of HCFA 1500)

Line 1, Initial Billing
Treatment Date: _5-18-04_ Bill Date: _5-18-04_

Charges: _100_ Adjustments: _0_ Amount Billed: _100_

Due from patient: _0_ Due from Insurance: _100-_

Patient Paid: _0_ Insurance paid: _0_

Line 1, Rebilling
Rebill Date: _6-18-04_ Rebilled to: _Ins._

Outstanding: _100-_ Interest: _0_ Amount Billed: _100-_

Rebill Date: _____ Rebilled to: _____

Outstanding: _____ Interest: _____ Amount Billed: _____

Line 2, Initial Billing
Treatment Date: _____ Bill Date: _____

Charges: ____ Adjustments: ____ Amount Billed: _____

Due from patient: _____ Due from Insurance: _____

Patient Paid: _____ Insurance paid: _____

Line 2, Rebilling
Rebill Date: _____ Rebilled to: _____

Outstanding: _____ Interest: _____ Amount Billed: _____

Rebill Date: _____ Rebilled to: _____

Outstanding: _____ Interest: _____ Amount Billed: _____

Line 3, Initial Billing
Treatment Date: _____ Bill Date: _____

Charges: ____ Adjustments: ____ Amount Billed: _____

Due from patient: _____ Due from Insurance: _____

Patient Paid: _____ Insurance paid: _____

Line 3, Rebilling
Rebill Date: _____ Rebilled to: _____

Outstanding: _____ Interest: _____ Amount Billed: _____

Rebill Date: _____ Rebilled to: _____

Outstanding: _____ Interest: _____ Amount Billed: _____

Line 4, Initial Billing
Treatment Date: _____ Bill Date: _____

Charges: ____ Adjustments: ____ Amount Billed: _____

Due from patient: _____ Due from Insurance: _____

Patient Paid: _____ Insurance paid: _____

Line 4, Rebilling
Rebill Date: _____ Rebilled to: _____

Outstanding: _____ Interest: _____ Amount Billed: _____

Rebill Date: _____ Rebilled to: _____

Outstanding: _____ Interest: _____ Amount Billed: _____

Line 5, Initial Billing
Treatment Date: _____ Bill Date: _____

Charges: ____ Adjustments: ____ Amount Billed: _____

Due from patient: _____ Due from Insurance: _____

Patient Paid: _____ Insurance paid: _____

Line 5, Rebilling
Rebill Date: _____ Rebilled to: _____

Outstanding: _____ Interest: _____ Amount Billed: _____

Rebill Date: _____ Rebilled to: _____

Outstanding: _____ Interest: _____ Amount Billed: _____

Line 6, Initial Billing
Treatment Date: _____ Bill Date: _____

Charges: ____ Adjustments: ____ Amount Billed: _____

Due from patient: _____ Due from Insurance: _____

Patient Paid: _____ Insurance paid: _____

Line 6, Rebilling
Rebill Date: _____ Rebilled to: _____

Outstanding: _____ Interest: _____ Amount Billed: _____

Rebill Date: _____ Rebilled to: _____

Outstanding: _____ Interest: _____ Amount Billed: _____

Wellness

Case Study: Lin Pak, a 38-year-old woman, is seeking bimonthly massage therapy for relaxation and stress reduction. She has type 1 diabetes and has been giving herself insulin injections 2 to 4 times per day since she was 12 years old. She has no health complications from her condition and wants to keep it that way. Her family has a history of heart disease, and she knows that diabetes further increases her chances of heart-related complications. She also knows that stress affects her blood sugar levels. Lin is hoping massage therapy will provide her with new ways of handling the stress in her life and keeping her heart strong and healthy.

Ms. Pak has informed her primary HCP of her intent to receive massage therapy and asks her massage therapist to keep her physician informed of the results of the sessions.

This flow chart demonstrates the forms that are recommended for use with patients seeking wellness care: who completes the form, how often the form is used, and any additional comments for using the form.

Wellness Care	Who	Frequency	Comments
INTAKE FORMS			
Fees and Policies	Patient	Initial visit	Update as needed
Health Information	—		
Health Info—Wellness	Patient	Initial visit	Update annually
Injury Information, Part 1	—		
Injury Information, Part 2	—		
Billing Information	—		
Prescription	HCP (optional)	As needed	A progress report should precede each renewal
PROGRESS SUMMARIES			
Health Report	Patient	Biannually	Patient reports current status
Pain Questionnaires	Patient	As needed	If Health Report indicates
Initial Report w/o Tx	MT	As needed	If referred by HCP but does not receive tx
Initial Report w/ Tx	MT	As needed	If referred by HCP
Progress Report	MT	As needed	If referred by HCP
Narrative Report	—		
TREATMENT NOTES			
Initial SOAP	—		
Subsequent SOAP	—		
Progress SOAP	—		
Discharge SOAP	—		
Wellness Chart	MT	Each visit	
Range of Motion	—		
BILLING FORMS			
Insurance Verification	—		
HCFA 1500 billing form	—		
Payment Log	—		

Naomi Wachtel
567 Sunnydale Dr.
Flat Irons, CO   80302
TEL   303 555 8866

A. Fee Schedules

My Fees For Services Are As Follows:

Massage Therapy	$45 for 1/2 hour
97124	$80 for 1 hour

B. Payment Policies

Payment at time of service only.

C. Office Policies

Cancellations

Cancellations must be made 24 hours in advance of the scheduled appointment time. If cancellations are not made within 24 hours, payment in full is required. This charge will be waived if a replacement can be found for your appointment time. Your insurance company will not be charged for your missed appointment; you will be responsible for payment out-of-pocket.

Right of Refusal

I reserve the right to refuse service to anyone. This includes but is not limited to anyone who requests treatment or services that are outside my scope of practice. I will exercise this right if anyone arrives for treatment under the influence of alcohol or recreational drugs; I reserve the right to charge for the session time, whether or not services were rendered, if I so choose.

Patient Agreement

I have read the policies stated above and agree to abide by them.

Signature   _Lin Pak_____   Date   _7-27-04_____

Naomi Wachtel
567 Sunnydale Dr.
Flat Irons, CO   80302
TEL   303 555 8866

PRESCRIPTION

Patient Name _Lin Pak_   Date _7-15-04_

Date of Injury _∅_   ID#/DOB _∅_

A. Diagnosis

(Include ICD-9 codes that specifically address Manual Therapy Treatment)

diabetes ŝ complications

↑ BP (boardline) no meds

Condition is related to
☐ Auto Accident
☐ Work Injury
☐ Illness
☒ Other: _stress_

B. Medically Necessary Treatment: Implement Plan as Prescribed Below

Application (Primary & Secondary)
☐ Head
☒ Neck
☒ Chest
☒ Shoulders
☐ Abdomen
☒ Back
☐ Lowback/Hips
☐ Upper extremities
☐ Lower extremities
☐ All of the above
☐ Other: _As needed_

Frequency & Duration
☐ 1× wk for _____ wks
☐ 2× wk for _____ wks
☐ 3× wk for _____ wks
☒ 2× month for _6_ months
☐ 1× month for _____ months

Specific Instructions/Precautions:
No cautions for Tx currently
Apply tx as needed

Treatment Type
☐ Manual Therapy
☐ Hot/Cold Packs
☐ Self-Care/Exercises
☐ Other

Treatment Goals
☐ Decrease Pain
☐ Decrease Inflammation
☐ Decrease Muscle Tension/Spasms
☐ Decrease Compensatory Patterns
☐ Increase Mobility
☐ Increase Strength
☐ Restore Function
☐ Restore Posture
☐ Patient Education
☐ All of the Above
☐ Other

C. Referring Health Care Provider (HCP)

Contact Information
HCP Name _Tami Chan OMD_
Address _675 Arapahoe Dr._
City _Flat Irons_   State _CO_ Zip _80302_
Phone _(303) 555-0202_
Fax _555-2020_
Email

Reporting—I will send an initial report after the first visit and a progress report after every 6–8 sessions. Please check how you would like to receive this information:
☒ Fax ☐ Mail ☐ Email
☐ Send Copies of Chart Notes with each report

HCP Signature: _Tami Chan OMD_   Date _7-15-04_

Revised and reprinted with permission, Adler ♦ Giersch, PS

338

Naomi Wachtel
567 Sunnydale Dr.
Flat Irons, CO   80302
TEL   303 555 8866

WELLNESS CHART

Name   _Lin Pak_   ID#/DOB   _5-31-63_   Date   _7-27-04_

Phone   _(303) 555-0033x253_   Address   _253 Boulder Rd., Flat Irons 80302_

1. What are your goals for health, and how may I assist you in achieving your goals?   _Limit_
   longterm complications of diabetes through relaxation and stress reduction

2. List typical daily activities—work, exercise, home.   _I sit a lot at work and watch movies_
   at home

3. Are you currently experiencing any of the following? If yes, please explain.

pain, tenderness	☒ No ☐ Yes: _____	stiffness ☒ No ☐ Yes: _____
numbness or tingling	☒ No ☐ Yes: _____	swelling ☒ No ☐ Yes: _____
allergies	☒ No ☐ Yes: _____	

4. List all illnesses, injuries, and health concerns you have now or have had in the past 3 years.
   (Examples: arthritis, diabetes, car crash, pregnancy)   _diabetes, borderline high_
   blood pressure

5. List medications and pain relievers taken this week.   _insulin_

6. I have provided all my known medical information. I acknowledge that massage therapy is
   not a substitute for medical diagnosis and treatment. I give my consent to receive treatment.

   Signature   _Lin Pak_   Date   _7-27-04_

   Tx: _F̶B̶ ̶S̶w̶ Ⓜ, LDT neck, chest, axillary_
         60 min.
   C: _HW-relaxation ex., ✓BP pre & post Ⓜ_

Legend:

℃ TP	• TeP	○ Ⓟ	⋇ Infl	≡ HT	≈ SP	initials _NW, LMT_
✕ Adh	≋ Numb	⟳ rot	╱ elev	⤛ Short	⟷ Long	

339

Naomi Wachtel
567 Sunnydale Dr.
Flat Irons, CO   80302
Tel   303 555 8866

HEALTH REPORT

Client Name ___Lin Pak___   Date ___7-27-04___

Date of Injury ___∅___   ID#/DOB ___5-31-63___

A. Draw today's symptoms on the figures.

1. Identify CURRENT symptomatic areas in your body by marking letters on the figures below. Use the letters provided in the key to identify the symptoms you are feeling today.
2. Circle the area around each letter, representing the size and shape of each symptom location.

Key
P = pain or tenderness
S = joint or muscle stiffness
N = numbness or tingling

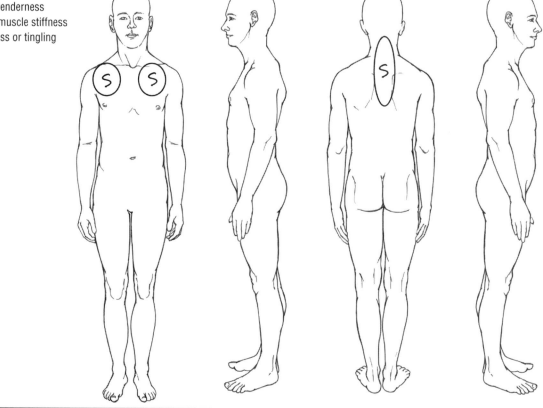

B. Identify the intensity of your symptoms.

1. Pain Scale: Mark a line on the scale to show the amount of pain you are experiencing today.

No Pain |⊕————————————————————————| Unbearable Pain

2. Activities Scale: Mark a line on the scale to show the limitations you are experiencing today in your daily activities.

Can Do Anything I Want |⊕————————————————————| Cannot Do Anything

C. Comments

___I get stiff in my chest, neck, and between my shoulder blades w/ long work days.___

___Tx: FB ⓂSW & LDT to ↓ stiffness ↑ circ & ↑ relaxation___
___M SH rot BL, HT chest, neck, midback L → L⁺, L Adh teres BL   NW, LMT___

Signature ___Lin Pak___   Date ___7-27-04___

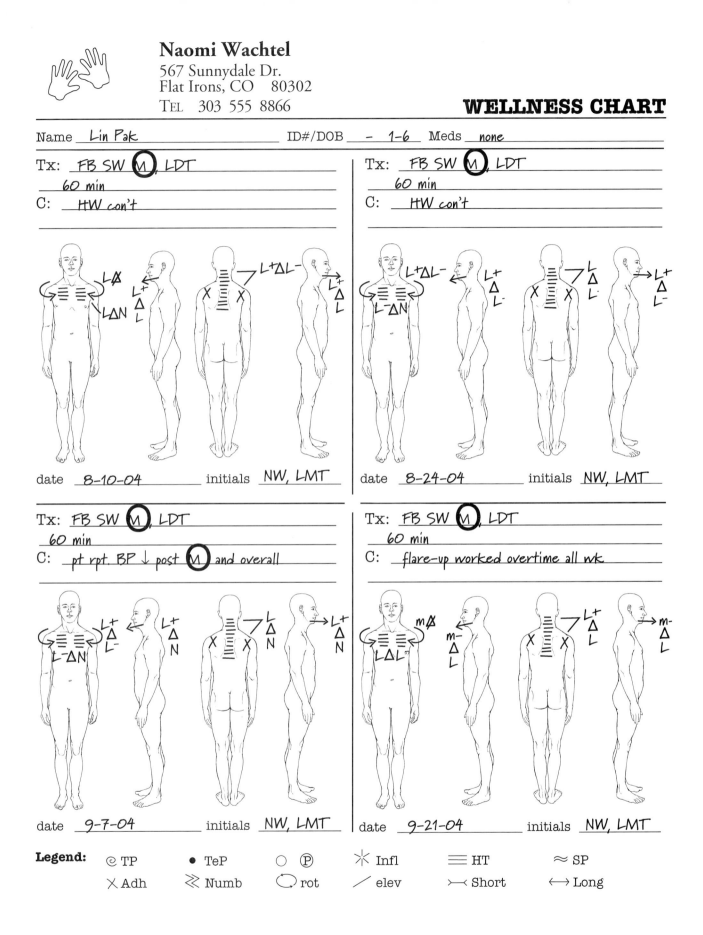

Naomi Wachtel
567 Sunnydale Dr.
Flat Irons, CO   80302
Tel   303 555 8866

WELLNESS CHART

Name   Lin Pak   ID#/DOB   - 1-6   Meds   none

Tx: FB SW Ⓜ, LDT
      60 min
C: HW con't

date   8-10-04   initials   NW, LMT

Tx: FB SW Ⓜ, LDT
      60 min
C: HW con't

date   8-24-04   initials   NW, LMT

Tx: FB SW Ⓜ, LDT
      60 min
C: pt rpt. BP ↓ post Ⓜ and overall

date   9-7-04   initials   NW, LMT

Tx: FB SW Ⓜ, LDT
      60 min
C: flare-up worked overtime all wk

date   9-21-04   initials   NW, LMT

Legend:

℮ TP	● TeP	○ Ⓟ	✳ Infl	≡ HT	≈ SP
✕ Adh	≋ Numb	↻ rot	╱ elev	≻─ Short	↔ Long

Naomi Wachtel
567 Sunnydale Dr.
Flat Irons, CO   80302
TEL   303 555 8866

Dr. Gregory Chandler
2323 Pill Hill
Flat Irons, CO 80309

Dear Dr. Chandler,

My client, Ms. Lin Pak, is a patient of yours. With her permission, I am writing to update you on her progress with massage therapy. Ms. Pak has been receiving bi-monthly massages for three months to promote relaxation and reduce the side effects of stress.

I have noted the following:
Posture—mild bilateral internal rotation of the shoulders and mild forward head position.
Tension—mild chest, neck and upper back.
Adhesions—mild shoulder.

I have used Swedish massage strokes and gentle lymphatic drainage to promote relaxation and enhance circulation and drainage. Ms. Pak has responded with a softening of her muscles, increased mobility in her shoulders, and her posture is returning to normal. Ms. Pak is doing breathing exercises at home which she finds very relaxing after a hard day at work. She tells me her blood pressure is lower for several days following her massages, which she'll be able to show you in her diary at her next appointment with you.

I will keep you informed of her progress with a short report every 6–8 sessions.

In health,
Naomi Wachtel

342

Appendix:
Abbreviations List

HANDS HEAL:
COMMUNICATION,
DOCUMENTATION,
AND INSURANCE BILLING
FOR MANUAL THERAPISTS

Symbols

ā, pre	before
@	at
&, +	and
~ , ≈	approximate
c̄, w/	with
Δ	change
↓	down, decrease
=	equals
♀	female
>	greater than
→	leading to, resulting in, through
<	less than
♂	male
–	minus, negative
#	number
Ø	no, none
p̄, post	after
//	parallel
/	per
1°	primary
+	plus, positive
s̄, w/o	without
2°	secondary, due to
x	times, repetitions
↑	up, increase

Symbols for figure drawing

✕	adhesion
╱	elevation
≡	hypertonicity, tension
⟷	longer than normal
⩾	numbness, tingling
Ⓟ	pain
↻	rotation
⟩⟨	shorter than normal
≈	spasm
✳	swelling, inflammation
•	tender points
⊚	trigger point

Anatomy (Sample list of common landmarks. Follow suit with additional terms by shortening words or using initials.)

abs	abdominals
AC	acromioclavicular
ACL	anterior crutiate ligament
AIIS	anterior inferior iliac spine
ASIS	anterior superior iliac spine
ATFL	anterior talofibular ligament
AW	abdominal wall
BBB	blood brain barrier
BEF	bioenergetic field
bi	biceps
BJM	bones, joints, and muscles
BR	breath
C, C 1-7	cervical, cervical vertebrae
CN 1-8	cervical nerves
CrN 1-12	cranial nerves
CSF	cerebral spinal fluid
ch	chest
Cl	clavicle
CM	carpometacarpal
CNS	central nervous system
coc	coccygeal
Cr	cranium
delt	deltoid
DH	dominant hand
dia	diaphragm
E	energy
elb	elbow
EMF	electromagnetic field
ES	erector spinae muscle group
FE	femur
gastroc	gastrocnemius
GHL	glenohumeral ligament
gluts	gluteal muscle group
GT	greater trochanter
hams	hamstring muscles
he	heart
hd	head
H&N	head and neck
hum	humerus
IC	ileocecal, iliococcygeal, intercarpal, intercostal, intracranial
IF	iliofemoral
IP	iliopsoas
ISF	interstitial fluid
ITB	iliotibial band
IT	ischial tuberosity
IVD	intervertebral disk
IVJC	intervertebral joint complex
J, jt	joint
JV	jugular vein
L, L 1-5	lumbar, lumbar vertebrae
LC	lymph capillaries
LCL	lateral collateral ligament
lats	latissimus dorsi
lev scap	levator scapula
LI	large intestine
LN	lymph node
LV	lymph vessel
mas	masseter
meta	metacarpal, metatarsal
mm	muscles
MN	median nerve
ms	musculoskeletal
nn	nerves
NR	nerve root
NS	nervous system
occ	occiput
OF	occipitofrontal
os	bone
PCx	paracervical
pecs M&m	pectoralis major and minor
PNS	parasympathetic nervous system
PSIS	posterior sacroiliac spine, posterior superior iliac spine
Q	radiant energy
QL	quadratus lumborum
quads	quadricep muscles
RC	rib cage
rhomb	rhomboids
SB	sternal border
SC	subclavian, sternoclavicular, sternocostal
sc	subcutaneous
SC	sternoclavicular
SCM	sternocleidomastoid
ScM	scalene muscle group
SCV	subclavian vein
SI	sacroiliac, small intestine
sh	shoulder
sol	soleus
ST	soft tissue
st	sternum
T, T 1-12	thoracic, thoracic vertebrae
TC	thoracic cage
TD	thoracic duct
TFA	tibiofemoral angle
TFL	tensor fascia lata
th	throat
tib	tibia, tibialis
tibfib	tibia and fibula
TMJ	temporal mandibular joint
traps	trapezius
tri	triceps
UN	ulnar nerve
vert	vertebrae
visc	viscera

Descriptive Terms

abn	abnormal
aux	auxiliary
avg	average
cons	constant
F	fair
freq	frequent
G	good
G&B	good and bad (days)
grad	gradual
interm	intermittent
L	light, low, mild
Ltd	limited, limitation
M	moderate
max	maximum
min	minimum
N	normal
OK	all right, acceptable
P	poor
QOL	quality of life
QWL	quality of working life
rig	rigid
S	severe
seg	segmented
seld	seldom
sm	smooth
sp	spastic
sym	symmetrical
VGH	very good health
WNL	within normal limits
xs	excessive

Directions and Positions

adj	adjacent, adjoining, adjunctive
ant	anterior
Ⓑ, BⓁ	bilateral, both
cd	caudal
ceph	cephalic
D/3	distal third
dist	distal
dp	deep
ext	external
glob	global
inf	inferior
int	internal
inter	between
intra	within
Ⓛ	left
L/3	lower third
lat	lateral
LE	lower extremities
LQ	lower quadrant
M/3	middle third
med	medial
ML	midline
OL	other location
P/3	proximal third
post	posterior
prox	proximal
pr	prone
Ⓡ	right

SL	sidelying
sup	superior, supine
super	superficial
U/3	upper third
UE	upper extremities
unilat	unilateral
univ	universal
UQ	upper quadrant

Movements and Planes of Movement

abd	abduction
act	activities
add	adduction
ADLs	activities of daily living
art	articulate
circ	circumduction
dep	depression
DF	dorsiflexion
ele	elevation
ever	eversion
ext	external
flex	flexion
FM	functional movement
front	frontal
inv	inversion
lat flex	lateral flexion
mob	mobility
mvmt	movement
opp	opposition
PF	plantarflexion
pro	pronation
Ptx	protraction
ROM	range of motion
AROM	active range of motion
AAROM	active assisted range of motion
PROM	passive range of motion
RROM	resistive range of motion
CPROM	complete and pain-free range of motion
rot	rotation
Rtx	retraction
sag	sagittal
SB	sidebending
sh	shear
sup	supination
tor	torsion
trans	transverse

Measurements and Medical Record Terminology

A:	assessment
a.c.	before meals
ACI	after care instructions
am	morning
AMAP	as much as possible
a.p.	before dinner
appt	appointment
ASAP	as soon as possible
b.i.d.	twice a day
bpm	beats per minute
cm	centimeter
CNT	could not test
c/o	complains of
COD	condition on discharge
cont	continue
cpm	counts or cycles per minute
CSR	CranioSacral rhythm
CSTx	continue same treatment
D	daughter
da	day
D/C	discharged or discontinued
DD	daily
DKA	did not keep appointment
DNT	did not test
DOB	date of birth
DOI	date of injury
dur	duration
ea	each
EOD	every other day
FB	full body
freq	frequency
ft	foot
GD	granddaughter
GF	grandfather
GM	grandmother
gm	gram
GS	grandson
h.d., h.s.	at bedtime
hr	hour
hgt	height
h.v.	this evening
Hx	history
i.c.	between meals
ID	identification
immed	immediately
in	inches
int	intensity
kg	kilogram
kph	kilometers per hour
l	liter
lb	pound
lpm	liter per minute
LTG	long-term goal
M	mother
m.d., m.g.	as directed
meds	medications
mg	milligrams
min	minutes
ml	milliliters
mm	millimeters
mo	month
mph	mile per hour
nv	next visit
O:	objective

ODAT	one day at a time
o.h., q.h.	every hour
o.m., q.m.	every morning
o.n., q.n.	every night
ons	onset
oz	ounce
P:	plan
p.c., p.p.	after meals
pg	page
pls	please
pm	afternoon, evening
POMR	problem-oriented medical record
ppm	pulses per minute
prn	as needed
PTD	prior to discharge
q2h	every two hours
q3h	every three hours
q.i.d	four times daily
q.l.	as much as desired
q.o.d	every other day
reps	repetitions
RR	respiratory rate
Rx	drugs, prescription, medication, therapy
S	son
S:	subjective
S/A	same as
SAA	same as above
SATx	same treatment
sched	schedule
sec	seconds
s.i.d., u.i.d	once a day
SOAP	Subjective, Objective, Assessment, Plan
stat	at once
STG	short-term goal
suc	success
t.d.d., t.i.d.	three times a day
t.i.w.	three times a week
TMTC	too many to count
TST	total sleep time
UFN	until further notice
unk	unknown

Symptoms and Maladies

Abr	abrasion
Acc	accident
Adh	adhesion
AE	acute exacerbation
AI	accidental injury
AIDS	autoimmune deficiency syndrome
ANI	acute nerve irritation
AOB	alcohol on breath
ASP	abnormal spine posture
atr	atrophy
BA	backache

CA	cancer
CFS	chronic fatigue syndrome
CHD	coronary heart disease
CHI	closed head injury
CHS	congestive heart failure
CHT	closed head trauma
CP	cerebral palsy
crep	crepitis
CTS	carpal tunnel syndrome
DDD	degenerative disk disease
DJD	degenerative joint disease
Dx	diagnosis
EC	energy cyst
ed	edema
EM	emotional, early memory
FB	foreign body
flac	flaccid
FLR	funny-looking rash
Flat	flatulence
Fl up	flare up
FOOSH	fell on outstretched hand
FM, FMS	fibromyalgia
FT	fibrous tissue
HA	headache
HD	heart disease, herniated disk
HI	head injury
HNP	herniated nucleus pulposus
Hnt	hypertension
HOH	hard of hearing
HT	hypertonicity, tension, tight muscles
HTR	hypertrophy
Infl	inflammation
AI	acute inflammation, phase I
SI	subacute inflammation, phase II
CI	chronic inflammation, phase III
JRA	juvenile rheumatoid arthritis
kyph	kyphosis
lax	laxity
LB	loose bodies
LD	learning disability
les	lesion
LJM	limited joint mobility
LOC	loss of consciousness

LOM	loss of movement
lord	lordosis
MAEW	moves all extremities well
MI	myocardial infarction
MPS	myofascial pain syndrome
NRI	nerve root irritation
NSI	no sign of infection, inflammation
OA	osteoarthritis
Ⓟ	pain
para	paraplegia
PCS	postconcussive syndrome
PD	perception disorder
PNP	peripheral neuropathy
POM	pain on motion
PTSD	posttraumatic stress disorder
Px	prognosis
RA	rheumatoid arthritis
RSS	repetitive stress syndrome
RTD	repetitive trauma disorder
SCI	spinal cord injury
SD	sleep disturbances
SFLE	stress from life experience
SL	subluxation
SOB	shortness of breath
SOBOE	shortness of breath on exercise
Sp	spasm, spastic
st	stiffness
STS	soft tissue swelling
STI	soft tissue injury
Sw	swelling
Sx	symptoms
TBI	traumatic brain injury
TeP	tender point
TJA	total joint arthrotomy or arthroplasty
THA	total hip arthrotomy or arthroplasty
TKA	total knee arthrotomy or arthroplasty
TJR	total joint replacement
TAR	total ankle replacement
TER	total elbow replacement
THR	total hip replacement
TKR	total knee replacement
TSR	total shoulder replacement
TOS	thoracic outlet syndrome
TP	trigger point
URI	upper respiratory infection
UTI	urinary tract infection
VGH	very good health
VV	vericose vein

Treatments, Modalities, Findings

AAS	active assisted stretching
AC	acupuncture, acupressure
AKS	arthroscopic knee surgery
aroma	aromatherapy
AT	adjunctive therapy
bal	balance
B&B	bowel and bladder function
BM	bowel movement
BJE	bone and joint exam
BP	blood pressure
BRS	breath sounds
BV	steam bath
C&E	consultation and examination
chak	chakra
contra	contraindicated
coord	coordinate
CP	cold packs
CST	CranioSacral therapy
DB	deep breathing
DBE	deep breathing exercise
detox	detoxification
DP	direct pressure
DT	deep tissue
eff	effleurage
erg	ergonomics consultation
EW	energy work
Ex	exercise
exam	examination
FS	facilitated stretching
FWB	full weight bearing
Fx	friction
HARPPS	signs of infection: heat, absence of use, redness, pain, pus, swelling
H&C	hot and cold
HEP	home exercise program
HMP	hot moist packs
HP	hot packs
HW	homework
hydro	hydrotherapy
ICES	ice, compression, elevation, support
IDM	indirect method
immob	immobilize
JM	joint mobility
jos	jostling
LAM	laminectomy
LAP	laproscopy
LBPQ	low back pain questionnaire
LDT	lymphatic drainage technique
LT	light touch
Ⓜ	massage
man	manipulation
mer	meridian
MET	muscle energy technique
MFT	muscle function test
MFR	myofascial release
MH	moist heat
MLD	manual lymphatic drainage
MT	manual therapy
NA	not attempted
N/A	not applicable
NMT	neuromuscular therapy
NP	not palpable
NWB	non–weight-bearing
OBE	out-of-body experience
obs	observation
O&E	observation and examination
OE	orthopedic examination
os adj	osseous adjustment
OTB	off the body
PA	postural analysis or assessment
palp	palpation
PB	parafin bath, postural balancing
pet	petrissage
PMP	pain management program
PNF	proprioceptive neuromuscular facilitation
PPR	passive positional release
PR	postural re-education
PRE	progressive resistive exercise
prev	prevention
proc	procedure
PT	physical therapy
PU	props utilized
PVD	percussion, vibration, drainage
PWB	partial weight-bearing
R&E	rest and exercise
re-ed	reeducation
reflex	reflexology
re-x	reexamination
ROS	review of symptoms, review of systems
RR	respiratory rate
RT	recreational therapy
RTW	return to work
SA	skeletal alignment
SAE	specific action exercise
SC	self-care
SDTx	sleeps during treatment
SE	somatic education
SER	somato-emotional release
SET	subtle energy techniques
SLR	straight leg raise
S&S	stretching and strengthening
str	stretching
SU	supports utilized
TENS	transcutaneous electrical nerve stimulation
Tx	treatment
tx	traction
Ptx	pelvic traction
Ltx	lumbar traction
Ttx	thoracic traction
Ctx	cervical traction
VAPS	visual analog pain scale
VS	vascular flush
WB	weight bearing
XFF	cross fiber friction

APPENDIX:
ICD-9 Coding for Self-Referred Patients

The International Classification of Diseases, Ninth Revision (ICD-9) is a statistical classification system that arranges diseases and injuries into groups according to established criteria. Most ICD-9 codes are numeric and consist of three, four, or five numbers and a description. The codes are revised approximately every 10 years by the World Health Organization, and annual updates are published by the Centers for Medicare and Medicaid Services (CMS).

Manual therapists without diagnostic scope rely on the referring HCP for correct diagnostic coding. At times, patients seek treatment without a prescription or referral—treatment covered by their insurance plan. Problems arise when the practitioner seeks reimbursement from a patient's insurance company and discovers that the majority of insurance carriers will refuse a bill submitted without ICD-9 codes. On page 348 are ICD-9 codes that are not considered diagnostic in scope; rather, they are codes that describe the patient's symptoms or require a simple assessment on behalf of the practitioner. Select one or more codes that adequately reflect the symptoms you are addressing in your treatment sessions, and record them on the HFCA 1500 billing form in section 21.

Before submitting a bill using any of the ICD-9 codes listed below, follow the guidelines in Chapter 8 and verify patient coverage. Every insurance plan is different, even within the same insurance company, so make sure the codes you select are covered under the patient's plan and that your services are a covered benefit for that condition. Also, confirm that you are able to bill for services when the patient doesn't have a referral or prescription from a primary HCP.

When selecting a code to describe your patients' symptoms, be as specific as possible. For example, a five-digit code is more specific that a four-digit code. Read through the entire code list before making your selection. If you have any concerns regarding the code selection, call the patient's HCP for a formal diagnosis.

348

HANDS HEAL:
COMMUNICATION,
DOCUMENTATION,
AND INSURANCE BILLING
FOR MANUAL THERAPISTS

LOCATION	PAIN	STIFFNESS	SWELLING
shoulder region	719.41	719.51	719.01
upper arm	719.42	719.52	719.02
forearm	719.43	719.53	719.03
hand	719.44	719.54	719.04
pelvis and thigh	719.45	719.55	719.05
lower leg	719.46	719.56	719.06
ankle and foot	719.47	719.57	719.07
other specified areas	719.48	719.58	719.08
multiple sites	719.49	719.59	719.09
TMJ	524.62		
neck	723.1		
thoracic spine	724.1		
intercostal muscles	786.59		
lumbar spine	724.2		
sciatica	724.3		
back pain, postural	724.5		
sacroiliac	724.6		
coccyx	724.79		
muscles of limbs: fingers, toes, etc.	729.5		
muscle tissue	729.1 (myalgia)	728.85 (spasm)	728.81 (myositis)
muscle weakness	728.87		
localized edema, traumatic origin			782.3
lymph nodes			785.6
lymphatic edema due to mastectomy			457.0
headache (HA), face	784.0		
tension HA	307.81		
cluster, allergic HA	346.2		
migraine HA	346.9		

APPENDIX:
Contact Information–
Offices of Insurance
Commissioners

Alabama Department of Insurance
Consumer Services Division
201 Monroe Street, Suite 1700
P.O. Box 303351
Montgomery, AL 36130-3351
(334) 269-3550
Fax: (334) 241-4192
http://www.aldoi.org/

Alaska Division of Insurance
Anchorage Office
Robert B. Atwood Building
550 W. 7th Avenue, Suite 1560
Anchorage, AK 99501-3567
(907) 269-7900
Fax: (907) 269-7910
http://www.dced.state.ak.us/insurance/

Arizona Department of Insurance
Phoenix Office
2910 N. 44th Street, Suite 210
Phoenix, AZ 85018
(602) 912-8444
(800) 325-2548 (In-State only)
http://www.state.az.us/id/

Arkansas Insurance Department
Consumer Services Division
Third and Cross Streets
Little Rock, AR 72201
(501) 371-2640
Fax: (501) 371-2749
(800) 852-5494 (In-State only)
http://www.state.ar.us/insurance/
    file_a_complaint.html

California Department of Insurance
Consumer Communications Bureau
300 S. Spring Street, South Tower
Los Angeles, CA 90013
(213) 897-8921
(800) 927-HELP (4357) (In-State only)
(800) 482-4833 TDD
http://www.insurance.ca.gov/docs/
    index.html

Colorado Division of Insurance
1560 Broadway, Suite 850
Denver, CO 80202
(303) 894-7499
Fax: (303) 894-7455
(800) 930-3745 (In-State only)
(303) 894-2512 TDD
http://www.dora.state.co.us/insurance/

Connecticut Insurance Department
153 Market Street
P.O. Box 816
Hartford, CT 06142-0816
(860) 297-3800
Fax: (860) 566-7410
(800) 203-3447 (In-State only)
http://www.state.ct.us/cid/

Delaware Insurance Department
841 Silver Lake Boulevard
Dover, DE 19904
(302) 739-4251
Fax: (302) 739-6278
(800) 282-8611 (In-State only)
http://www.state.de.us/inscom/index.html

350

HANDS HEAL:
COMMUNICATION,
DOCUMENTATION,
AND INSURANCE BILLING
FOR MANUAL THERAPISTS

District of Columbia Department of
Insurance
810 First Street, NE, Suite 701
Washington, DC 20002
(202) 727-8000
(202) 727-1000 (In-District only)
http://disr.washingtondc.gov/disr/site/
default.asp

Florida Department of Insurance
200 E. Gaines Street
Tallahassee, FL 32399-0300
(850) 413-3100
Fax: (850) 488-2349
(800) 342-2762 (In-State only)
http://www.doi.state.fl.us/

Georgia Insurance and Fire
Commissioner
Two Martin Luther King, Jr. Drive
West Tower, Suite 704
Atlanta, GA 30334
(404) 656-2070
Fax: (404) 657-8542
(800) 656-2298 (In-State only)
http://www.inscomm.state.ga.us/

Hawaii Insurance Division
King Kalakaua Building
335 Merchant Street, Room 213
P.O. Box 3614
Honolulu, Hawaii 96813
(808) 586-2790 or
(808) 586-2799
Fax: (808) 586-2806
http://www.state.hi.us/dcca/ins/

Idaho Department of Insurance
700 W. State Street
P.O. Box 83720
Boise, ID 83720-0043
(208) 334-4250
Fax: (208) 334-4398
http://www.doi.state.id.us/

Illinois Department of Insurance
320 W. Washington Street
Springfield, IL 62767-0001
(217) 782-4515
Fax: (217) 782-5020
(217) 524-4872 TDD
James R. Thompson Center
100 W. Randolph Street, Suite 9-301
Chicago, IL 60601-3395
(312) 814-2420
Fax: (312) 814-5416
(312) 814-2603 TDD
http://www.ins.state.il.us/default2.htm

Indiana Department of Insurance
311 W. Washington Street, Suite 300
Indianapolis, IN 46204-2787
(317) 232-2385
Fax: (317) 232-5251
http://www.state.in.us/idoi

Iowa Insurance Division
330 Maple Street
Des Moines, IA 50319-0065
(515) 281-5705
Fax: (515) 281-3059
(877) 955-1212 (In-State only)
http://www.iid.state.ia.us/

Kansas Insurance Department
420 SW 9th Street
Topeka, KS 66612-1678
(785) 296-3071
Fax: (785) 296-2283
(800) 432-2484 (In-State only)
http://www.ksinsurance.org/

Kentucky Office of Insurance
215 W. Main Street
Frankfort, KY 40601
(502) 564-3630
(800) 595-6053 (In-State only)
(800) 462-2081 TDD
http://www.doi.state.ky.us/

Louisiana Department of Insurance
1702 N. 3rd Street
P.O. Box 94214
Baton Rouge, LA 70802
(225) 342-5900 or (225) 342-0895
(800) 259-5300 or (800) 259-5301
    (In-State only)
http://www.ldi.la.gov/

Maine Bureau of Insurance
#34 State House Station
Augusta, ME 04333-0034
(207) 624-8475
Fax: (207) 624-8599
(800) 300-5000 (In-State only)
http://www.state.me.us/pfr/ins/
    inshome2.htm

Maryland Insurance Administration
525 St. Paul Place
Baltimore, MD 21202-2272
(410) 468-2000
Fax: (410) 468-2020
(800) 492-6116 (In-State only)
(800) 735-2258 TTY
http://www.mdinsurance.state.md.us/

Massachusetts Division of Insurance
One South Station, 5th Floor
Boston, MA 02110-2208
(617) 521-7794
Fax: (617) 521-7575
(617) 521-7490 TTD/TDD
http://www.state.ma.us/doi/

Michigan Division of Insurance
Consumer Services
P.O. Box 30220
Lansing, MI 48909
(517) 373-0220
Fax: (517) 335-4978
(877) 999-6442 (In-State only)
http://www.michigan.gov/cis

Minnesota Department of Commerce
85 7th Place East, Suite 500
St. Paul, MN 55101
(651) 296-4026
Fax: (651) 297-1959
651-297-1959 TTY
http://www.commerce.state.mn.us/

Mississippi Department of Insurance
P.O. Box 79
Jackson, MS 39205
(601) 359 3569
(800) 562 2957 (In-State only)
http://www.doi.state.ms.us/

Missouri Department of Insurance
301 West High Street, Room 530
P.O. Box 690
Jefferson City, MO 65102
(573) 751-4126
Fax: (573) 751-1165
(573) 526-4536 TDD
http://www.insurance.state.mo.us/

Montana State Auditor's Office
840 Helena Ave.
Helena, MT 59601
(406) 444-2040
(800) 332-6148 (In-State only)
(406) 444-3246 TDD
http://www.state.mt.us/sao/

Nebraska Department of Insurance
Terminal Building
941 "O" Street, Suite 400
Lincoln, NE 68508-3639
(402) 471-2201
(800) 833-7352 TDD
http://www.nol.org/home/NDOI/

Nevada Insurance Division
788 Fairview Drive, Suite 300
Carson City, NV 89701
(775) 687-4270
Fax: (775) 687-3937
2501 East Sahara Avenue, Suite 302
Las Vegas, NV 89104
(702) 486-4009
Fax: (702) 486-4007
http://doi.state.nv.us/

New Hampshire Insurance Department
21 S. Fruit Street, Suite 14
Concord, NH 03301
(603) 271-2261
(603) 271-1406
(800) 852-3416 (In-State only)
http://www.state.nh.us/insurance/

New Jersey Department of Banking
   and Insurance
P.O. Box 325
Trenton, NJ 08625
(609) 292-5360
Fax: (609) 292-3144
http://www.state.nj.us/dobi/

New Mexico Department of Insurance
P.E.R.A. Building
1120 Paseo de Peralta
P.O. Box 1269
Santa FE, NM 87504-1269
(505) 827-4601
Fax: (505) 827-4734
http://www.nmprc.state.nm.us/insurance/
   inshm.htm

New York State Insurance Department
25 Beaver Street
New York, NY 10004
(212) 480-6400
(800) 342-3736 (In-State only)
(800) 220-9250 TDD
http://www.ins.state.ny.us/

North Carolina Department of Insurance
1201 Mail Service Center
Raleigh, NC 27699-1201
(919) 733-2032
(800) 546-5664 (In-State only)
http://www.ncdoi.com/

352

HANDS HEAL:
COMMUNICATION,
DOCUMENTATION,
AND INSURANCE BILLING
FOR MANUAL THERAPISTS

North Dakota Insurance Department
State Capitol, Fifth Floor
600 E. Boulevard Avenue
Bismarck, ND 58505-0320
(701) 328-2440
Fax: (701) 328-4880
(800) 247-0560 (In-State only)
http://www.state.nd.us/ndins/

Ohio Department of Insurance
2100 Stella Court
Columbus, OH 43215-1067
(614) 644-2658
Fax: (614) 644-3743
(800) 686-1526 (In-State only)
http://www.ohioinsurance.gov/

Oklahoma Insurance Department
2401 N.W. 23rd, Suite 28
P.O. Box 53408
Oklahoma City, OK 73152-3408
(405) 521-2828
(800) 522-0071 (In-State only)
http://www.oid.state.ok.us/

Oregon Insurance Division
350 Winter St. NE Room 440
P.O. Box 14480
Salem, OR 97309-0405
(503) 947-7980
Fax: (503) 378-4351
(888) 877-4894 (In-State only)
(503) 947-7280 TTY
http://www.cbs.state.or.us/external/ins/
    index.html

Pennsylvania Insurance Department
1321 Strawberry Square
Harrisburg, PA 17120
(717) 787-2317
(877) 881-6388 (In-State only)
Fax: (717) 787-8585
(717) 787-3898 TTY/TDD
http://www.ins.state.pa.us/ins/site

**Rhode Island Department of Business
    Regulation**
233 Richmond Street
Providence, RI 02903
(401) 222-2246
Fax: (401) 222-6098
http://www.dbr.state.ri.us/

South Carolina Department of Insurance
300 Arbor Lake Drive, Suite 1200
Columbia, SC 29223
P.O. Box 100105
Columbia, SC 29202-3105
(803) 737-6212
Fax: (803) 737-6229
http://www.doi.state.sc.us/

South Dakota Division of Insurance
445 E. Capitol Avenue
Pierre, SD 57501
(605) 773-3563
Fax: (605) 773-5369
http://www.state.sd.us/drr2/reg/insurance/

**Tennessee Department of Commerce and
    Insurance**
500 James Robertson Parkway
Davy Crockett Tower
Nashville, TN 37243-0565
(615) 741-2241
http://www.state.tn.us/commerce/

Texas Department of Insurance
333 Guadalupe
Austin, TX 78701
P.O. Box 149104
Austin, TX 78714-9104
(512) 463-6169
(800) 578-4677 (In-State only)
http://www.tdi.state.tx.us/

Utah Insurance Department
3110 State Office Building
Salt Lake City, UT 84114-6901
(801) 538-3800
Fax: (801) 538-3829
(800) 439-3805 (In-State only)
(801) 538-3826 TDD
http://www.insurance.state.ut.us/

Vermont Department of Insurance
(BISHCA)
89 Main Street, Drawer 20
Montpelier, VT 05620-3101
(802) 828-3301
Fax: (802) 828-3306 (Fax)
http://www.bishca.state.vt.us/InsurDiv/
insur_index.htm
Virginia State Bureau of Insurance
Tyler Building
1300 E. Main Street
Richmond, VA 23219
P.O. Box 1157
Richmond, VA 23218
(804) 371-9741
(800) 552-7945 (In-State only)
(804) 371-9206 TDD
http://www.state.va.us/scc/division/boi/
index.htm

Washington State Insurance
Commissioner
5000 Capitol Boulevard
Tumwater, WA 98501
P.O. Box 40255
Olympia, WA 98504-0255
(360) 725-7000
(800) 562-6900 (In-State only)
http://www.insurance.wa.gov/

West Virginia Insurance Commission
Consumer Services Division
1124 Smith Street
P.O. Box 50540
Charleston, WV 25305-0540
(304) 558-3386
(888) 879-9842 (In-State only)
http://www.wvinsurance.gov/

Wisconsin Office of the Commissioner
of Insurance
125 South Webster Street
Madison, WI 53702
(608) 266-3585
Fax: (608) 266-9935
(800) 236-8517 (In-State only)
(800) 947-3529 TDD (ask for 608-266-3586)
http://oci.wi.gov/oci_home.htm

Wyoming Insurance Department
Herschler Bldg. 3rd Floor East
122 West 25th Street
Cheyenne, WY 82002
(307) 777-7401
Fax: (307) 777-5895
(800) 438-5768 (In-State only)
http://www.insurance.state.wy.us/

American Samoa Insurance
Commissioner
Office of the Governor
American Samoa Government
Pago Pago, American Samoa 96799
011 (684) 633-4116
Fax: 011-684-633-2269
http://www.emystic.com/state/as.html

APPENDIX:
Contact Information–
Workers' Compensation

For more information, please contact the office below and request the phone number of the specific department you are seeking (for example, provider information, claims authorization, or billing).

ALABAMA
Jim Bennett, Commissioner
Department of Labor
100 North Union Street
Montgomery, AL 36130-3500
(334) 242-3460
Fax: (334) 240-3417
http://www.alalabor.state.al.us/contact1/htm

ALASKA
Greg O'Claray, Commissioner
Department of Labor
P.O. Box 21149
Juneau, AK 99802-1149
(907) 465-2700
Fax: (907) 465-2784
http://www.labor.state.ak.us

ARKANSAS
James Salkeld, Director
Department of Labor
10421 West Markham
Little Rock, AR 72205
(501) 682-4500
Fax: (501) 682-4535
http://www.state.ar.us/labor

CALIFORNIA
Department of Industrial Relations
Office of the Director
455 Golden Gate Avenue
San Francisco, CA 94102
(415) 703-5070
http://www.dir.ca.gov

COLORADO
Jeff Wells, Executive Director
Department of Labor and Employment
Tower 2, Suite 400
1515 Arapahoe Street
Denver, CO 80202
(303) 318-8000
http://cdle.state.co.us

CONNECTICUT
Commissioner
Department of Labor
200 Folly Brook Blvd.
Wethersfield, CT 06109
(860) 263-6000
(860) 263-6074 (TTY/TDD)
http://www.ctdol.state.ct.us

DELAWARE
Harold E. Stafford, Secretary
Department of Labor
4425 North Market Street
Wilmington, DE 19802
(302) 761-8085
Fax: (302) 761-6621
http://www.delawareworks.com

356

HANDS HEAL:
COMMUNICATION,
DOCUMENTATION,
AND INSURANCE BILLING
FOR MANUAL THERAPISTS

DISTRICT OF COLUMBIA
Director
Department of Employment Services
64 New York Avenue NE
Washington, DC 20002
(202) 724-7000
Fax: (202) 724-5683
(202) 673-6994 TDD/TYY
http://does.ci.washington.dc.us

FLORIDA
Division of Workers' Compensation
Office of the Director
200 East Gaines St.
Tallahassee, FL 32399-4220
(850) 413-1601
http://www.fldfs.com/wc/

GEORGIA
Michael Thurmond, Commissioner
Department of Labor
Sussex Place, Room 600
148 International Blvd. NE
Atlanta, GA 30303
(404) 656-3011
Fax: (404) 656-2683
http://www.dol.state.ga.us/

HAWAII
Nelson Befitel, Director
Dept. of Labor & Industrial Relations
830 Punchbowl Street, Room 321
Honolulu, HI 96813
(808) 586-8842
Fax: (808) 586-9099
http://www.dlir.state.hi.us

IDAHO
Roger Madsen, Director
Department of Labor
317 W. Main Street
Boise, ID 83735-0001
(208) 334-6110
Fax: (208) 334-6430
http://cl.idaho.gov/portal/

ILLINOIS
Arthur Ludwig, Director
Department of Labor
160 North LaSalle Street
13th Floor, Suite C-1300
Chicago, IL 60601
(312) 793-1808
Fax: (312) 793-5257
http://www.state.il.us/agency/idol

INDIANA
Nancy Guyott, Commissioner
Department of Labor
402 West Washington Street, Room W195
Indianapolis, IN 46204-2739
(317) 232-2378
Fax: (317) 233-5381
http://www.state.in.us/labor or
   http://www.teenworker.org

IOWA
Richard Running, Director
Division of Labor Services
1000 East Grand Avenue
Des Moines, IA 50319
(515) 281-3447
Fax: (515) 281-4698
http://www.state.ia.us/iwd/

KANSAS
Jim Garner, Secretary
Department of Human Resources
401 S.W. Topeka Blvd.
Topeka, KS 66603
(785) 296-7474
Fax: (785) 368-6294
http://www.dol.ks.gov/index.html

KENTUCKY
Joe Norsworthy, Secretary
Labor Cabinet
1047 US Highway 127 South, Suite 4
Frankfort, KY 40601
(502) 564-3070
Fax: (502) 564-5387
http://www.labor.ky.gov/

LOUISIANA
John Warner Smith, Secretary
Department of Labor
1001 North 23rd Street
Baton Rouge, LA 70804-9094
(225) 342-3011
Fax: (225) 342-3778
http://www.ldol.state.la.us/

MAINE
Laura Fortman, Commissioner
Department of Labor
20 Union Street, P.O. Box 309
Augusta, ME 04332-0309
(207) 287-3788
Fax: (207) 287-5292
http://www.workerscompensation.com/
   maine/

MARYLAND
James D. Fiedler, Secretary
Department of Labor, Licensing,
    and Regulation
500 N Calvert St., Room 401
Baltimore, MD 21202
(410) 230-6020
Fax: (410) 333-0853
http://www.dllr.state.md.us

MASSACHUSETTS
Angelo Buonopane, Director
Department of Labor & Workforce
    Development
1 Ashburton Place, Rm. 2112
Boston, MA 02108
(617) 727-6573
Fax: (617) 727-1090
http://www.mass.gov/dlwd/

MICHIGAN
David Hollister, Director
Department of Consumer and Industry
    Services
525 West Ottawa, P.O. Box 30004
Lansing, MI 48909
(517) 373-7230
Fax: (517) 373-2129
http://www.michigan.gov/cis

MINNESOTA
Scott Brener, Commissioner
Department of Labor and Industry
443 Lafayette Road, N.
St. Paul, MN 55155
(651) 296-2342
Fax: (651) 282-5405
http://www.doli.state.mn.us/

MISSOURI
Catherine B. Leapheart, Director
Department of Labor and Industrial
    Relations
3315 West Truman Boulevard Room 213
P.O. Box 504
Jefferson City, MO 65102
(573) 751-9691
Fax: (573) 751-4135
http://www.dolir.state.mo.us

MONTANA
Wendy Keating, Commissioner
Department of Labor and Industry
1327 Lockey, P.O. Box 1728
Helena, MT 59624
(406) 444-9091
Fax: (406) 444-1394
http://dli.state.mt.us/

NEBRASKA
Fernando "Butch" Lecuona,
    Commissioner
Department of Labor
550 South 16th Street, Box 94600
Lincoln, NE 68509-4600
(402) 471-9792
Fax: (402) 471-2318
http://www.dol.state.ne.us

NEVADA
Michael Tanchek, Labor Commissioner
555 East Washington Ave., Suite 4100
Las Vegas, NV 89101
(702) 486-2650
Fax: (702) 486-2660
http://www.laborcommissioner.com/

NEW HAMPSHIRE
George M. Copadis
Commissioner of Labor
95 Pleasant Street
Concord, NH 03301-3838
(603) 271-3171
Fax: (603) 271-6852
http://www.state.nh.us/dol

NEW JERSEY
Thomas Carver, Acting Commissioner
New Jersey Department of Labor
John Fitch Plaza
PO Box 110, 13th Floor, Suite D
Trenton, NJ 08625-0110
(609) 292-2323
Fax: (609) 633-9271
http://www.state.nj.us/labor/

NEW MEXICO
Conroy Chino, Secretary
Department of Labor
401 Broadway, NE, P.O. Box 1928
Albuquerque, NM 87103-1928
(505) 841-8406
Fax: (505) 841-8491
http://www.dol.state.nm.us/

358

HANDS HEAL:
COMMUNICATION,
DOCUMENTATION,
AND INSURANCE BILLING
FOR MANUAL THERAPISTS

NEW YORK
Linda Angelo, Commissioner
New York State Department of Labor
State Office Campus, Building 12
Albany, NY 12240
(518) 457-2741
Fax: (518) 487-6908
http://www.labor.state.ny.us

NORTH CAROLINA
Cherrie Berry, Commissioner
Department of Labor
4 West Edenton Street
Raleigh, NC 27601-1092
(919) 733-0360
Fax: (919) 733-6197
http://www.dol.state.nc.us

NORTH DAKOTA
Leann K. Bertsch, Commissioner
Department of Labor
State Capitol, 13th Floor
Bismarck, ND 58505
(701) 328-2660
Fax: (701) 328-2031
http://www.state.nd.us/labor

OHIO
Gordon Gatien, Superintendent
Division of Labor & Worker Safety
50 West Broad Street, 28th floor
Columbus, Ohio 43216
(614) 644-2239
Fax: (614) 728-8639
http://www.state.oh.us.objfs/

OKLAHOMA
Brenda Reneau, Commissioner
Department of Labor
4001 North Lincoln Boulevard
Oklahoma City, OK 73105
(405) 528-1500
Fax: (405) 528-5751
http://www.state.ok.us/~okdol

OREGON
Dan Gardner, Commissioner
Bureau of Labor and Industries
800 NE Oregon Street, #32, Suite 1045
Portland, OR 97232
(503) 731-4070
Fax: (503) 731-4103
http://www.boli.state.or.us

PENNSYLVANIA
Stephen M. Schmerin, Secretary
Department of Labor and Industry
1700 Labor and Industry Building
7th and Forster Streets
Harrisburg, PA 17121
(717) 787-3756
Fax: (717) 787-8826
http://www.dli.state.pa.us/landi/site/
default.asp

PUERTO RICO
Roman Valesco Gonzalez, Secretary
Department of Labor and Human
Resources
505 Munoz Rivera Avenue
GPO Box 3088
Hato Rey, PR 00918
(787) 754-2119
Fax: (787) 753-9550
http://www.osha.gov/oshdir/stateprogs/
Puerto_Rico.html

RHODE ISLAND
Adelita S. Orefice, Director
Department of Labor and Training
610 Manton Avenue
Providence, RI 02909
(401) 462-8870
Fax: (401) 462-8872
http://www.det.state.ri.us

SOUTH CAROLINA
Adrienne Riggins Youmans, Director
Department of Labor, Licensing &
Regulation
110 Centerview Drive
Columbia, SC 29211-1329
(803) 896-4300
Fax: (803) 896-4393
http://www.llr.state.sc.us

SOUTH DAKOTA
Pamela Roberts, Secretary
Department of Labor
700 Governors Drive
Pierre, SD 57501-2291
(605) 773-3101
Fax: (605) 773-4211
http://www.state.sd.us/dol/dol.html

TENNESSEE

James Neeley, Commissioner
Department of Labor
710 James Robertson Parkway, 8th Floor
Nashville, TN 37243-0655
(615) 741-6642
Fax: (615) 741-5078
http://www.state.tn.us/labor-wfd/

TEXAS

Larry Temple, Executive Director
Texas Workforce Commission
101 East 15th Street, Room 618
Austin, Texas 78778
(512) 463-0735
Fax: (512) 475-2321
http://www.twc.state.tx.us

UTAH

Richard E. Kendell, Commissioner
Labor Commission, State of Utah
160 East 300 South, 3rd Floor
P.O. Box 146600
Salt Lake City, UT 84114-6600
(801) 530-6880
Fax: (801) 530-6390
http://www.labor.state.ut.us

VERMONT

Laura Collins, Commissioner
Department of Labor and Industry
National Life Building
Montpelier, VT 05620-3401
(802) 828-2288
Fax: (802) 828-0408
http://www.state.vt.us/labind

VIRGIN ISLANDS

John Sheen, Acting Commissioner
Department of Labor
2203 Church St.
Christiansted, St. Croix
US Virgin Islands 00820-4612
(340) 773-1994
Fax: (340) 773-0094
http://www.vidol.org

WASHINGTON

Paul Trause, Director
Department of Labor & Industries
PO Box 44001
Olympia, WA 98504-4001
(360) 902-4213
Fax: (360) 902-4202
http://www.lni.wa.gov/

WEST VIRGINIA

James R. Lewis, Commissioner
Division of Labor
Bureau of Commerce
State Capitol Complex, Building 3,
    Room 319
Charleston, WV 25305
(304) 558-7890
Fax: (304) 558-3797
http://www.labor.state.wv.us/

WISCONSIN

Roberta Gassman, Secretary
Department of Workforce Development
201 East Washington Avenue
P.O. Box 7946
Madison, WI 53707
(608) 267-9692
Fax: (608) 266-1784
http://www.dwd.state.wi.us

WYOMING

Cindy Pomeroy, Director
Department of Employment
122 W. 25th Street
Cheyenne, WY 82002
(307) 777-7672
Fax: (307) 777-5805
http://wydoe.state.wy.us/

U.S. DEPARTMENT OF LABOR

Office of the Secretary
200 Constitution Avenue, NW
Washington, DC 20210
(202) 219-8271
Fax: (202) 219-8822

SECRETARIAT

The Council of State Governments
Dave Scott, Policy Analyst
444 North Capitol Street, NW, Suite 401
Washington, DC 20001
(202) 624-5460
Fax: (202) 624-5452
E-mail: dscott@csg.org

Index

Page numbers in *italics* indicate figures. *Blank Forms* are designated as such.